MIRACLES THROUGH PRANIC HEALING

(formerly "The Ancient Science and Art of Pranic Healing")

Third Edition

Master Choa Kok Sui

INSTITUTE FOR INNER STUDIES, INC.
Room 206, Evekal Building
855 Pasay Road corner Amorsolo St.
Makati City 1200, Philippines
Tel. Nos.: 819-1874; 813-2562; 812-2326
Fax No.: (63) (2) 731-3828

MIRACLES THROUGH PRANIC HEALING
(Formerly "The Ancient Science and Art of
Pranic Healing")

First edition 1987
Second edition 1990
Third edition 1997

Philippine Copyright © 1987, 1990, 1997
by Choa Kok Sui

ISBN 971-91106-4-3

All rights reserved. No part of this book may be reproduced in any form whatsoever without the written permission of the author, except for brief quotations or passages with proper acknowledgements.

Cover Design and Illustrations by
Benny Gantioqui

Lay-out and Typeset in
11.5 pts. Goudy Old Style by
Rodney Tejares and *Steven Martin*

Printed in the Philippines by
Quality Bookbinding and Printing
32 Hyacinth St., Roxas District
Quezon City, Metro Manila
Philippines

BOOKS WRITTEN BY CHOA KOK SUI

Miracles Through Pranic Healing (formerly The Ancient Science and Art of Pranic Healing)

Advanced Pranic Healing

Pranic Psychotherapy

The Ancient Science and Art of Pranic Crystal Healing

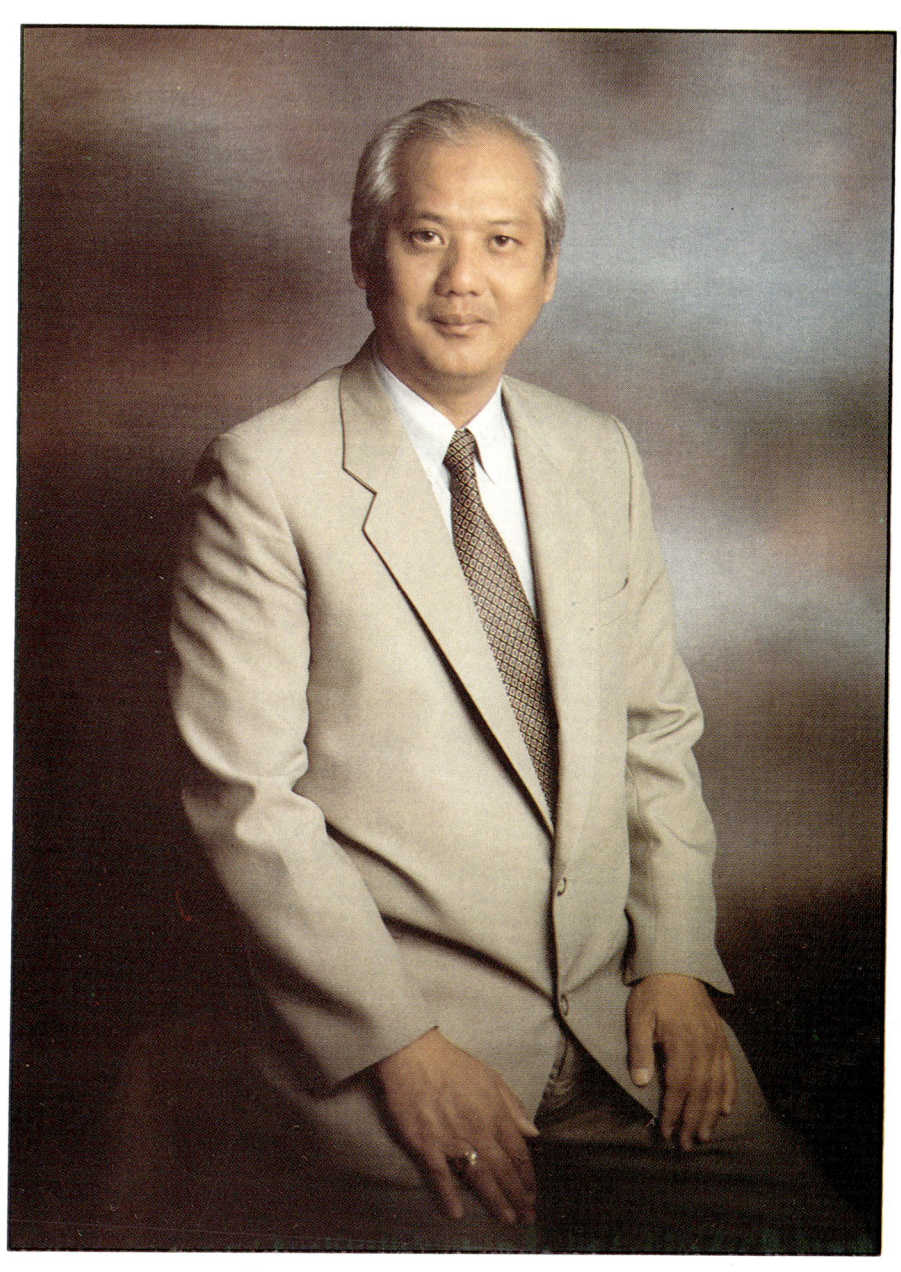

Grand Master Choa Kok Sui
Modern Founder of Pranic Healing
and Arhatic Yoga

ACKNOWLEDGEMENT

To my Respected Teacher Mei Ling and others for their instructions and blessings.

To Mike Nator and others for spending their time with the author in esoteric experiments and in clairvoyantly monitoring them.

To Dr. Rolando Carbonell, Marilou Guillen, and Lynn Payno for making valuable advice and for editing the work.

To Benny Gantioqui, the artist, for his wonderful air brush paintings and illustrations.

To all others not mentioned for their help and support.

**Dedicated
to my parents,
to my Respected Teachers,
especially Teacher Mei Ling,
and to my countries,
the Philippines and China.**

MIRACLES THROUGH PRANIC HEALING

(formerly "The Ancient Science and Art of Pranic Healing")

Miracles do not happen in contradiction to nature, but only to that which is known to us in nature.

– St. Augustine

Foreword

Just so you know my credentials and biases at the outset, let me say that I am a practicing urologist in Los Angeles, California. I truly love the practice of standard allopathic medicine. I love being in the operating room and I enjoy immensely being a physician. It was this very passion for medicine and the health of my patients that led me to realize that there was something lacking in both my training and my practice. I came to this discovery when it became clear that allopathic medicine was not providing cures for a significant percentage of my patients. I grew tired of giving medications which would treat my patients' symptoms but would not cure the underlying problem.

This caused me to challenge the most basic principle underpinning allopathic medicine: The body needs medicines or surgery to heal itself. I came to find working within the confines of this principle to be terribly frustrating, principally because it does not place the emphasis — and more importantly, the responsibility — for healing on the patient. After all, doctors don't really heal people. People heal themselves. As a physician, I may diagnose a bacterial infection and give you an antibiotic to combat it, but that's only to give your body's own immune system a "fighting chance" to swing into action and do the real work of healing.

When I discovered Pranic Healing a little over a year ago, I was immediately excited because here was a system that "filled in the gaps" that I saw in my own training and practice. Here was a system that addressed the source of ailments, offered a well-reasoned complement to my medical practice and most importantly, demonstrated how a Pranic Healing practitioner could clearly assist the body in healing itself.

As I began to use pranic healing on some of my patients, my success rate in curing acute and chronic illnesses improved dramatically. And as word got out in the hospital of my "work," some of my colleagues began to send their more difficult patients to me after a complete workup and standard medical care had failed to produce results. Invariably after several pranic treatments, these patients improved.

Prior to my exposure to Pranic Healing, I used to do a fair amount of medical hypnosis. What became obvious to me as I studied this field is that negative emotions are stored in the body. Think about it. Whenever someone tells you he or she is angry or depressed, he or she only knows these emotions as feelings, tensions or discomforts — in the body! What I have come to learn as a result of studying and practicing Pranic Healing is that stress and negative emotions stored in the body create blockages in the body's energy system. When the body's healing energy becomes blocked and cannot flow properly, then disease occurs. What Pranic Healing did for me was to make the connection between bodily ailments and these energy blocks more evident. And then of course, to offer very simple, easy-to-use techniques to heal them. Let me detail for you some of the successes I've had with pranic healing.

I saw a woman in my clinic who was complaining of urinary frequency and urgency. I did a full workup on her — as I always do — to rule out any serious problems such as urinary tract infection, tumor or neurologic disease. When the entire workup came back negative, I told her that her problem represented the physical manifestations of stress in her body. She went on to tell me of some significant problems at home, including an abusive alcoholic ex-husband, and the fact that she was a single mother trying to raise three small kids. As I was feeling her aura, I noted a lot of energy congestion over her heart chakra, which I proceeded to sweep away. When I was done, she said that she felt a lot more comfortable and relaxed. Then she said, "All of the heaviness is gone from my heart." In the language of Pranic Healing, what she was feeling as an emotion, I was feeling as an energy congestion.

One of my colleagues referred to me a lady with a complex of symptoms, including urinary frequency and bladder pain, irritable bowel syndrome, headaches, insomnia and constipation. Nothing within the realm of standard medicine had been able to give her any relief. After one 15-minute pranic treatment, she walked out of the office calmer, saying that she felt 50 % better. We then gave her some anti-inflammatory agents for her bladder, and within one month she reported feeling 100 % better. She has had no problems for the last six months.

Another case involved a family friend who has advanced scleroderma, an autoimmune disease affecting the connective tissues of the body. The skin of the hands get thick and tight. The esophagus can scar and become blocked, making swallowing difficult. The lungs can also develop scar tissue, making breathing difficult. When I first started seeing M.G. for pranic healing, she was experiencing marked shortness of breath with minimal exertion. After walking up one flight of stairs to her second floor apartment, she would literally collapse on the floor for half an hour to catch her breath. Additionally, she had stiff and painful joints, making extended walking difficult. After one pranic treatment, she experienced dramatic relief in her joint pain and her fatigue. It was easier to breathe, and her energy level exploded. She remarked to me after the first treatment that her life had changed to such an extent that she now runs up the stairs to her second floor apartment and then turns on the music to dance!

Perhaps my most dramatic case was that of J.M. He wasn't my patient nor was he referred to me, but I had seen his name up on the roster of our surgical ward for so long that I decided to introduce myself. He had had a surgery to remove his gallbladder many months before this, and unfortunately had suffered some significant complications, including an injury to his common bile duct. After this injury, he required several more major explorations. As frequently happens with complex cases, once things start going really wrong with the body, they seem to escalate. The patient developed multiple enterocutaneous fistulae (This means that intestinal fluid was leaking out through the skin of his abdominal wall.); yeast sepsis (a very serious condition that is fatal nearly 70 % of the time, in which yeast grows in the blood); and a pulmonary embolism (a blood clot in the lungs, fatal nearly 60 % of the time). He also had daily fever spikes for the past six weeks, and months of constant nausea and vomiting. No one thought that he was going to live past Christmas. It seemed to me in simplistic terms that the patient's energy level was low, his batteries were depleted, and he could no longer heal himself. Most of what was going wrong was a symptom of this. I began to apply pranic healing daily. Within two days, his fever and nausea disappeared. Within one week, his pulse rate decreased from the 150 range to the 120 range. He eventually got strong enough to tolerate a final surgery to repair his fistulae, and went on to make a full recovery. Occasionally, he stops by after work to visit me and shoot the bull.

"It is almost as if they forgot to teach us this stuff in medical school" is how one of my physician colleagues described the philosophy behind Pranic Healing after he became more acquainted with it. And he is right. With Pranic Healing, what we are doing is assisting the body's energy system to normalize so that the body can heal itself. If there are blockages in the energy field, we remove these; if there is depletion of energy, we give some back. We are continuously working with the whole person — not just a single organ system — to facilitate self-healing. And we are not taught these concepts in Western medical schools. Fortunately, Master Choa has revealed these concepts and has made them available to everyone — physician and lay person alike — in an easy-to-understand fashion.

What was most striking to me when I first started reading this book was the simple, cookbook approach that the author uses. If you have enough initial faith to try what is offered here, you will get results. As your success accumulate, your confidence will increase. You will eventually get to the point where you will know that you can help facilitate healing in almost anyone. On the energy level, beliefs affect physiology. What this means is that as your belief system expands in pace with your successes, you will be able to flow more and more healing energy.

Master Choa Kok Sui's work has had an enormous impact on my medical practice, my life and my personal philosophy. It will have the same impact on your life if you allow it.

I close by wishing you much success, health, love and blessings on your journey towards healing with prana.

Eric B. Robins, M.D.
Board Certified Urologist
Los Angeles, California, USA

Table Of Contents

INTRODUCTION

1 THE NATURE OF PRANIC HEALING — 1

2 THE NATURE OF THE ENERGY BODY — 11

3 ELEMENTARY PRANIC HEALING — 47

4 INTERMEDIATE PRANIC HEALING — 129

5 PRANIC SELF-HEALING AND PRANIC INVOCATIVE HEALING — 213

6 PRANIC DISTANT HEALING — 249

7 TESTIMONIALS — 257

8 MEDITATION ON TWIN HEARTS — 325

9 APPENDICES
   Courses on the Inner Sciences — 359
   Pranic Healing Centers
      and Organizations — 360
   Recommended Readings — 381

Introduction

> *The most beautiful experience we can have is the mysterious. It is the fundamental emotion which stands at the cradle of true art and science. Whoever does not know it and can no longer marvel, is as good as dead, and his eyes are dimmed.*
>
> – Albert Einstein

This book basically deals with paranormal healing, not so much on its speculative aspect, but rather more on how and why. The approach in this book is simplified and mechanistic and, at the same time, spiritual. It is mechanistic in the sense that all that one has to do is to follow the instructions step-by-step and the predetermined results will follow. It is spiritual in the sense that, by praying or by invoking, one becomes a divine healing channel. This book teaches, within a week or two, how to heal simple ailments; and within a month or two how to heal difficult cases. One does not have to spend 10 to 20 years just to learn how to perform paranormal healing. Neither does one need any "special inborn healing power" nor be a clairvoyant to heal. All that one needs is the willingness to heal and to follow the instructions given in this book.

The author, at a very young age, was already very interested in yoga, psychic phenomena, mysticism, Chinese ki kung (the art of generating internal power) and other esoteric sciences. Because of his strong interest, he has spent more than 18 years researching and studying books and literatures on esoteric sciences. He has also made close association with yogis, healers, clairvoyants, practitioners of Chinese ki kung and a few extraordinary persons who are in telepathic contact with their Spiritual Gurus. The author and his clairvoyant friends have spent several years experimenting to determine the effectivity and the mechanisms of the healing techniques commonly known and used by healers and students of esoteric sciences. This book is the distillation and synthesis of energy healing, minus the superstitious beliefs and practices. Some of the techniques have been revealed in books by other writers or other healing practitioners for quite sometime, while some were "rediscovered" by the author. The more advanced techniques that were privately taught to him are now revealed in another book entitled *Advanced Pranic Healing*. This will help uplift the suffering of humanity as a result of diseases. Many of the advanced healing techniques and concepts were taught to him by his Respected Teacher Mei Ling. The author is not a clairvoyant nor was he born with any healing ability. If the author can learn how to heal effectively, then you can also!

The instructions in this book have been arranged in such a way that an ordinary person can easily and gradually learn how to perform paranormal healing. Instructions on how to paranormally diagnose a patient without using clairvoyance is also given.

The term "paranormal healing" may not be the proper description. What is considered paranormal healing today may become quite common and normal a few decades from now. This is exactly the purpose of this book: to make paranormal healing quite common in the near future. The appropriate term should be pranic or ki healing since life energy or ki is used in healing. This will give proper recognition to its ancient origin and to all esoteric students who have greatly contributed to its development.

It is very advantageous for everyone to learn pranic healing, especially for parents, since it is very fast and effective in treating simple and severe ailments such as headache, toothache, fever, sore throat, bumps, mumps, gas pain, arthritis, lung infection, heart problems, hearing problems and others.

An advice to students of Pranic Healing: When doing pranic healing, please open the book and follow carefully the instructions on how to treat a specific ailment or disorder. Following the instructions step by step will ensure that the patient gets the proper pranic treatment. You will be amazed by the many cases of miraculous healing. Therefore, do not be embarrassed to heal with the book open. Simply explain to the patient that you want to heal him thoroughly.

— Choa Kok Sui

NOTE:

PRANIC HEALING IS NOT INTENDED TO REPLACE ORTHODOX MEDICINE, BUT RATHER TO COMPLEMENT IT. IF SYMPTOMS PERSIST OR THE AILMENT IS SEVERE, PLEASE CONSULT IMMEDIATELY A MEDICAL DOCTOR AND A CERTIFIED PRANIC HEALER.

An intelligent person is not closed-minded. He does not behave like an ostrich burying his head in the ground trying to avoid new ideas and developments.

An intelligent person is not gullible. He does not accept ideas blindly.

He studies and digests them thoroughly, then evaluates them against his reason; he tests these new ideas and developments through experiments and his experiences.

An intelligent person studies these ideas with a clear objective mind.

— Choa Kok Sui

How To Practice Simplified Pranic Healing Immediately

In situations where you have to heal somebody immediately, and you have no time to gradually learn pranic healing and no access to a qualified pranic healer, you may go directly to the following sections:

1. Eleven Major Chakras (Chapter 2)
2. Increasing One's Energy Level by Connecting the Tongue to the Palate (Chapter 3)
3. Bioplasmic Waste Disposal Unit (Chapter 3)
4. General Sweeping (Chapter 3)
5. Localized Sweeping (Chapter 3)
6. Avoiding Diseased Energy Contamination: Washing the Hands (Chapter 3)
7. Increasing the Receptivity of the Patient (Chapter 3)
8. Energizing with Prana: Hand Chakras Technique (Chapter 3)
9. Stabilizing the Projected Prana (Chapter 3)
10. Releasing the Projected Pranic Energy (Chapter 3)
11. Five Things to Avoid in Pranic Healing (Chapter 3)
12. Pranic Treatment for the Specific Ailment or Disorder (Chapters 3 and 4)

Studying and practicing sections 1-11 will take about one to two hours. The pranic treatment will take about 20 minutes to one hour. In general, you will be amazed that the patient will either be relieved almost immediately or within a few hours. In severe cases, the patient may experience relief after a day or two or maybe even sooner.

This set of instructions is not applicable to the following people:

   a. heavy smokers
   b. alcoholics
   c. drug addicts,
   d. people who are under stress
   e. people experiencing anger or irritation at the moment when healing is required.

The patient may get worse after being healed since the energy bodies of these people are very dirty and may contaminate the patient.

If you want to become a good pranic healer, you have to study the book thoroughly and practice regularly. It is important to avoid eating pork and eventually become semi-vegetarian in order to have a clean energy body.

The pronoun 'he' will be used in this book as a general term for both the masculine and feminine genders.

CHAPTER ONE

The Nature of Pranic Healing

Then the Lord God formed man out of the dust of the ground and breathed into his nostrils the breath of life, and man became a living being.

— Genesis 2:7

We get most of our ki or life energy from the air we breathe. Every living thing depends upon breathing and cessation of breathing is cessation of life itself. From the first cry of an infant to the last gasp of a dying man, there is nothing but a series of breaths. We constantly drain our life energy or ki by our every thought, every act of will or motion of muscles. In consequence, constant replenishment is necessary, which is possible through breathing and other healthful practices.

What is Pranic Healing?	2
Prana or Ki	2
Bioplasmic or Energy Body	5
Meridians or Bioplasmic Channels	6
Prana or Ki Used in Acupuncture, Acupressure, and Reflexology	6
Two Basic Laws of Pranic Healing	7
What Can Pranic Healing Do?	8
Pranic Healing is Easy to Learn	9

Pranic Healing is based on the overall structure of the human body. Man's whole physical body is actually composed of two parts: the visible physical body, and the *invisible energy body* called the *bioplasmic body*. The visible physical body is that part of the human body that we see, touch, and are most acquainted with. The bioplasmic body is that invisible luminous energy body which interpenetrates the visible physical body and extends beyond it by four or five inches. Traditionally, clairvoyants call this energy body the etheric body or etheric double.

WHAT IS PRANIC HEALING?

Pranic healing is an ancient science and art of healing that utilizes *prana* or *ki* or *life energy* to heal the whole physical body. It also involves the manipulation of ki and bioplasmic matter of the patient's body. It has also been called *medical qigong* (ki kung or ki healing), *psychic healing, vitalic healing, therapeutic touch, laying of the hand, magnetic healing, faith healing, and charismatic healing.*

PRANA OR KI

Prana or ki is that life energy which keeps the body alive and healthy. In Greek it is called *pneuma*, in Polynesian *mana*, and in Hebrew *ruah*, which means "breath of life." The healer projects prana or life energy or "the breath of life" to the patient, thereby healing the patient. It is through this process that this so-called "miraculous healing" is accomplished.

Basically, there are three major sources of prana: solar prana, air prana, and ground prana. Solar prana is prana from sunlight. It invigorates the whole body and promotes good health. It can be obtained by sunbathing or exposure to sunlight for about five to ten minutes and by drinking water that has been exposed to

THE NATURE OF PRANIC HEALING

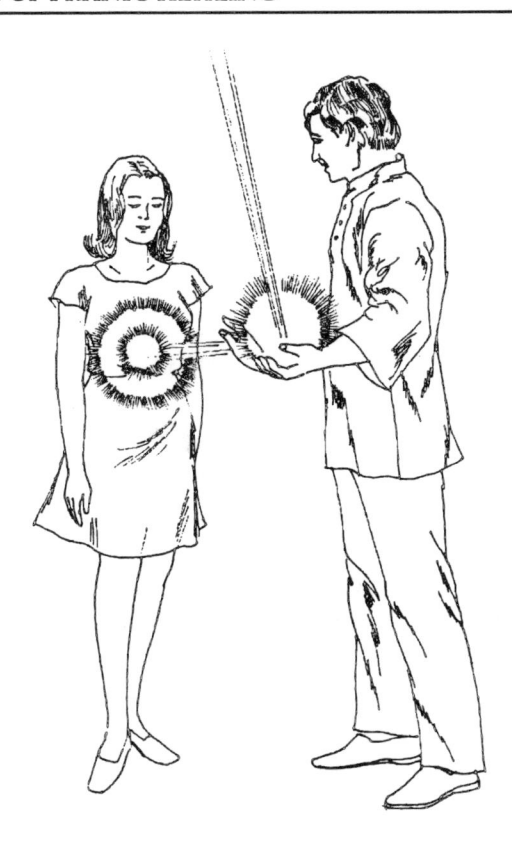

Fig. 1-1 *Pranic healing involves the transference of life energy (ki or prana) to the patient.*

sunlight. Prolonged exposure or too much solar prana would harm the whole physical body since it is quite potent.

Prana contained in the air is called *air prana* or air vitality globule. Air prana is absorbed by the lungs through breathing and is also absorbed directly by the energy centers of the bioplasmic body. These energy centers are called *chakras*. More air prana can be absorbed by deep slow rhythmic breathing than by short shallow breathing. It can also be absorbed through the pores of the skin by persons who have undergone certain training.

Prana contained in the ground is called *ground prana* or ground vitality globule. This is absorbed through the soles of the feet. This is done automatically and unconsciously. Walking barefoot increases the amount of ground prana absorbed by the body. One can learn to consciously draw in more ground prana to increase one's vitality, capacity to do more work, and ability to think more clearly.

Water absorbs prana from sunlight, air, and ground that it comes in contact with. Plants and trees absorb prana from sunlight, air, water, and ground. Men and animals obtain prana from sunlight, air, ground, water, and food. Fresh food contains more prana than preserved food.

Prana can also be projected to another person for healing. Persons with a lot of excess prana tend to make other people around them feel better and livelier. However, those who are depleted tend to unconsciously absorb prana from other people. You may have encountered persons who tend to make you feel tired or drained for no apparent reason at all.

Certain trees, such as pine trees or old and gigantic healthy trees, exude a lot of excess prana. Tired or sick people benefit much by lying down or resting underneath these trees. Better results can be obtained by verbally requesting the being of the tree to help the sick person get well. Anyone can also learn to consciously absorb prana from these trees through the palms, such that the body would tingle and become numb because of the tremendous amount of prana absorbed. This skill can be acquired after only a few sessions of practice.

Certain areas or places tend to have more prana than others. Some of these highly energized areas tend to become healing centers.

THE NATURE OF PRANIC HEALING

During bad weather conditions, many people get sick not only because of the changes in temperature but also because of the decrease in solar and air prana (life energy). Thus, a lot of people feel mentally and physically sluggish or become susceptible to infectious diseases. This can be counteracted by consciously absorbing prana or ki from the air and the ground. It has been clairvoyantly observed that there is more prana during daytime than at night. Prana reaches a very low level at about three or four in the morning.

BIOPLASMIC OR ENERGY BODY

Clairvoyants, with the use of their psychic faculties, have observed that every person is surrounded and interpenetrated by a luminous energy body called the bioplasmic body. Just like the visible physical body, it has a head, two eyes, two arms, etc. In other words, the bioplasmic body looks like the visible physical body. This is why clairvoyants call it the etheric double or etheric body.

The word *"bioplasmic"* comes from *bio* which means life and *plasma* which is the fourth state of matter, the first three being solid, liquid, and gas. Plasma is ionized gas or gas with positive and negative charged particles. This is not the same as blood plasma. Bioplasmic body means a living energy body made up of invisible subtle matter or etheric matter. *To simplify the terminology, the term "energy body" will be used to replace the word "bioplasmic body."* Science, with the use of kirlian photography, has rediscovered the energy body. With the aid of Kirlian photography, scientists have been able to study, observe, and take pictures of small bioplasmic articles like bioplasmic fingers, leaves, etc. It is through the energy body that prana or life energy is absorbed and distributed throughout the whole physical body.

MERIDIANS OR BIOPLASMIC CHANNELS

Just as the visible physical body has blood vessels through which the blood flows, the energy body has fine invisible bioplasmic channels or meridians through which ki and bioplasmic matter flow and are distributed all over the body. There are several major bioplasmic or energy channels and thousands of minor ones. In yoga, these are called the major and minor nadis. Through these channels flow prana or ki that nourishes and invigorates the whole body.

PRANA OR KI USED IN ACUPUNCTURE, ACUPRESSURE, AND REFLEXOLOGY

Acupuncture is an ancient Chinese form of medicine which uses needles to manipulate the life energy within the patient's body, thereby curing the patient's ailment. This is accomplished by using needles to redistribute excess prana or ki in the patient's body to the affected part. Congested prana in the diseased part is redistributed to other parts of the body. Blocked meridians or bioplasmic channels are cleansed or opened by directing ki to them.

In acupressure or in reflexology, the principle is the same as acupuncture's except that the healer intentionally or unintentionally uses his own excess prana. This excess prana is directed towards the acupressure point which then goes to the meridian or energy channel then to the affected part. Some acupuncturists use and direct their own ki or life energy to the needle in order to reach the diseased part. This is done especially with patients who are very weak or depleted. The author has met a practicing acupuncturist and a practicing acupressurist who is also a master of Tai Chi. Both of them are proficient in transferring ki to their patients.

TWO BASIC LAWS OF PRANIC HEALING

Pranic healing is based on two laws: The law of self-recovery and the law of prana or life energy. These laws are quite obvious but strangely they are usually the least noticed or least remembered by most people. It is through these basic laws that rapid or miraculous healing occurs.

1. Law of Self-Recovery

In general, the body is capable of healing itself at a certain rate. If a person has a wound or burn, the body will heal itself and recover within a few days to a week. In other words, even if you do not apply antibiotic on the wound or burn, the body will repair or heal itself. At the present moment, there is no medicine available for the treatment of viral infection. But even if a person has cough or colds due to viral infection, the body will recover generally in one or two weeks without medication.

2. Law of Life Energy

For life to exist, the body must have prana, chi or life energy. The healing process can be accelerated by increasing life energy on the affected part(s) and on the entire body.

In chemistry, electrical energy is sometimes used as a catalyst to increase the rate of chemical reaction. Light can affect chemical reaction. This is the basis for photography. In electrolysis, electricity is used to catalyze or produce chemical reaction. In pranic healing, prana or life energy serves as the catalyst to accelerate the rate of biochemical reactions involved in the natural healing process of the body. When pranic energy is applied to the affected part of the body, the rate of recovery or healing increases tremendously.

What we call miraculous healing is nothing more than increasing the rate of self-recovery of the body. There is nothing supernatural or paranormal about pranic healing. It is simply based on natural laws that most people are not aware of.

Although science is not able to detect and measure life energy or prana, it does not mean that prana does not exist or does not affect the health and well-being of the body. In ancient times, people were not aware of the existence of electricity, its properties and practical uses. But this does not mean that electricity does not exist. One's ignorance does not change reality; it simply alters the perception of reality, resulting in misperception and misconception of what is and what is not, what can be done and what cannot be done.

Children have more life energy than elderly people. You notice that they move a lot from morning to night, hardly getting tired at all. When suffering from a fracture, who heals faster - the child or the elderly? The broken bone of a child heals very fast while that of an elderly heals very slowly; sometimes, it will not even heal at all.

WHAT CAN PRANIC HEALING DO?

1. It can help parents bring down the temperature of their children suffering from high fever in just a few hours and heal it in a day or two in most cases.

2. It can relieve headaches, gas pains, toothaches, and muscle pains almost immediately in most cases.

3. Cough and colds can usually be cured in a day or two. Loose bowel movement can be healed in a few hours in most cases.

THE NATURE OF PRANIC HEALING

4. Major illnesses such as eye, liver, kidney, and heart problems can be relieved in a few sessions and healed in a few months in many cases.

5. It increases the rate of healing by three times or more than the normal rate of healing.

These are some of the few things that pranic healing can do. All of these assume that the healer has attained a certain degree of proficiency.

PRANIC HEALING IS EASY TO LEARN

Any healthy person with an average intelligence, an average ability to concentrate, an open but discriminating mind, and a certain degree of persistence can learn pranic healing in a relatively short period. Learning pranic healing is easier than learning to play the piano or painting. It is as easy as learning to drive. Its basic principles and techniques can be learned in a few sessions. Like driving, pranic healing requires much practice and time to achieve a certain degree of proficiency.

A time will come when science will make tremendous advances, not because of better instruments for discovering and measuring things, but because a few people will have at their command great spiritual powers, which at the present are seldom used. Within a few centuries, the art of spiritual healing will be increasingly developed and universally used.

— *Gustaf Stromberg*
Mount Wilson Astronomer
Man, Mind, and the Universe

CHAPTER TWO

The Nature of the Energy Body

> *The idea of a human aura, a radiating luminous cloud surrounding the body, is an ancient one. Sacred images from early Egypt, India, Greece, and Rome used this convention before it became so popular in Christian art, and before the aura was considered an attribute of ordinary everyday mortals.... For centuries it has been believed that clairvoyant people could actually see an aura surrounding ordinary individuals, and this aura differed from person to person in color and character, expressing the health, emotional and spiritual attributes of the subject. The visionary Swedenborg wrote in his Spiritual Diary: There is a spiritual sphere surrounding everyone as well as a natural and corporeal one.*
>
> – W.J. Kilner
> The Human Aura

The Intimate Relationship Between the Energy Body and the Physical Body	15
Diseases First Appear in the Energy Body and can be Prevented from Manifesting	16
The Mind can Influence to a Certain Degree the Pattern of the Energy Body	17
Chakras or Energy Centers	18
Eleven Major Chakras	19
The Mechanism Behind Psychosomatic Diseases	30
The External and Internal Factors of Diseases	32
What are the Functions of the Energy Body?	33
Basic Problems and Treatments in Pranic Healing	34
Levels in Pranic Healing	35
Levels of Certification	37
Recommended Readings	38
Modern Findings	40

The energy body interpenetrates the visible physical body and extends beyond it by four to five inches. This invisible luminous energy field which follows the contour of the visible physical body is called the inner aura. When the energy body becomes sick, it may be caused partially by general or localized depletion of prana in the energy body. This is called pranic depletion. The inner aura of the affected part is reduced to about two inches or less. For example, nearsighted persons usually have pranic depletion around the eye areas. The inner aura around the eye area may be smaller than two inches. However, there are cases in which an eye may suffer pranic depletion and congestion simultaneously. The more severe the sickness, the smaller is the affected inner aura. There are cases in which the affected inner aura has been reduced to half an inch or less. You can learn to feel the inner auras with your palms in two to four sessions by following the instructions in this book. Feeling the aura is called scanning.

Sickness may also be caused by excess prana in localized area or areas for a prolonged period of time. This is called pranic congestion. The affected areas may protrude to about seven inches or more. In more severe cases, the affected inner aura may protrude to two and a half feet or more. An example is a person suffering from heart enlargement who has pranic congestion around the heart, left shoulder, and upper left arm. The affected areas may protrude to about one foot in thickness.

In pranic depletion and congestion, the surrounding fine meridians or bioplasmic channels are partially or severely blocked. It means prana cannot flow freely in and out around the affected area. Clairvoyantly, the affected areas are seen as light gray to dark gray in color. If these are inflamed, then they appear muddy red; with some cases of cancer, they appear muddy yellow-red; with appendicitis, muddy green; and with some cases of ear problems, muddy orange.

THE NATURE OF THE ENERGY BODY 13

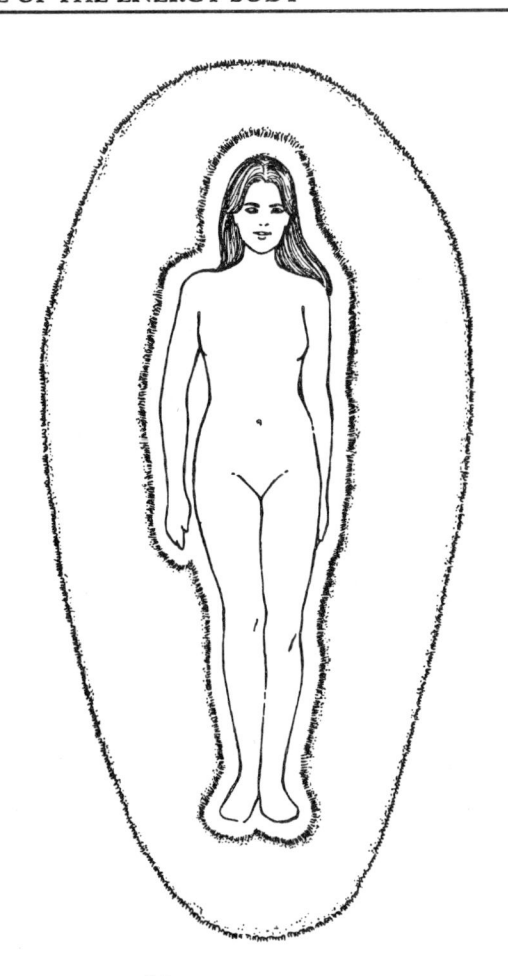

Fig. 2-1 *The outer and inner auras*

From the surface of the physical body are bioplasmic rays perpendicularly projecting from it. These rays are called health rays which interpenetrate the inner aura. The sum of these health rays is called the health aura. The health rays and the health aura are roughly two or three feet in length. The health aura follows the contour of the visible physical body and functions as a protective force field which shields the whole body from germs and diseased energy in the surroundings. Toxins, wastes, germs, and diseased energy are expelled by the health rays predominantly through the

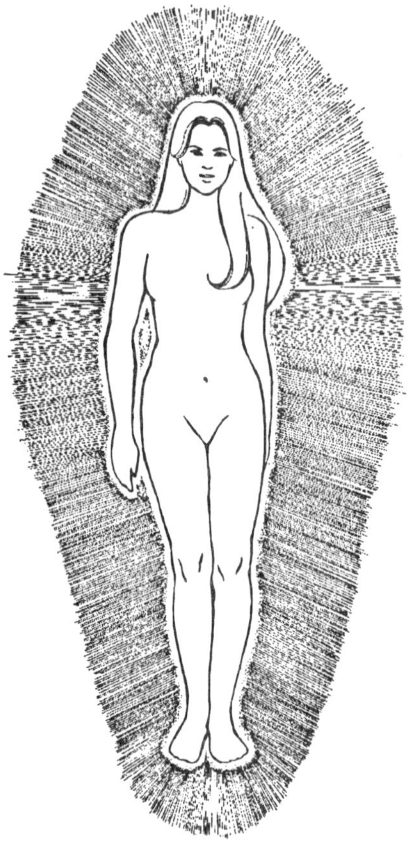

Fig. 2-2 *The health aura and its health rays*

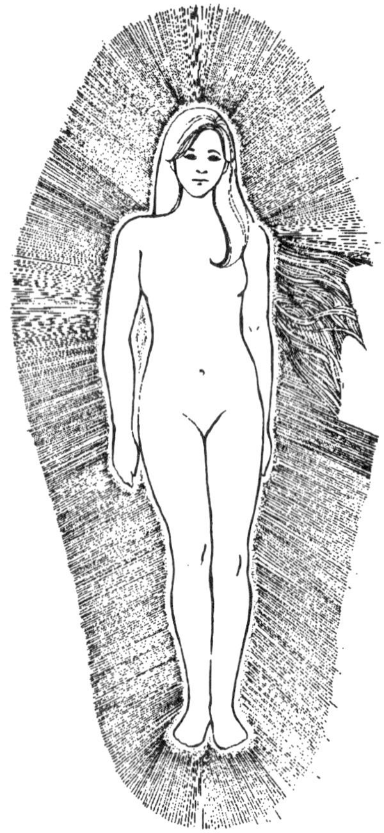

Fig. 2-3 *Drooping and entangled health rays of a sick person*

pores. If a person is weakened, the health rays droop and are partially entangled. Then the whole body becomes susceptible to infection. The capacity of the health rays to expel toxins, wastes, germs, and diseased energy is also greatly diminished. Healing is facilitated by strengthening and disentangling the health rays.

Beyond the health aura is another luminous energy field called the outer aura. It interpenetrates the inner and health auras and usually extends about one meter away from the visible physical body. It is usually multicolored and shaped like an inverted egg. Its colors are influenced by the physical, emotional, and mental states of the person. Clairvoyantly, some sick persons have been observed to have holes in their outer auras through which prana leaks out. Therefore, the outer aura can be considered as a force field that contains or prevents the leaking out of pranic energy. In a sense, it acts as a container for the subtle energies.

The size of the chakras, inner aura, health rays, health aura, and outer aura may considerably increase as the human race evolves to a higher level.

THE INTIMATE RELATIONSHIP BETWEEN THE ENERGY BODY AND THE PHYSICAL BODY

Both the energy body and the visible physical body are so closely related that what affects one affects the other and vice-versa. For instance, if the bioplasmic throat is weakened, then this may manifest on the visible physical body as cough, cold, sore throat, tonsillitis or other throat-related problems. Should a person accidentally cut his skin, there is a corresponding pranic leak in the area where there is bleeding. Initially, the affected area where there is a cut or sprain would become temporarily brighter due to pranic leak but would inevitably become grayish because of pranic depletion. If any part of the energy body is weakened either because of pranic congestion or depletion, the visible physical counterpart would either malfunction or become susceptible to infection. For example, a depleted solar plexus and liver may manifest as jaundice or hepatitis.

From the given examples, it becomes quite clear that the energy body and the visible physical body affect each other. By healing the energy body, the visible physical body gets healed in the process. This is called the Law of Correspondence. By regularly cleansing and energizing with prana, the nearsighted eyes would gradually improve and heal. A person with heart enlargement can be relieved in one or two sessions by simply decongesting the affected heart, shoulder, and upper left arm areas. Complete cure would take at least several months. By decongesting and energizing the head area, headaches can be removed in a few minutes.

DISEASES FIRST APPEAR IN THE ENERGY BODY AND CAN BE PREVENTED FROM MANIFESTING

Through clairvoyant observation, a disease can be seen in the energy body even before it manifests itself on the visible physical body. Non-clairvoyants may scan or feel that the inner aura of the affected part is either smaller or bigger than usual. For instance, before a person suffers from cough and colds, the bioplasmic throat and lungs are pranically depleted and can be observed clairvoyantly as grayish. These areas when scanned can be felt as hollows in the inner aura. Another example: A person who is about to suffer from jaundice can be observed clairvoyantly as having a gray solar plexus and liver. Physical tests or diagnoses will show the patient as normal or healthy. Unless the patient is treated, the disease will manifest inevitably on the visible physical body.

The author had a patient who was a habitual drinker. Based on scanning, his solar plexus chakra (energy center) was depleted, a part of the liver was depleted and another part of it congested. He told his patient that he had a liver problem and that it should be treated as soon as possible. The patient had a blood test and the medical finding showed that his liver was fine. As a result, he was hesitant to be treated. After several months, the patient had severe pain in the liver and the medical findings showed that he had hepatitis. The disease must be treated before it manifests on the visible physical body. The emphasis is on prevention. It is a lot easier and faster to heal the disease when it is still in the energy body and has not yet manifested on the visible physical body. Manifestation of the disease can also be prevented by taking proper medication. In cases where the disease has manifested, healing should be applied as early as possible. The earlier pranic treatment is applied, the faster is the rate of healing. Healing becomes more difficult if the disease has developed fully since it takes more time and more pranic energy. It is important that the disease must be treated as early as possible to insure speedy recovery.

THE MIND CAN INFLUENCE TO A CERTAIN DEGREE THE PATTERN OF THE ENERGY BODY

Clairvoyants have observed that the visible physical body is patterned or molded after the energy body. The mind can intentionally or unintentionally influence the pattern of the energy body. Men well-versed in esoteric studies encourage their pregnant wives to look at beautiful things, listen to harmonious music, feel and think positively, engage in serious studies, and avoid the opposites. These activities affect not only the features of the unborn baby but also his emotional and mental potentialities and tendencies. If the influences are positive, then the effects are positive. If the influences are negative, then the effects are negative. Pregnant women should take note of this so that they would be able to bear better children.

This idea that the mind can influence and actually mold the energy body to a certain degree is not new. There is a Biblical story in Genesis that illustrates this point. This concerns the manner in which Jacob was able to successfully build up his own flock. Jacob had been working for his father-in-law, Laban, for approximately twenty years and yearned to establish himself financially. An agreement was made between Laban and Jacob that all goats born speckled, spotted, and striped and all lambs born black would belong to Jacob. Laban, being a shrewd businessman, that same day removed all the male goats that were streaked or spotted, and all the speckled or spotted female goats (all that had white on them), including all the dark-colored lambs. Genetically, it would be very difficult, if not unlikely, to breed the types of goats and lambs promised to him.

Jacob, through divine guidance, "took fresh-cut branches from poplar, almond and plane trees and made white stripes on them by peeling the bark and exposing the white inner wood of the branches. Then he placed the peeled branches in all the watering troughs, so that they would be directly in front of the flocks when they came to drink. When the flocks were in heat and came to drink, they mated in front of the branches. And they bore young that were streaked or speckled or spotted" (Genesis 30:37-39). In this way, Jacob became very prosperous. As to the outcome concerning the black lambs, the Holy Bible was not clear about it.

From this story, it becomes clear that what we see, feel, and think can influence the energy body, especially that of the unborn baby.

CHAKRAS OR ENERGY CENTERS

Chakras or whirling energy centers are very important parts of the energy body. Just as the visible physical body has vital and minor organs, the energy body has major, minor, and mini chakras. Major chakras are whirling energy centers which in general are about three to four inches in diameter. They control and energize the major and vital organs of the visible physical body. Major chakras are just like power stations that supply life energy to major and vital organs. When the power stations malfunction, the vital organs become sick or diseased because they do not have enough life energy to operate properly! Minor chakras are about one to two inches in diameter. Mini chakras are smaller than one inch in diameter. Minor and mini chakras control and energize the less important parts of the visible physical body. The chakras interpenetrate and extend beyond the visible physical body.

They have several important functions as follows:

1. They absorb, digest, and distribute prana to the different parts of the body.

2. The chakras control, energize, and are responsible for the proper functioning of the whole physical body and its different parts and organs. The endocrine glands are controlled and energized by some of the major chakras. The endocrine glands can be stimulated or inhibited by controlling or manipulating the major chakras. A lot of ailments are caused partially by the malfunctioning of the chakras.

3. Some chakras are sites or centers of the psychic faculties. Activation of certain chakras (energy centers) may result in the development of certain psychic faculties. For example, among the easiest and safest chakras to activate are the hand chakras. These are located at the center of the palms. By activating the hand chakras, one develops the ability to feel subtle energies and the ability to feel the outer, health, and inner auras. This can simply be accomplished by regularly concentrating on them. In this book, it is called sensitizing the hands.

ELEVEN MAJOR CHAKRAS

1. *Basic Chakra.* This chakra is located at the base of the spine or the coccyx area. The basic chakra controls, energizes and strengthens the whole visible physical body. It controls and energizes the muscular and skeletal systems, the spine, the production and the quality of the blood produced, the adrenal glands, the tissues of the body and of the internal organs. It also affects and

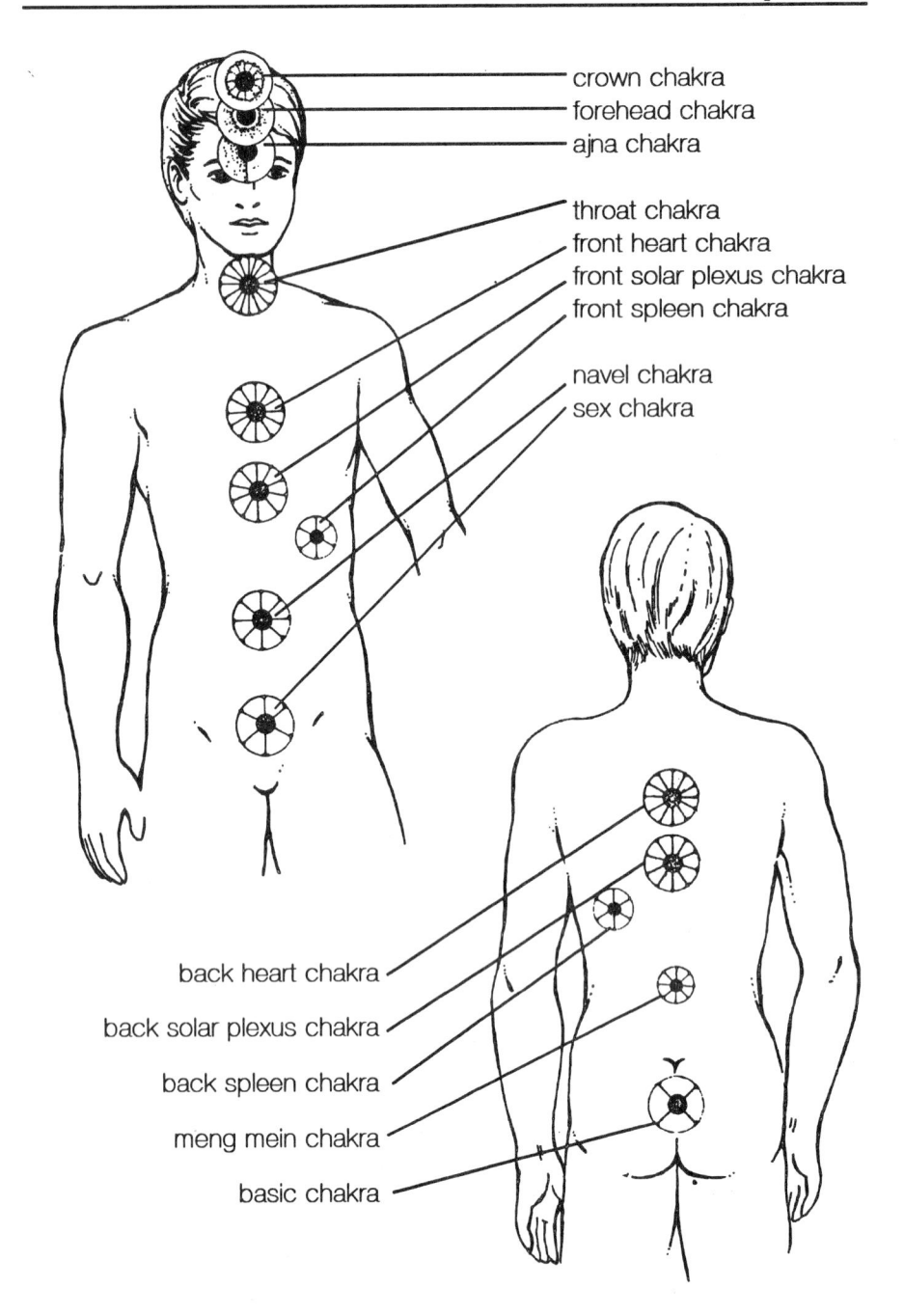

Fig. 2-4 *Eleven major chakras (energy centers)*

THE NATURE OF THE ENERGY BODY 21

energizes the sexual organs. The basic chakra affects body heat, the general vitality, and the growth of infants and children. Malfunctioning of this chakra manifests as arthritis, spinal ailments, blood ailments, cancer, bone cancer, leukemia, allergy, growth problem, low vitality, and slow healing of wounds and broken bones.

Persons with highly activated basic chakras tend to be robust and healthy, while those with less active basic chakras tend to be fragile and weak.

Old people usually have depleted or very depleted basic chakras. This is why their bodies are weak and become smaller; their spine tend to curve, and they tend to develop arthritis.

The basic chakra is like the root of a tree. If the root is weak, the tree is weak. If the basic chakra is very weak, the body is also very weak. Another term for the basic chakra is "root chakra".

2. *Sex Chakra.* This chakra is located on the pubic area. It controls and energizes the sexual organs and the bladder. Malfunctioning of this chakra manifests as sex-related problems. The ajna chakra, throat chakra and basic chakra have a strong influence on the sex chakra. Malfunctioning of any of these chakras may result in malfunctioning of the sex chakra.

3. *Meng Mein Chakra.* This chakra is located at the back of the navel. It serves as a "pumping station" in the spine; thus, it is responsible for the upward flow of subtle pranic energies coming from the basic chakra. It controls and energizes the kidneys and adrenal glands. It also controls the blood pressure.

Malfunctioning of this chakra manifests as kidney problems, low vitality, high blood pressure and back problems.

The meng mein chakra of infants, children, pregnant women and very old people should not be energized because of the

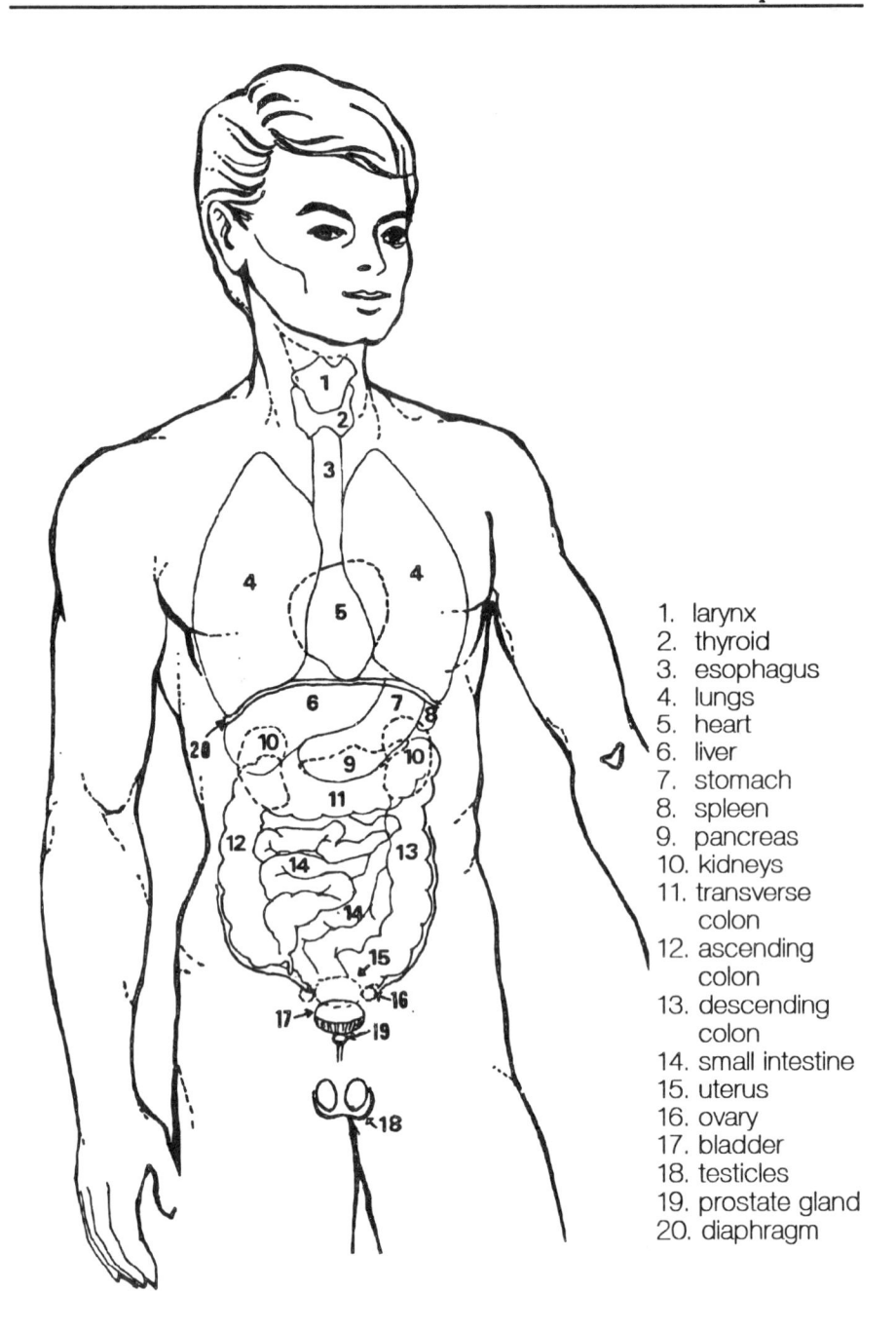

1. larynx
2. thyroid
3. esophagus
4. lungs
5. heart
6. liver
7. stomach
8. spleen
9. pancreas
10. kidneys
11. transverse colon
12. ascending colon
13. descending colon
14. small intestine
15. uterus
16. ovary
17. bladder
18. testicles
19. prostate gland
20. diaphragm

Fig. 2-5 *Internal organs*

THE NATURE OF THE ENERGY BODY 23

possible adverse effects that will be produced (please read *Advanced Pranic Healing* by Choa Kok Sui.). The meng mein chakra is about 1/3 to 1/2 the size of the other major chakras. This chakra should be treated only by experienced or advanced pranic healers.

The meng mein chakra and the sex chakra control and energize the urinary system.

4. *Navel Chakra.* This chakra is located on the navel. It controls and energizes the small intestine, large intestine, and appendix. It affects the general vitality of a person. Malfunctioning of the navel chakra manifests as constipation, appendicitis, difficulty in giving birth, low vitality and other diseases related to the intestines.

The word "ki" is used quite loosely to mean subtle energies. Ki is sometimes used to mean air prana, ground prana, red prana and other types of prana. It is also used to mean a type of "biosynthetic ki" produced by the navel chakra. This "biosynthetic ki" is quite different from prana or life energy. It affects one's ability to draw in, distribute, and assimilate prana. During bad weather conditions, the quantity of air prana is quite scarce. Persons with lesser "biosynthetic ki" have greater difficulty drawing in air prana; therefore, they tend to feel more tired or low than the average person.

The body gets nutrients by drinking and eating and, in the process, produces hormones through the endocrine glands. The food, water and juices correspond to the different types of pranic energies that is absorbed by the energy body. The hormones produced by the body correspond to the biosynthetic ki produced by the energy body. The biosynthetic ki produced by the navel chakra is golden in color.

5. *Spleen Chakra.* The front spleen chakra is located on the left part of the abdomen between the front solar plexus chakra and

the navel chakra. It is located at the middle part of the left bottom rib. The back spleen chakra lies at the back of the front spleen chakra. The spleen chakra is about 1/3 to 1/2 the size of the other major chakras.

The front and back spleen chakras control and energize the spleen. The spleen purifies the blood of diseased-causing germs. It also destroys worn-out blood cells. The front and back spleen chakras are the major entry points of air prana or air vitality globules. Air prana is digested by the spleen chakra; the digested prana is distributed to the other major chakras and the entire body, thereby energizing them. The spleen chakra apparently plays a vital part in man's general well-being. A weak spleen chakra means a weak physical body and low pranic energy level.

It is not advisable to energize the spleen chakra of infants and children because they may faint as a result of pranic congestion. Should this happen, just apply general sweeping (this is a general cleansing technique which is fully explained in Chapter Three). Also, it is not advisable to energize the spleen chakra of patients with hypertension or a history of hypertension because this may increase the blood pressure. However, this chakra is used to treat patients who are very weak or very depleted. In cases of severe infection, the spleen chakra should be treated to facilitate the rate of healing. Only experienced or advanced pranic healers should energize the spleen chakra.

6. *Solar Plexus Chakra.* There are two solar plexus chakras: the one located at the solar plexus area or the hollow area between the ribs is called the front solar plexus chakra, and the one at the back is called the back solar plexus chakra. The term "solar plexus chakra" shall mean both the front and back solar plexus chakras. This chakra controls and energizes the diaphragm, pancreas, liver, stomach and, to a certain degree, energizes the large and small intestines, appendix, lungs, heart and other parts of the body. This chakra also affects the quality of the blood because it controls and

THE NATURE OF THE ENERGY BODY

energizes the liver which detoxifies the blood. The solar plexus, through the liver, controls the cholesterol level of the body. It therefore affects the condition of the heart.

The solar plexus chakra is the energy clearing house center. Subtle energies from the lower chakras and from the higher chakras pass through it. The whole body can be energized through the solar plexus chakra. On rare occasions, overenergizing this chakra without first thoroughly cleansing may result in pranic congestion, thereby partially paralyzing the diaphragm, resulting in difficulty in breathing. Congested prana should be removed immediately. The solar plexus chakra also controls the heating and cooling system of the body. Malfunctioning of this chakra may manifest as diabetes, ulcer, hepatitis, heart ailments and other illnesses related to the organs mentioned.

The solar plexus chakra and the navel chakra control and energize the gastrointestinal system.

7. *Heart Chakra.* The front heart chakra is located at the center of the chest. It energizes and controls the heart, the thymus gland and the circulatory system. Malfunctioning of the front heart chakra manifests as heart and circulatory ailments. The solar plexus chakra is quite sensitive to emotion, tension and stress, and has a strong influence on the physical heart and the front heart chakra. Malfunctioning of the solar plexus chakra may cause the front heart chakra and the physical heart to also malfunction. The front heart chakra is closely connected to the front solar plexus chakra by several big energy channels, and is also energized by the front solar plexus chakra to a certain degree. Patients with heart problems usually have malfunctioning solar plexus chakra.

The back heart chakra is located at the back of the heart. It primarily controls and energizes the lungs and, to a lesser degree, the heart and the thymus gland. Malfunctioning of the back heart chakra manifests as lung problems such as asthma, tuberculosis, and others.

CHAKRA	LOCATION	FUNCTIONS AND CORRESPONDING ORGANS	DISEASES
1. Basic Chakra	Base of the Spine	Adrenal glands and sex organs. Energizes the whole physical body – bones, muscles, blood, and the internal organs. Affects general vitality, body heat, and the growth of infants and children. Center of self-survival or self-preservation.	Cancer, leukemia, low vitality, allergy, asthma, sexual ailments, arthritis, back problems, blood ailments, growth problem and psychological problems.
2. Sex Chakra	Pubic Area	Sexual organs, bladder and legs. Lower or physical creative center.	Sex-related problems and bladder ailments.
3. Meng Mein Chakra	Back of the navel	Kidneys, adrenal glands. Energizes to a certain degree other internal organs. Controls blood pressure.	Kidney problems, low vitality, high blood pressure and back problems.
4. Navel Chakra	Navel	Small and large intestines.	Constipation, difficulty in giving birth, appendicitis, low vitality and other diseases related to the intestines.
5. Spleen chakra a) Front Spleen	Left part of the abdomen between the front solar plexus chakra and the navel chakra. It is located at the middle part of the left bottom rib.	Spleen Major entry point for air prana or vitality globule. Energizes the other major chakras and the entire body.	

THE NATURE OF THE ENERGY BODY

b) Back Spleen	Back of the front spleen chakra.	Has similar functions as the front spleen chakra.	Low vitality, general weakness, and blood ailments.
6. Solar Plexus Chakra:		Acts as an energy clearing house center. Also controls the heating and cooling system of the body.	
a) Front Solar Plexus	Solar plexus area or the hollow area between the ribs.	Diaphragm, pancreas, liver, stomach and to a certain degree, large and small intestines, appendix and other internal organs.	High cholesterol level, diabetes, ulcer, hepatitis, rheumatoid arthritis, heart ailments and other diseases related to these organs.
b) Back Solar Plexus	Back of the front solar plexus chakra.	Has the same functions as the front solar plexus chakra.	
7. Heart Chakra:			
a) Front Heart	Center of the chest	Heart, thymus gland, and the circulatory system.	Heart and circulatory ailments.
b) Back Heart	Back of the heart	Lungs, heart, and thymus gland.	Lung ailments.
8. Throat Chakra	Center of the throat	Throat, thyroid and parathyroid glands, and the lymphatic system.	Throat-related illnesses like goiter, sore throat, asthma, etc.
9. Ajna Chakra	Between the eyebrows	Pituitary gland and endocrine glands. Controls the other major chakras.	Cancer, allergy, asthma, and diseases related to the endocrine glands.
10. Forehead Chakra	Center of the Forehead	Nervous system and pineal gland.	Diseases related to the nervous system.
11. Crown Chakra	Crown of the head	Brain and pineal gland.	Diseases related to the pineal gland and the brain (physical or psychological illnesses).

Energizing of the heart is done through the back heart chakra. Energizing the front heart chakra directly and immediately energizes the physical heart. However, the pranic energy tends to localize, or does not spread easily to other parts of the body. This may result in serious heart pranic congestion. It is not therefore advisable to intensely energize the front heart chakra for a prolonged period of time. Experienced pranic healers energize through the back heart chakra. This does not have a localized effect on the physical heart. Excess prana can easily flow to the lungs and to other parts of the body. The whole body could be energized through the back heart chakra.

8. *Throat Chakra.* This chakra is located at the center of the throat. It controls and energizes the throat, the thyroid glands, parathyroid glands and the lymphatic system. To a certain degree, it also influences the sex chakra. Malfunctioning of the throat chakra manifests as throat-related ailments such as goiter, sore throat, loss of voice, asthma, sterility, etc.

9. *Ajna Chakra.* This chakra is located at the area between the eyebrows. It controls and energizes the pituitary gland, the endocrine glands, and energizes the brain to a certain extent. It is also called the master chakra because it directs and controls the other major chakras and their corresponding endocrine glands and vital organs. It also affects the eyes and the nose. Malfunctioning of this chakra manifests as diseases related to the endocrine glands like diabetes. This requires not only treating the solar plexus chakra which controls the pancreas, but also the ajna chakra. Energizing this chakra also causes the whole body to be energized. The mechanism is different from the crown and the forehead chakra. Instead of the usual funneling effect, energizing the ajna chakra causes the other chakras to light up in a certain rapid sequence, thereby, energizing the whole body. That is why in charismatic healing or invocative healing, the healers touch with their fingers or palms either the crown or the forehead or the ajna chakra of the patients. The sudden intense rushing in of prana into the head area causes some patients to lose consciousness.

THE NATURE OF THE ENERGY BODY 29

The ajna, throat, back heart and solar plexus chakras control and energize the respiratory system.

10. *Forehead Chakra.* This is located at the center of the forehead. It controls and energizes the pineal gland and the nervous system. Malfunctioning of the forehead chakra may manifest as loss of memory, paralysis and epilepsy. Energizing this chakra has a similar funneling effect like the crown chakra, causing the whole body to be flooded with prana.

11. *Crown Chakra.* This is located at the crown of the head. It controls and energizes the pineal gland, the brain and the entire body. It is one of the major entry points of prana. Energizing the crown chakra has the effect of energizing the whole body. It is similar to pouring water on a funnel causing the whole body to be flooded with prana. Some healers proceed to energize the crown chakra even though the affected part is somewhere else. Malfunctioning of the crown chakra may manifest as diseases related to the pineal gland and brain. These may manifest as physical or psychological illnesses.

The crown and forehead chakra facilitates the harmonizing and normalizing of the other chakras, just as the pineal gland facilitates the harmonizing and normalizing of the other endocrine glands of the body. Modern scientific research shows that the pineal gland is connected with the aging and anti-aging process.

The whole body can be energized through the crown, forehead, ajna, back heart, solar plexus, navel, spleen, basic, hand, and foot chakras. An affected part can be energized directly or through the nearest chakra. Some healers may energize through a farther chakra, like the ajna or the crown chakra, to treat a heart or abdominal problem. Therefore, one can deduce that there are so many possible healing techniques to treat one type of ailment. But the basic principles are the same: cleansing and energizing.

Acupuncture points and chakras are gates through which prana can easily go in and out. By energizing through the nearest chakra, the projected prana will have easy and direct access to the affected part. While energizing directly, the affected part has a filtering action on the projected prana; therefore, energizing takes more time and more prana.

In energizing the whole body, the solar plexus chakra is usually used because of its proximity to the many important organs in the body. It is located at the center of the trunk which contains many essential organs. When energizing the solar plexus chakra, it should be done slowly and gently. Too much and too intense energizing can cause difficulty in breathing.

Many ancient esoteric books reveal only seven chakras or less. Although a few of them hint on the existence of more than seven, only in this book is the closely-guarded secret of the 11 major chakras explicitly revealed and explained in detail.

A thorough knowledge of the 11 major chakras is important. Just as learning physical anatomy is necessary for a person to become a good medical doctor, a full understanding of the 11 major chakras, which correspond to the anatomy of the energy body, is necessary to become a highly proficient pranic healer or energy healer.

THE MECHANISM BEHIND PSYCHOSOMATIC DISEASES

Uncontrolled and suppressed emotions and feelings such as anger, worry, prolonged irritation and frustrations have undesirable potent effects on the energy body. For instance, anger and frustration may result in pranic depletion around the solar plexus chakra and abdominal areas or may manifest as pranic congestion around the solar plexus chakra and the front heart chakra. In the first case, it manifests itself as indigestion or loose bowel movement. In the long run, it may manifest itself as an ulcer or a gall bladder problem. In the second case, it may manifest as heart enlargement or some other heart-related problems. It seems that negative emotion may manifest as a certain type of disease in one patient but may manifest as another type of disease in another patient.

Anger and intense worry devitalize the whole energy body so that the body becomes susceptible to all kinds of diseases. Negative emotions cause disturbances in the energy body so that the whole physical body becomes sick. You may have experienced that after intense anger or an altercation, you felt physically exhausted or became sick. This is because both the energy and visible physical bodies had been drained of prana or life energy and become susceptible to infection.

If the ailment is of emotional origin, the patient must not only be given pranic healing but also psychological counseling. He should be asked to undergo a course in character-building and to meditate regularly to help him overcome his negative emotional tendencies. Through daily inner reflection and meditation, the patient will develop greater self-awareness and emotional maturity, greatly improving his ability to control and channel his emotions, and consequently, vastly improving his health. It should be noted that in this case, pranic healing will not produce a permanent cure unless there is a corresponding emotional change. It is like extinguishing a fire caused by an arsonist without bothering to catch the culprit. What is to prevent the arsonist from burning the house again once it has been rebuilt? The root cause of the disease must be removed so that permanent healing can take place.

THE EXTERNAL AND INTERNAL FACTORS OF DISEASES

In the understanding of diseases, one should take into consideration the external and internal factors or the seen and unseen causes. External factors mean those physical factors which contribute to diseases like germs, malnutrition, toxins, pollutants, lack of exercise, poor breathing habits, insufficient water intake, etc. Internal factors mean the emotional and energy factors which contribute to diseases like negative emotions, blocked meridians, pranic depletion and congestion, chakral malfunctioning, etc.

For instance, an emotional factor may lead to the weakening of the solar plexus chakra and the liver, and the attack by a virus will lead to an inflammation of the liver. The external factor is the virus. The internal factors are the negative emotion and weakening of the solar plexus chakra and the liver, which make the liver vulnerable to viral infection.

If the person's solar plexus chakra and liver are in good condition, and if he is a person of higher vitality, then his probability of contracting the disease is lesser. His body's defense mechanism or detoxifying and eliminating system would likely overcome the virus or the toxin.

The application of pranic healing would cleanse, strengthen, and gradually restore the solar plexus chakra and the liver to their normal conditions. This can be done with or without the aid of drugs.

Diseases may manifest under the following conditions:

1. The presence of external and internal factors

2. The presence of an overwhelming internal factor only. For example, a person harboring intense anger and

frustration may cause severe pranic congestion around the solar plexus chakra and, in the long run, the heart. Even if he were to watch his diet, he would still end up with a heart problem like heart enlargement. Also, habitual tension or stress may result in pranic congestion around the eye area and, in the long run, may result in glaucoma. (NOTE: Not all glaucomae are of emotional origin.)

3. The presence of an overwhelming external factor only. For instance, taking a large dose of poison would certainly be fatal even if your energy body is in perfect condition. Poor reading habits would also eventually result in eye defects.

WHAT ARE THE FUNCTIONS OF THE ENERGY BODY?

1. It absorbs, distributes, and energizes the whole physical body with prana or ki. Prana or ki is that life energy which nourishes the whole body so that it could, together with its different organs, function properly and normally. Without prana, the body would die.

2. It acts as a mold or pattern for the visible physical body. This allows the visible physical body to maintain its shape, form and feature despite years of continuous metabolism. To be more exact, the visible physical body is molded after the energy body. If the energy body is defective, then the visible physical body is defective. They are so closely related that what affects one affects the other. If one gets sick, the other also gets sick. If one gets healed, the other also gets healed. This may manifest gradually or almost instantaneously, assuming there are no interfering factors.

3. The energy body, through the chakras or whirling energy centers, controls and is responsible for the proper functioning of the whole physical body and its different parts and organs. This includes the endocrine glands, which are external manifestations of some of the major chakras. A lot of sicknesses are caused partially by the malfunctioning of one or more chakras.

4. The energy body, through its health rays and health auras, serves as a protective shield against germs and diseased energy. Diseased energy, used-up energy, toxins, wastes, and germs are expelled by the health rays predominantly via the pores, thereby purifying the whole physical body.

BASIC PROBLEMS AND TREATMENTS IN PRANIC HEALING

Pranic healing involves the use of prana and the manipulation of bioplasmic matter of the patient's body. The following are the basic problems and treatments encountered in pranic healing:

1. In areas where there is pranic depletion, cleansing and energizing are applied to the affected areas. The emphasis is on energizing.

2. In areas where there is pranic congestion, diseased and congested energy is removed or extracted from the affected areas. This is followed by projecting prana to the treated area. The emphasis is on cleansing or decongesting.

3. A malfunctioning chakra is restored by simply cleansing and energizing it with prana.

THE NATURE OF THE ENERGY BODY

4. Drooping and entangled health rays are disentangled and strengthened.

5. Blocked meridians or energy channels are cleansed and energized.

6. Prana which leaks out through holes in the outer aura are sealed.

7. Specific types of prana are applied to produce specific results. Certain illnesses need a specific type or types of prana to produce faster results. This is taught in advanced pranic healing.

LEVELS IN PRANIC HEALING

Pranic healing has several levels gradating from simple to more complicated concepts, and from easy to difficult techniques.

Level One: Elementary Pranic Healing

At this level, the concepts and techniques are easy to learn. Tactile concentration is required. It takes about three to five sessions to learn the basic principles and techniques and to be able to do simple pranic healing. About a few days, a few weeks or a few months of regular practice and application are required to become proficient, depending on the attitude of the student.

Level Two: Intermediate Pranic Healing

This level is still easy. Pranic breathing is used at this level. Visual concentration is optional but still not required. Just as in level one, this takes about three to five sessions to learn the basic principles and techniques to be able to start healing more difficult cases. To become proficient takes about a few weeks to about two months of regular practice and application, depending on the attitude of the student.

Level Three: Distant Pranic Healing

This level involves a gradual development of one's psychic faculty. It may take several weeks or months to a year or two of regular practice and application to become very accurate in diagnosis and to produce specific, accurate, predetermined results.

Level Four: Advanced Pranic Healing

The use of visualization techniques is definitely required and a more thorough knowledge on the nature of diseases and the properties of different types of prana is necessary. Advanced pranic healers are expected to have a strong energy body and a big inner aura. This is taught in the book *Advanced Pranic Healing* by Choa Kok Sui. Advanced pranic healing uses color prana and advanced healing techniques to produce rapid healing results. To become proficient in advanced pranic healing would require at least one to two years of regular practice.

Level Five: Pranic Psychotherapy

Pranic psychotherapy is advanced pranic healing applied in the field of psychological ailments. The practitioner should be at least proficient in intermediate pranic healing. This is taught in the book *Pranic Psychotherapy* by Choa Kok Sui.

Level Six: Pranic Crystal Healing

Pranic Crystal Healing is using crystals as instruments to facilitate pranic treatment.

LEVELS OF CERTIFICATION

Associate Pranic Healer

Proficient in elementary and intermediate pranic healing. In the process of becoming proficient in distant healing, advanced pranic healing and pranic psychotherapy. An associate pranic healer is just like a medical intern or an apprentice.

Certified Pranic Healer

Proficient in advanced pranic healing, pranic psychotherapy, and pranic crystal healing.

Certified Pranic Psychotherapist

A certified pranic healer who has specialized in pranic psychotherapy.

Certified Senior Pranic Healer

Very experienced and proficient in advanced pranic healing, pranic psychotherapy, and pranic crystal healing. At the moment, relatively rare.

Certified Assistant Master Pranic Healer

Proficient in using powerful and very advanced pranic healing techniques not revealed at the moment to the public. A certified assistant master pranic healer has been trained under the guidance of a master or grand master pranic healer. Also, should have a track record of producing many rapid miraculous healing that other pranic healers in general will find difficult to duplicate. At the moment, rare.

Certified Master Pranic Healer

Much more skillful and powerful than an assistant master pranic healer. Has trained several students to become a certified assistant master pranic healer. At the moment, very rare.

Certified Grand Master Pranic Healer

Can heal very difficult cases in one or two sessions if karmically permissible and if patient is receptive. The high level of healing skill achieved is extremely rare.

The standards set in Pranic Healing are relatively high. As a matter of fact, an associate pranic healer is usually more skillful and competent in healing than another healer with the title of a master belonging to some other schools.

Many healers of other schools are adapting techniques from pranic healing. This is good. However, pranic healing is not given proper acknowledgement. Credit should be given where it is due.

RECOMMENDED READINGS

The Chakras by C.W. Leadbeater. 1927. The Theosophical Publishing House. Adyar, Madras.

This book deals with the different types of prana. It also discusses the negative effects of alcohol, drugs, and tobacco on the etheric body. It contains 10 colored illustrations of the chakras based on the clairvoyant observations of Mr. Leadbeater.

Esoteric Healing by Alice Bailey. 1953. New York. Lucis Publishing Company.

THE NATURE OF THE ENERGY BODY

The Aura by W. J. Kilner. 1911. York Beach, Maine. Samuel Weiser, Inc.

The Etheric Double by A. E. Powell. 1969. Wheaton, Ill. The Theosophical Publishing House, Quest Books.

Essentially, this book is a treatise on the etheric body and etheric phenomena. Its contents are largely based on the writings of Madame Blavatsky, C. W. Leadbeater, and Annie Besant. These highly developed clairvoyants conducted clairvoyant researches and experiments. They recorded their observations and conclusions in their writings during the years 1897-1923.

The following is a summation of the main points relevant to the study of pranic healing:

1. The whole physical body is actually composed of two bodies: the visible physical body and the invisible etheric body which is made up of finer substances called etheric matter (Chap. 1, p. 3). This etheric body corresponds to what is now called the bioplasmic body.

2. The etheric body is the vehicle of prana or ki (Chap. 1, p. 4).

3. The etheric body has many nadis or etheric channels through which prana or ki flows (Chap. 3, p. 22). These etheric channels are the equivalent of the meridians or bioplasmic channels.

4. The etheric body is the mold or pattern of the visible physical body (Chap. 2, p. 13).

5. The etheric body has several chakras or etheric whirling centers which absorb, digest, and distribute prana and is responsible for the proper functioning of the whole body (Chap. 3, p. 22;

Chap. 4, p. 32).

6. Some chakras are psychic faculty centers or the sites of our psychic faculties (Chaps. 3-13, pp. 22-62).

7. Prana can be obtained from sunlight, air, and trees (Chap. 2, pp. 8, 16-21).

8. The visible physical body and its etheric body are so closely interrelated that what affects one also affects the other (Chap. 1, p. 6). Healing is brought about by removing the diseased etheric matter from the patient's etheric body and by transferring or projecting prana from the healer's etheric body to that of the patient's etheric body (Chap. 17, pp. 74-83).

9. A strong health aura acts as a protective shield against germs and infection (Chap. 4, p. 33).

10. Persons whose limbs have been amputated sometimes complain that they still feel the limb in place. The reason for this is that the etheric counterpart or the etheric mold is still intact (Chap, 1, p. 6).

It should be noted that the existence of the etheric body and other important points mentioned in the preceding items were later verified or rediscovered by Russian scientists!

MODERN FINDINGS

Theories of the Chakras: Bridge to Higher Consciousness by Hiroshi Motoyama. 1981. Wheaton, Ill. The Theosophical Publishing House.

This book deals with the scientific experiments and personal experience of Dr. Hiroshi Motoyama on the chakras. It also gives instructions on how to activate the chakras. The Chinese acupuncture meridians are compared with the Indian nadis. This book is quite interesting and very informative.

Psychic Discoveries Behind the Iron Curtain by Sheila Ostrander and Lynn Schroeder. Englewood Cliffs: Prentice Hall, 1970. Bantam edition, 1971.

This book describes the extensive scientific investigations on psychic phenomena being conducted in the Soviet Union. Many of the findings merely reconfirm what have been known by esoteric students since ancient times. All references are made to the Bantam edition.

1. In 1939, Semyon Davidovich Kirlian and his wife developed Kirlian photography based on high-frequency electric field which is used to take pictures of a portion of the invisible energy body or the bioplasmic body (Chap. 16, pp. 202-06).

2. Based on the studies of the Kirlians, it has been observed that disease first manifests on the bioplasmic body before it appears on the visible physical body (Chap. 16, pp. 207-10).

3. At the highly respected Kirov State University in Alma-Ata, a group of biologists, biochemists and biophysicists declared that the bioplasmic body is not merely some sort of plasma-like constellation of ionized, excited electrons, protons and possibly some other particle but is a whole unified organism in itself which acts as a unit that gives off its own electromagnetic fields (Chap. 17, p. 217).

4. Emotions, states of mind, and thoughts affect the bioplasmic body (Chap. 16, p. 209).

5. Based on the findings of the State University of Kazakhstan, the energy body has a specific organizing pattern that

determines the form of the organism. For instance, Dr. Alexander Studitsky of the Institute of Animal Morphology in Moscow minced up muscle tissue and packed it into a wound in a rat's body. An entirely new muscle was grown. From this they concluded that there is some sort of an organizing pattern (Chap. 17, p. 218).

6. If a man loses a finger or an arm, he still retains the bioplasmic finger or arm so that sometimes he still feels it is still there (Chap. 17, p. 216).

7. Dr. Mikhail Kuzmich Gaikin, a Leningrad scientist, confirmed the existence of bioplasmic channels and centers that correspond to the meridians and the acupuncture points described in ancient Chinese medicine (Chap. 18, pp. 226-29). With the aid of the tobiscope, he accurately pinpointed the location of the acupuncture points. Later, a young physicist, Victor Adamenko, invented an improved version of the tobiscope and called it the CCAP — Conductivity of the Channels of Acupuncture Points, which locates not only acupuncture points but also numerically graphed reactions and changes in the bioplasmic body (Chap. 18, p. 232).

8. The acupuncture points correspond to the bright spots in the bioplasmic body (Chap. 18, p. 226).

9. The Russians also seriously considered the possibility of stimulating certain points in the bioplasmic body to activate latent psychic abilities (Chap. 18, pp. 231-33).

10. Researches done on Russian psychic healers indicate that psychic healing involves a transfer of energy from the bioplasmic body of the healer to the bioplasmic body of his patient (Chap. 18, p. 224).

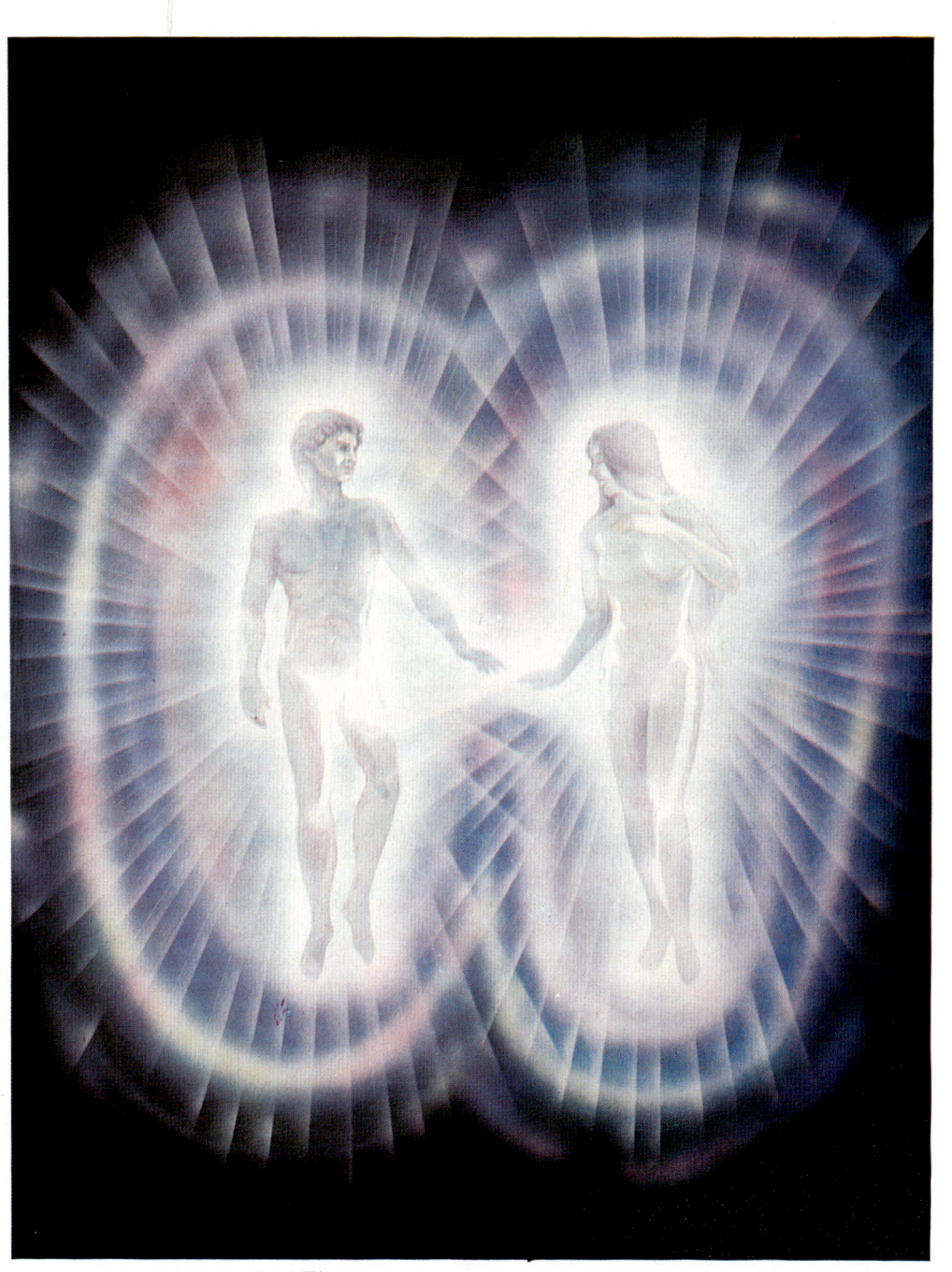

Inner *and* Outer Auras *of a Loving Couple*

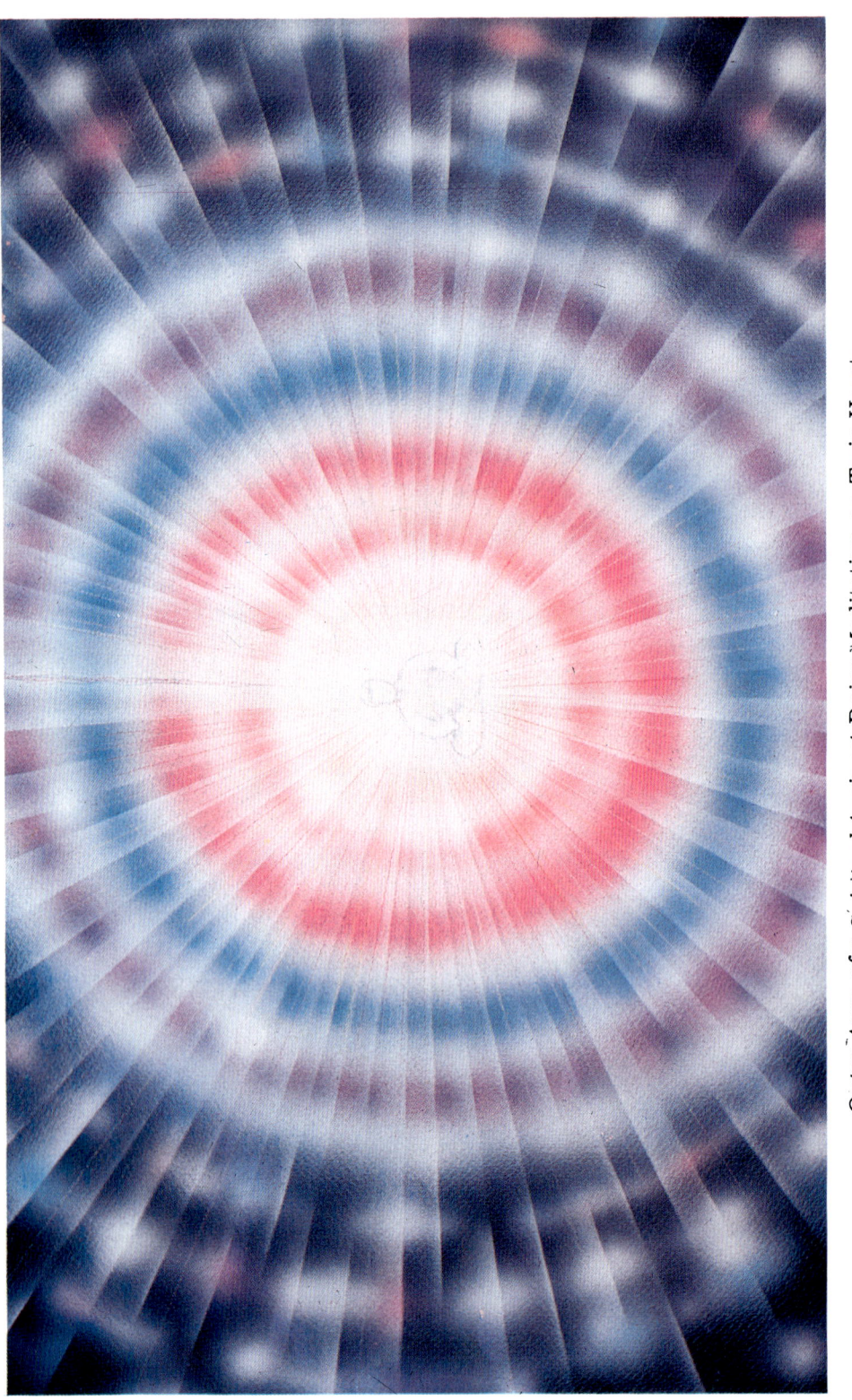

Outer Aura of a Spiritual Aspirant Doing Meditation on Twin Hearts

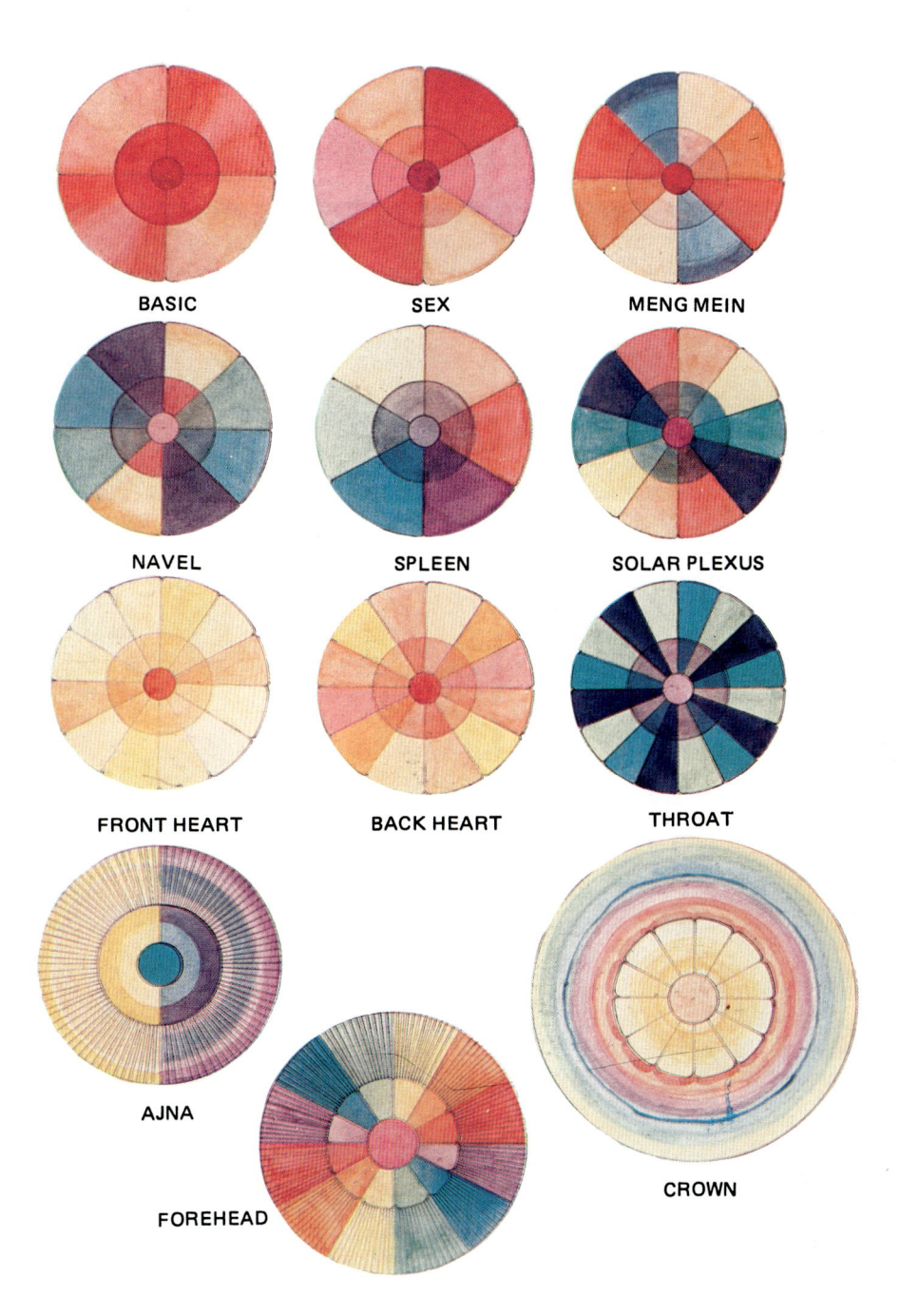

BASIC	SEX	MENG MEIN
NAVEL	SPLEEN	SOLAR PLEXUS
FRONT HEART	BACK HEART	THROAT
AJNA	FOREHEAD	CROWN

Eleven Major Chakras

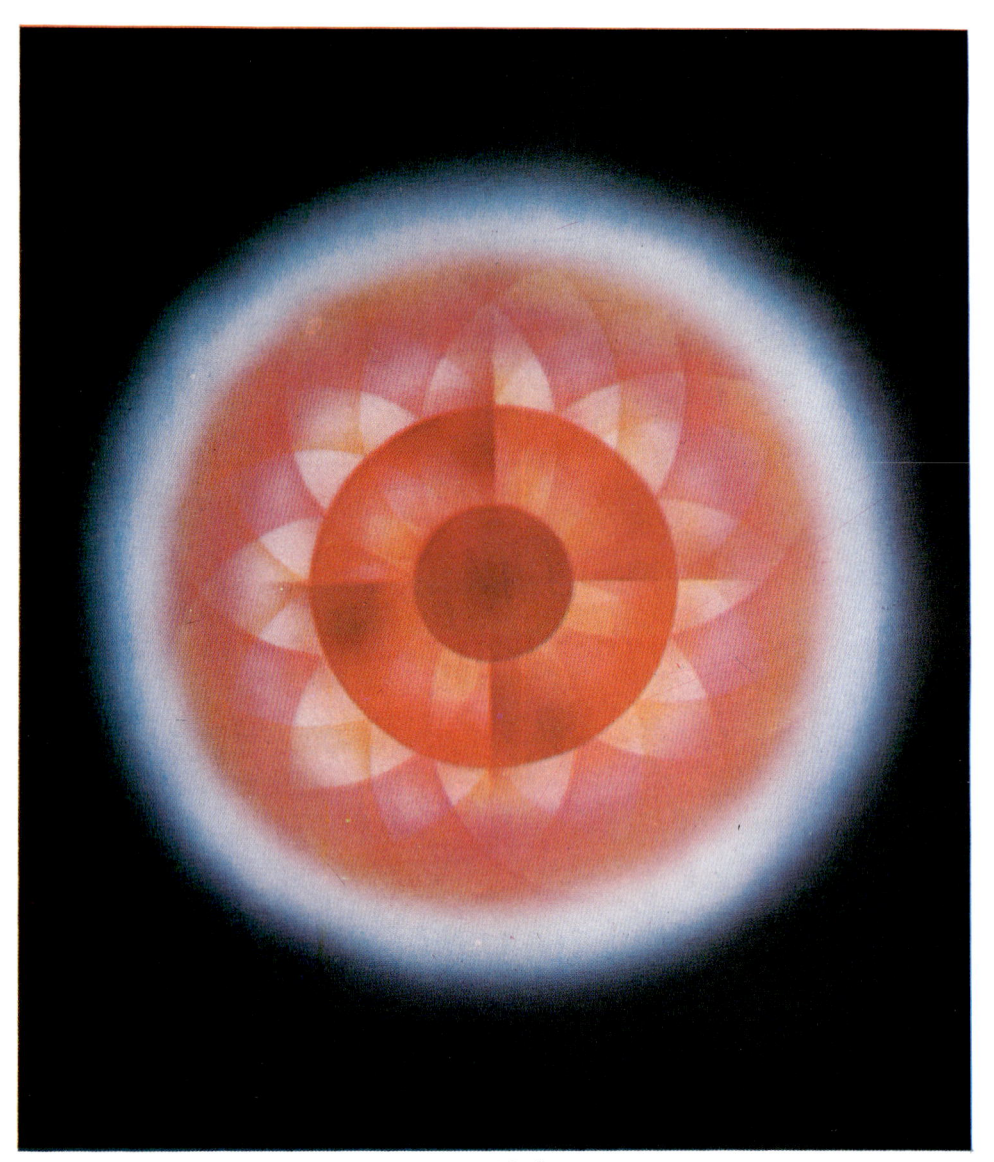

Basic Chakra

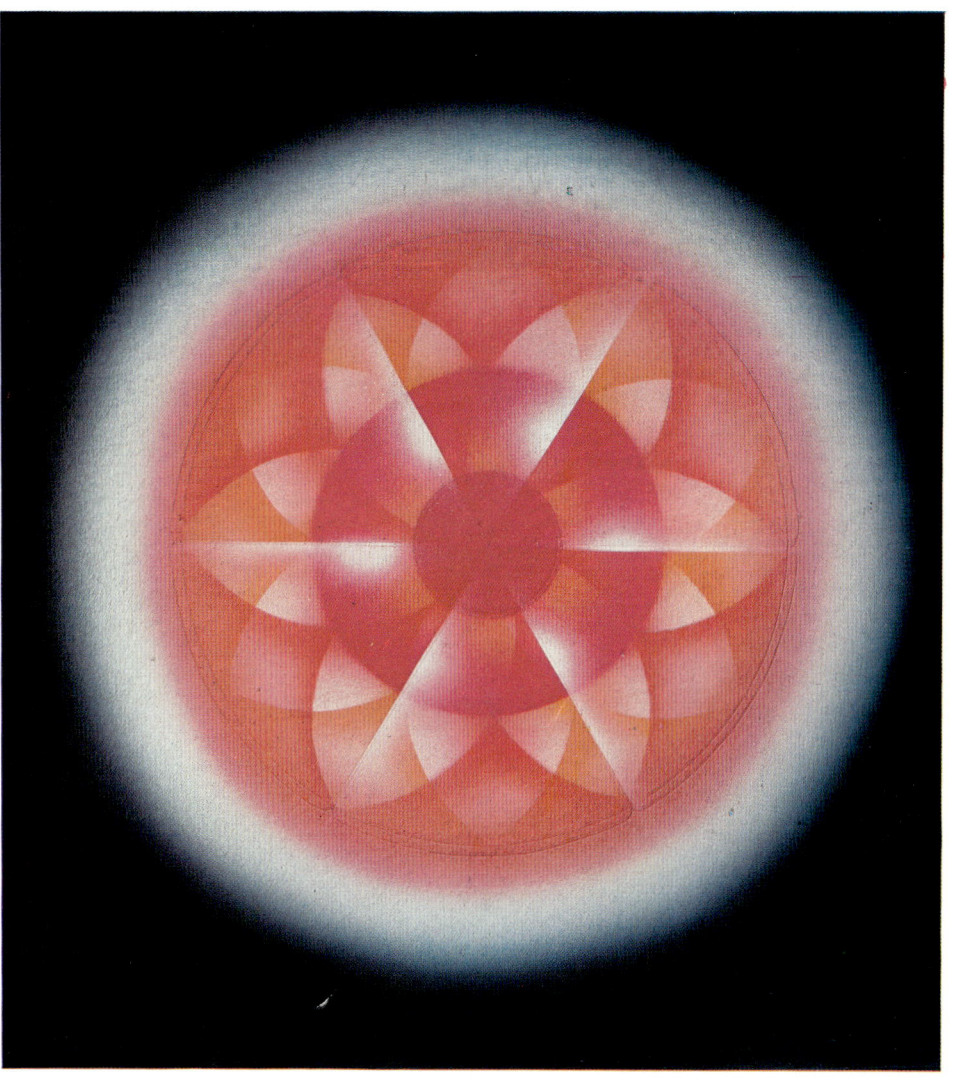

Sex Chakra

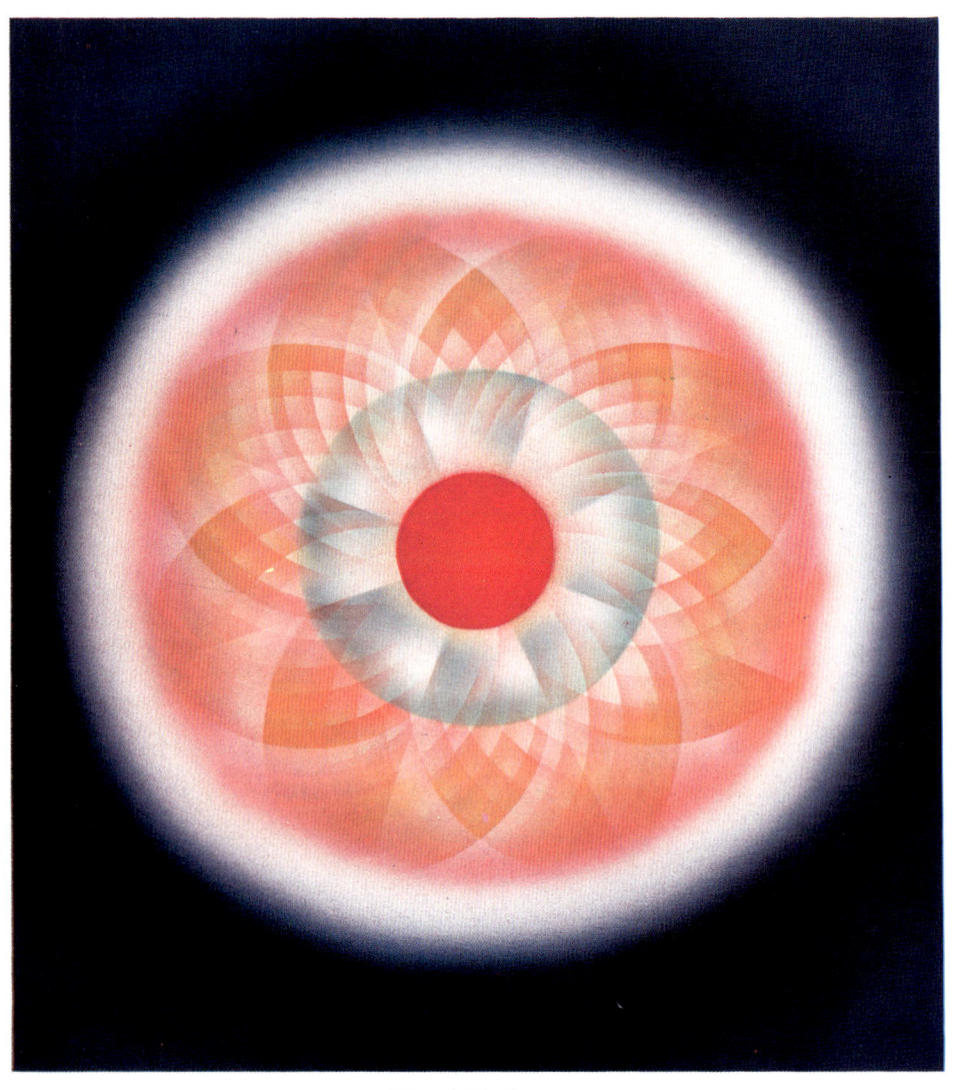

Navel Chakra

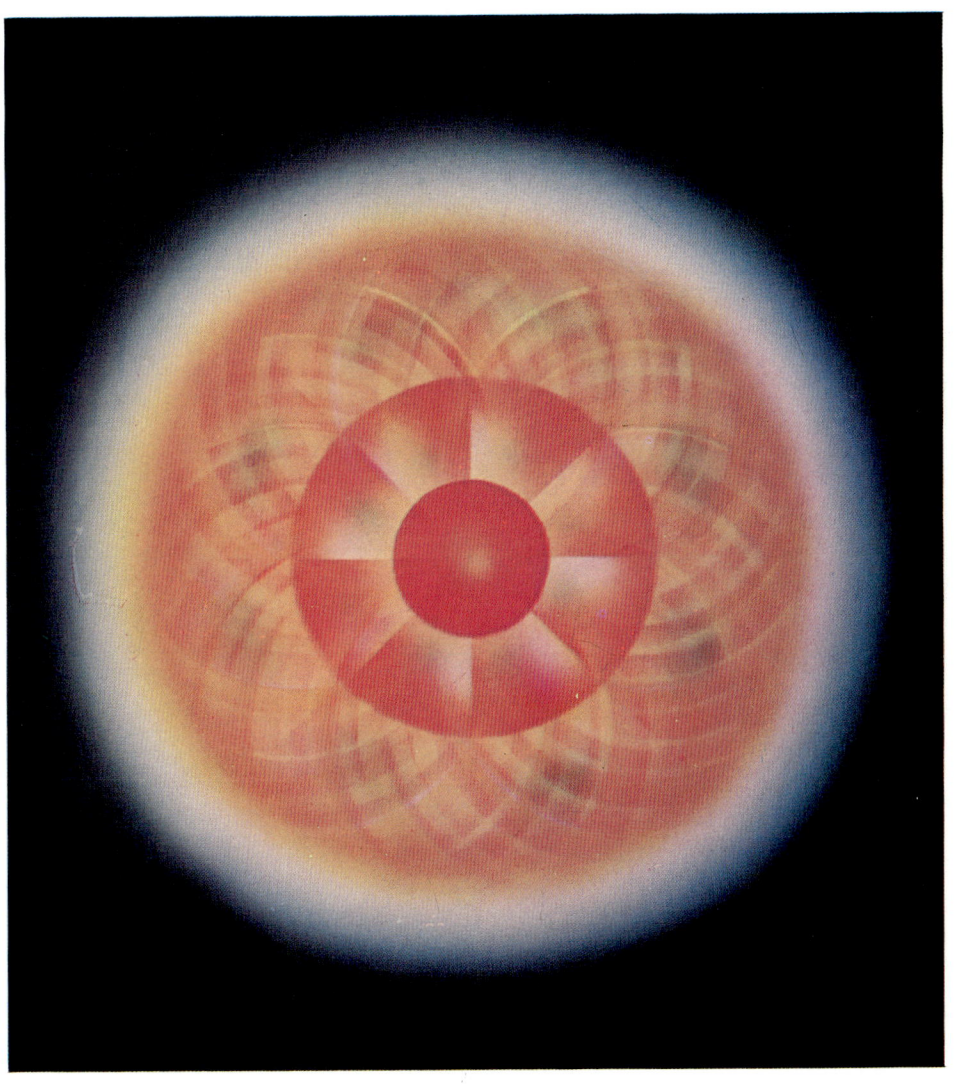

Meng Mein Chakra

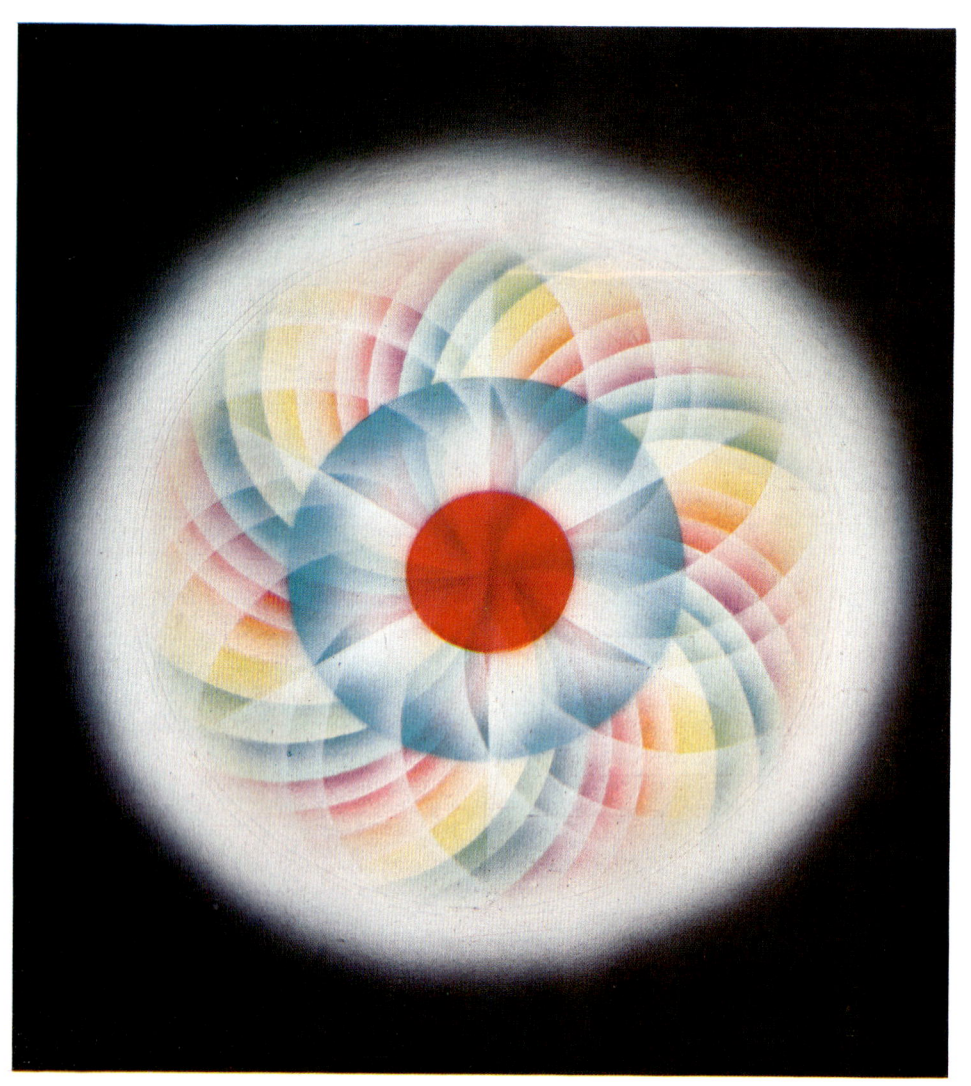

Spleen Chakra

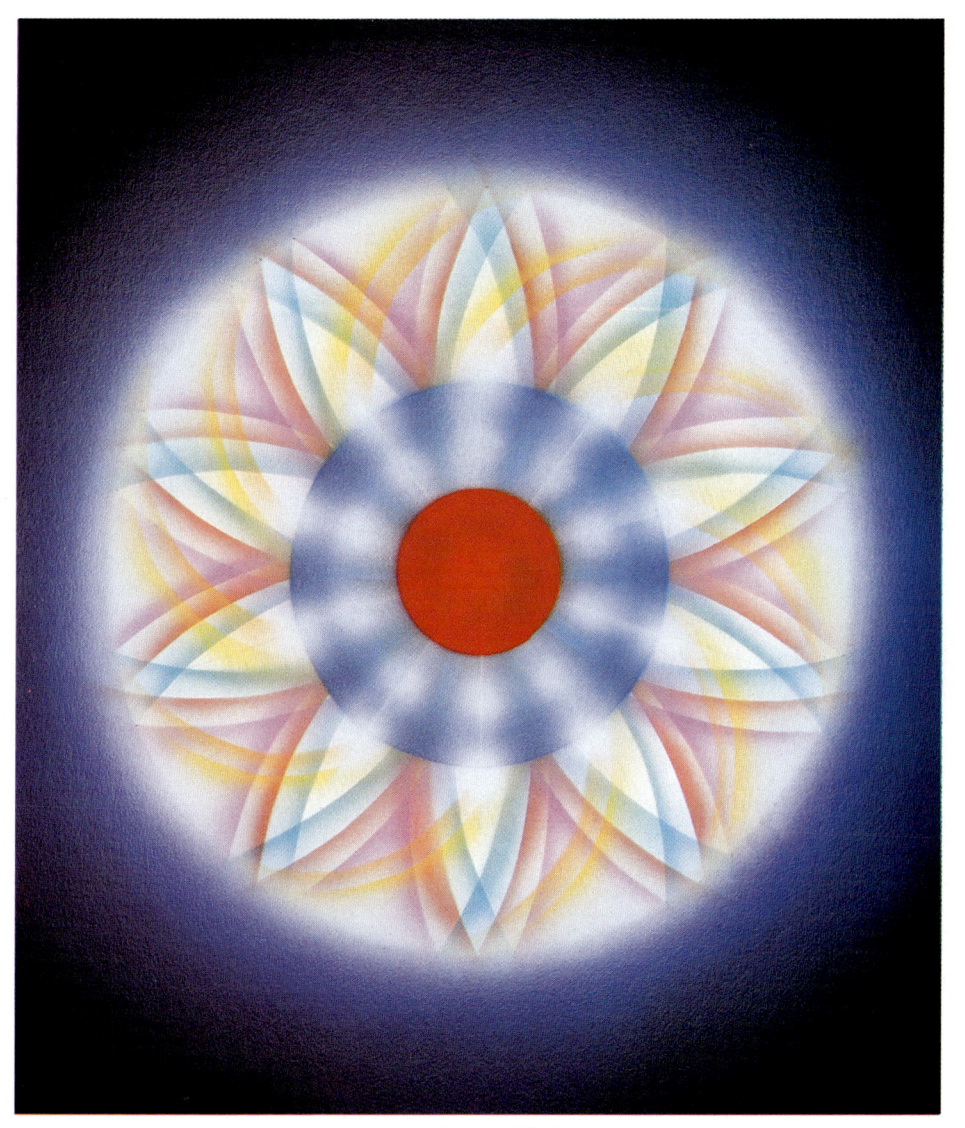

Solar Plexus Chakra

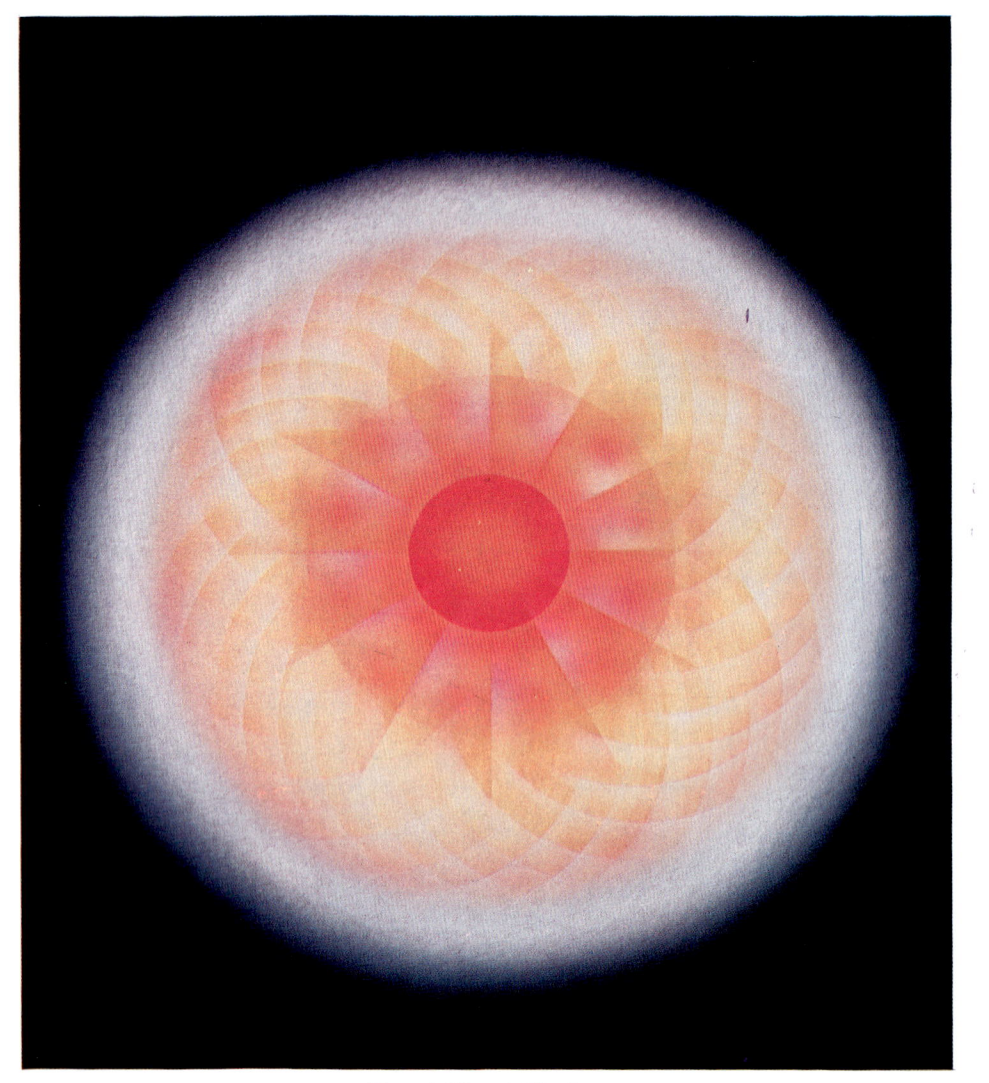

Front Heart Chakra

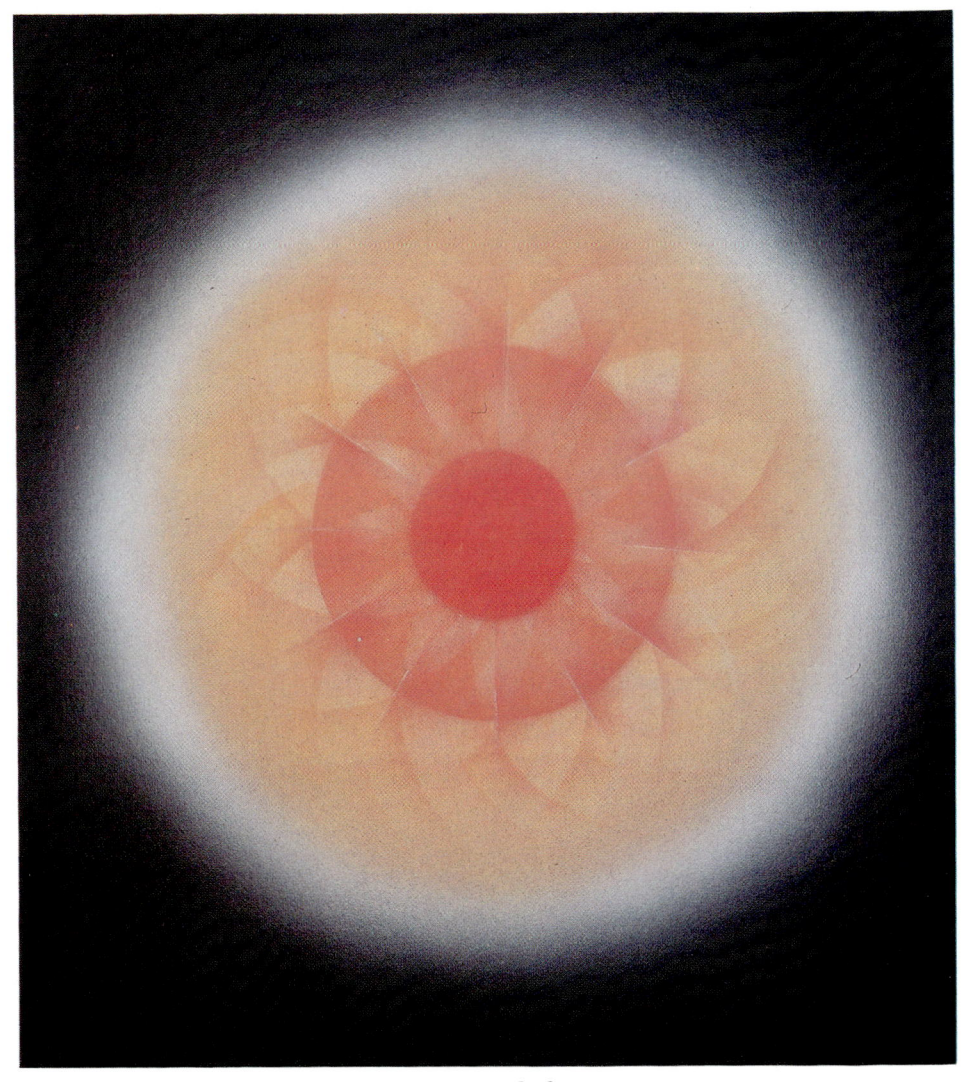

Back Heart Chakra

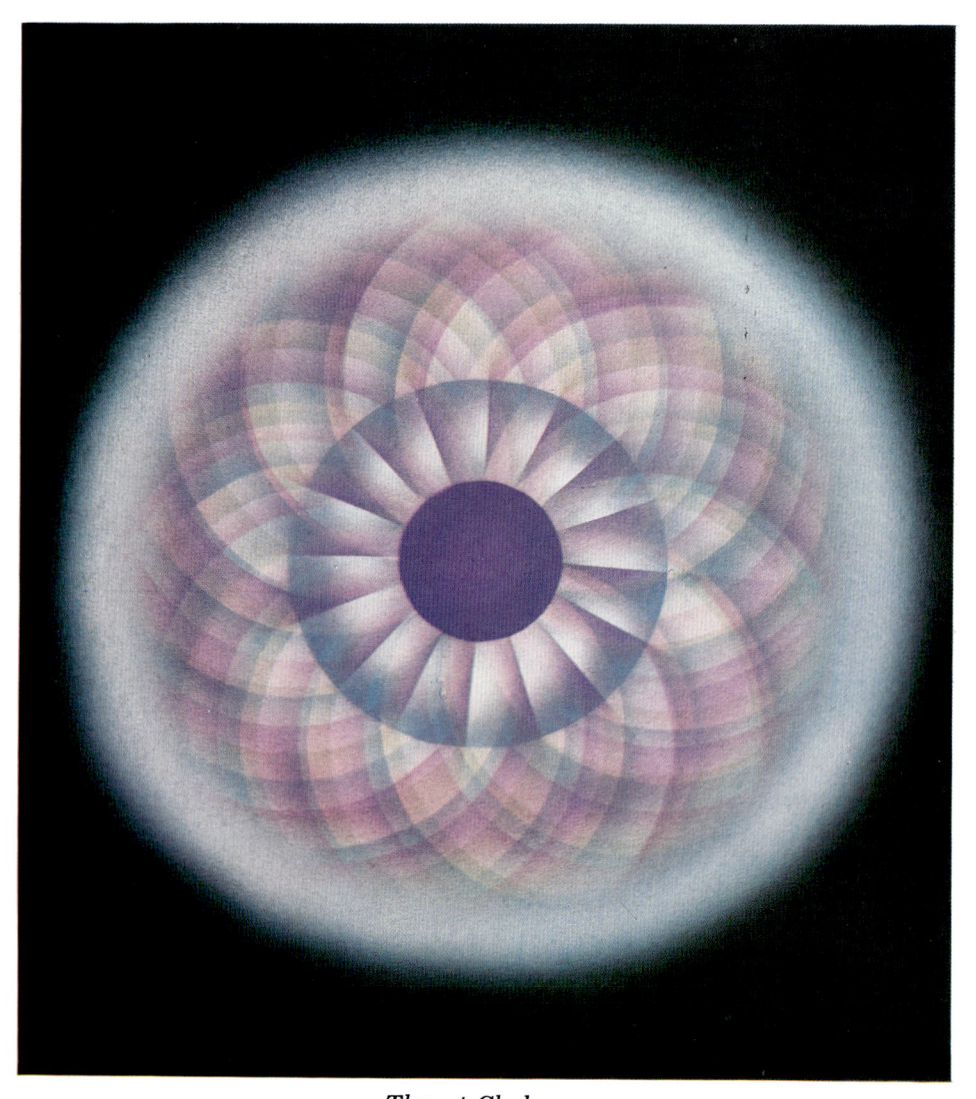

Throat Chakra

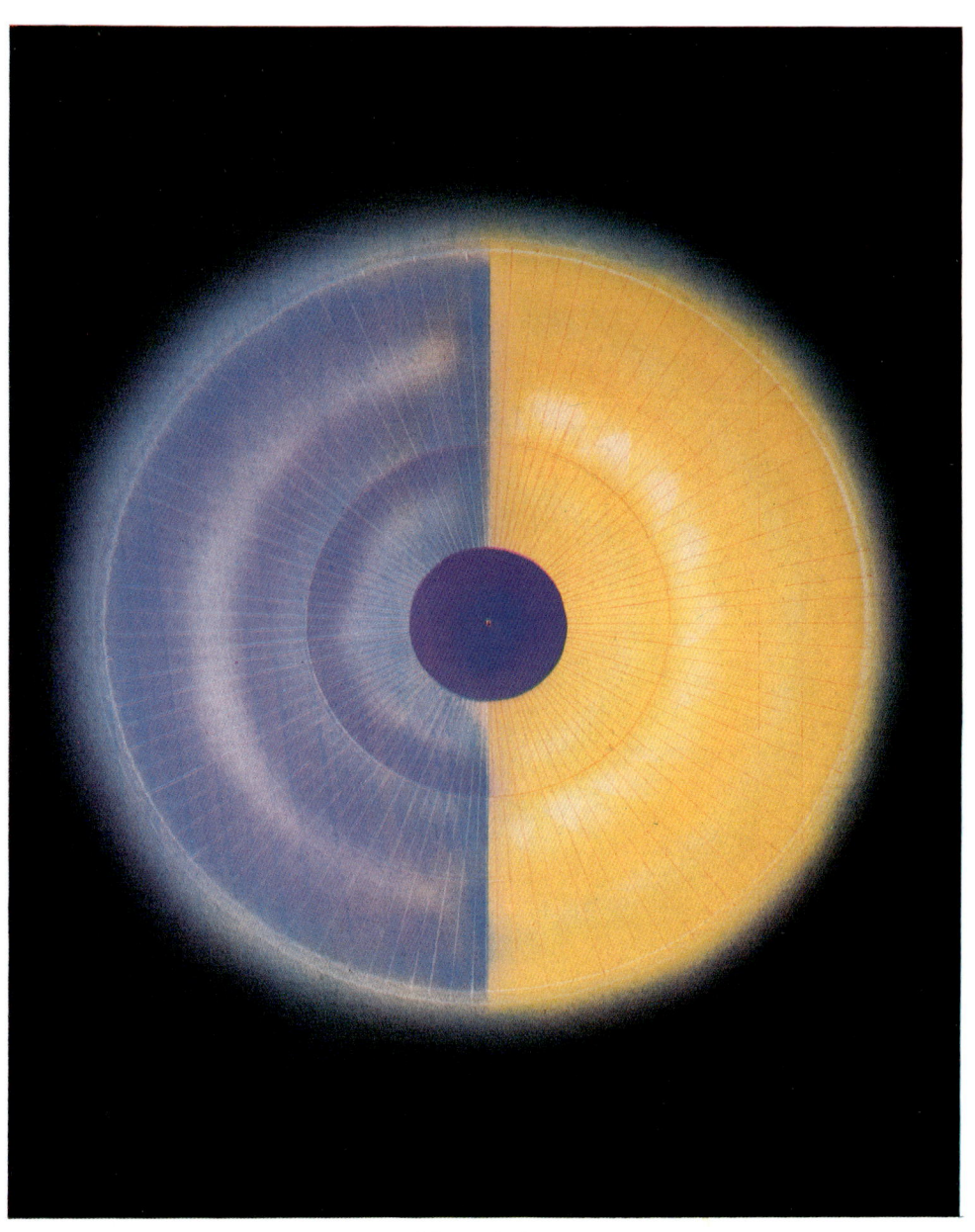

Ajna Chakra

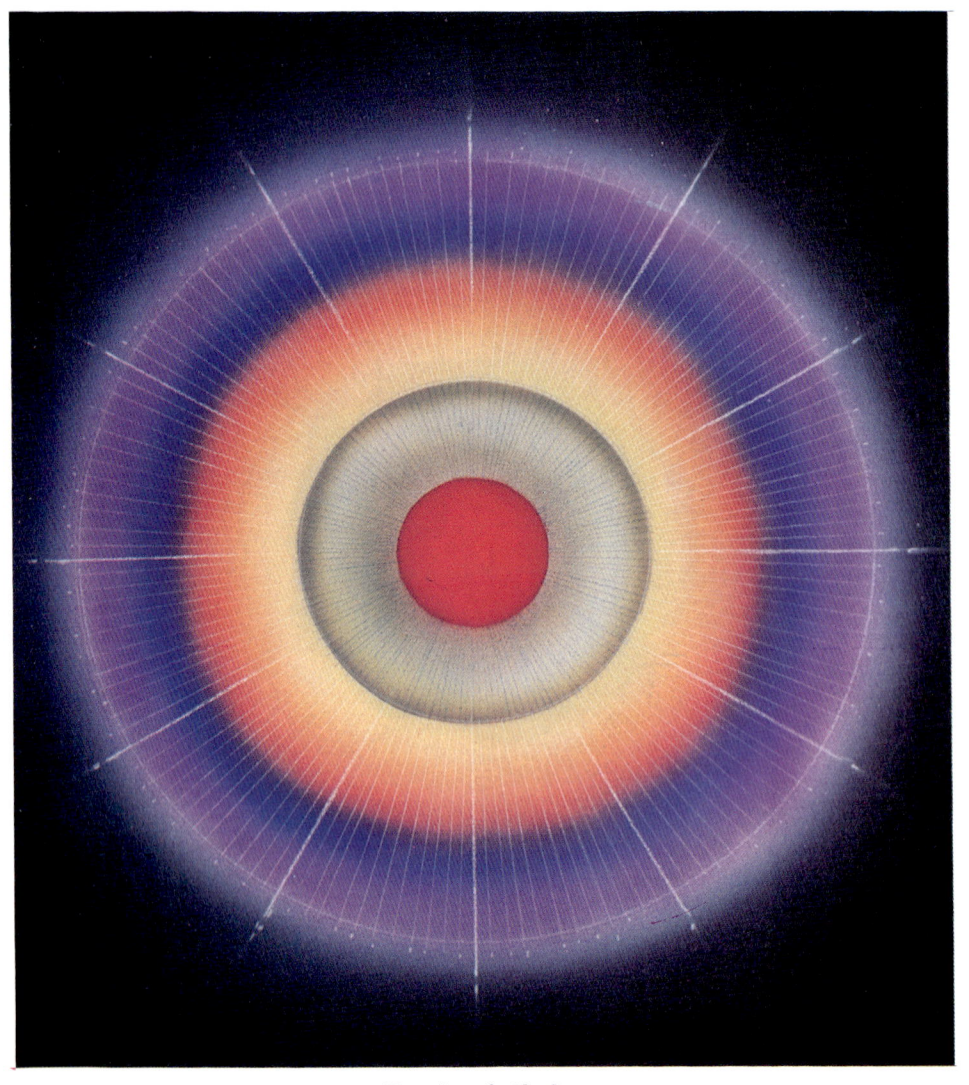

Forehead Chakra

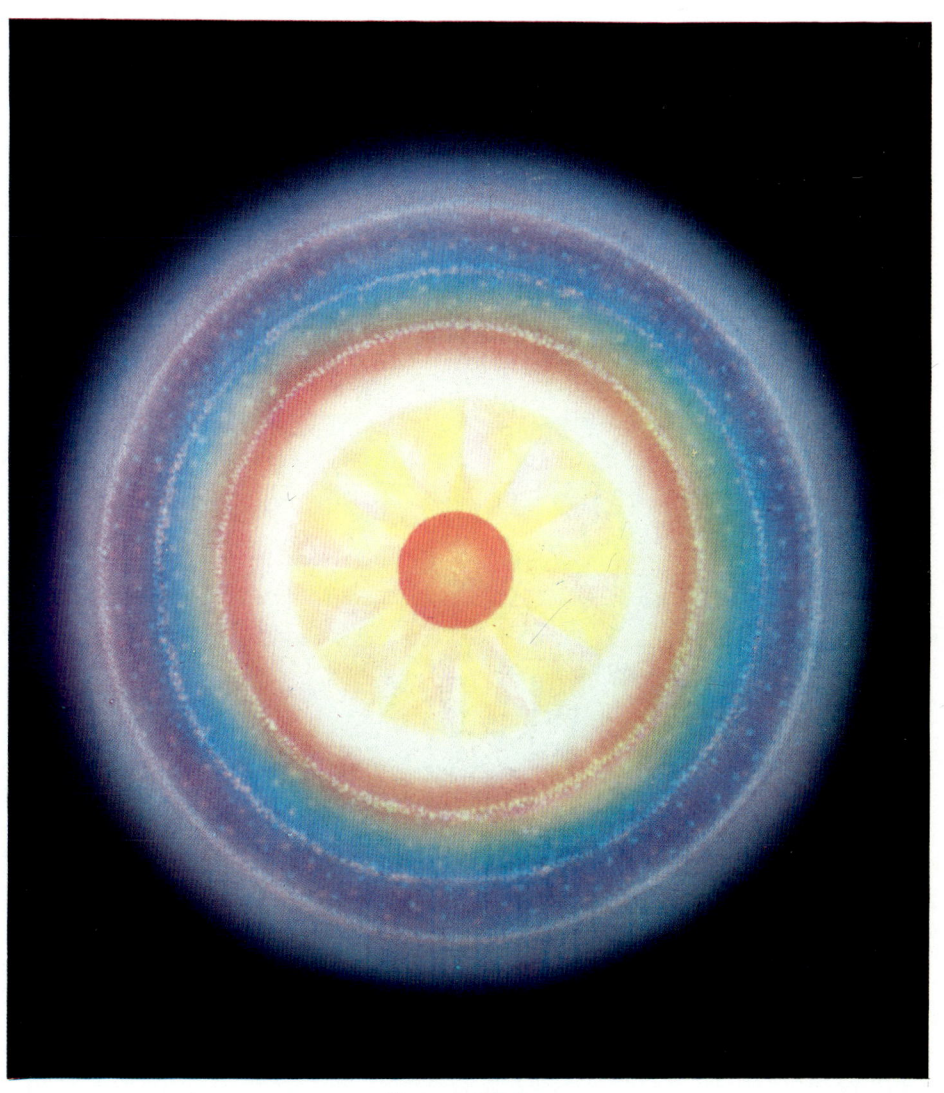

Crown Chakra

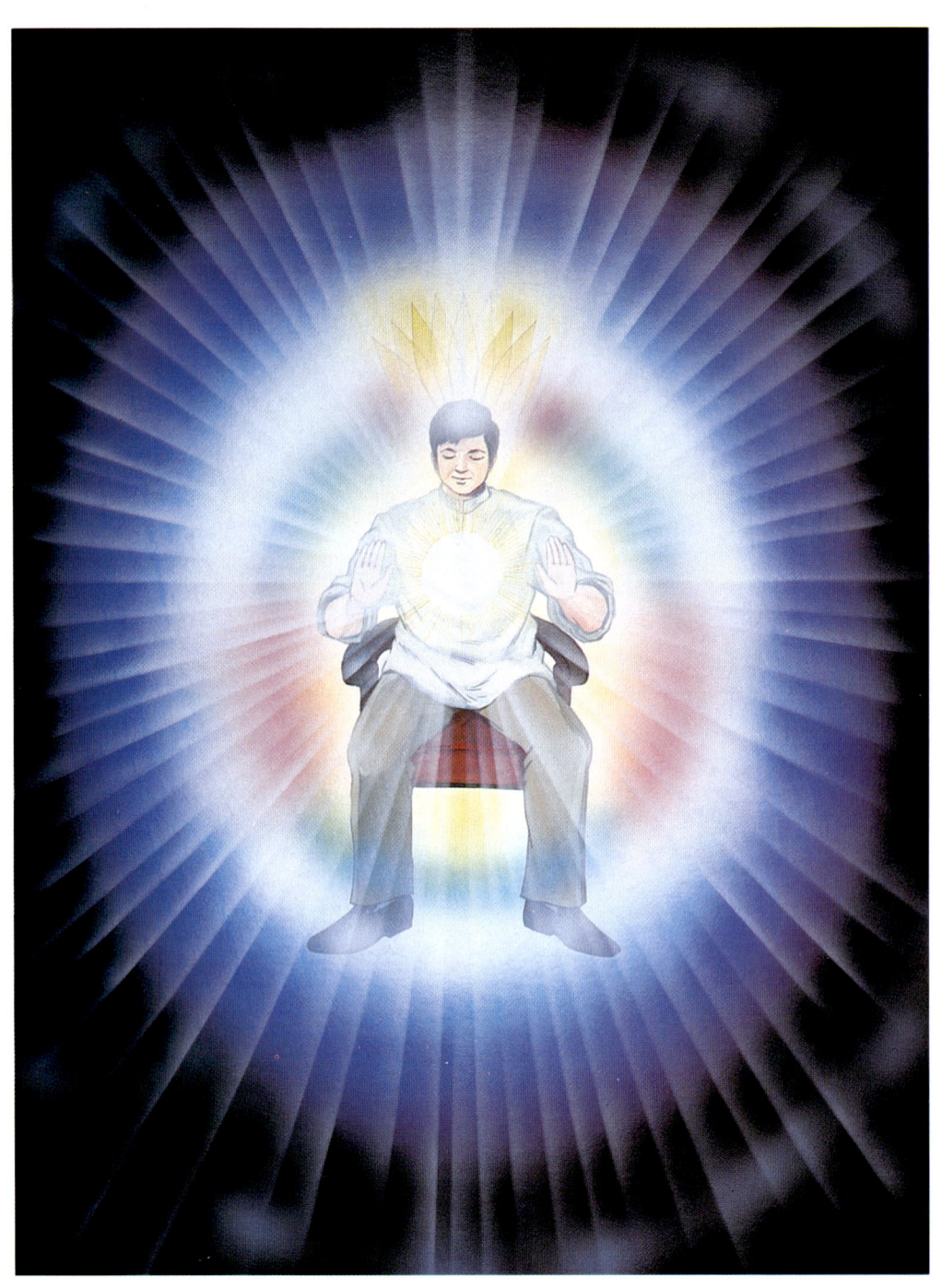

Activated Crown Chakra of a Spiritual Aspirant Doing
Meditation on Twin Hearts

The First World Conference for Academic Exchange of Medical Qigong (Abstracts of Presentations). Beijing, China. 1988.

As a matter of interest, it is further noted that in 1988, written papers (128 abstracts) were presented at the first world conference for the academic exchange of medical qigong in Beijing, China. It is noteworthy that the application of qigong to a wide range of illnesses and diseases was demonstrated in technical papers presented at the conference. A summary of a few selected abstracts is given below so that the reader can obtain some form of appreciation for the potential and far-ranging application of qigong therapy.

1. *A Study of the Effects of the Emitted Qi (Life Energy) of Qigong on Human Carcinoma Cells* by Feng Lida, Qian Juqing, Chen Suqing, et al. (China Immunology Research Center, Beijing, China); page 1.

The effects of emitted qi (life energy) on Hale cells, and SGC-7901 human gastric adenocarcinoma cells and chromosomes of the gastric adenocarcinoma cells were studied using the techniques of tissue culture, cytogenetics, and electronmicroscope.

The results of these studies revealed that:
- the average destruction rate of the Hale cells by the emitted qi was 30.72%, with the highest destruction reaching 59.61% as contrasted with a 0% destruction rate of the untreated cells.

- in 41 experiments, the average destruction rate of the gastric adenocarcinoma cells was 25.02% after receiving emitted qi for 60 minutes compared with 0% destruction rate of the untreated cells. A scanning electronmicroscope was used to observe the cells.

- the rate of exchange, breaking, and dicentromere in the

structure of the chromosomes of the gastric adenocarcinoma cells increased after receiving the emitted qi.

Tabled results are given for each of the above cells tested, and between each of the groups, a statistical difference between the experimental group and the control group was established (P < 0.01).

2. *The Use of the Emitted Qi in Qigong and Acupuncture in the Treatment of Food Allergies* by Chu Chow (Canada Qigong Health Clinic); page 157.

Treatment of 52 patients with a medical diagnosis of food allergy for a duration of one to 25 years was reported. The treatment consisted of qigong therapy supported by acupuncture techniques, with acupuncture being used in the earlier stages of treatment, and qigong in the later stages of treatment. Acupuncture points were disclosed and generally referred to the areas for the strengthening of the spleen, liver, stomach, and lung systems. The use of the emitted qi of qigong in combination with acupuncture, increased qi, which in turn helped the function of the internal organs and improved the immune system. The result was a decreased intensity of allergic reactions and a cessation of the food substances as allergens.

3. *The Effects of the Emitted Qi on the Immune Functions of Mice* by Wang Yunsheng, Feng Lida, Chen Shuying, and Chen Haixing (China Immunology Research Center, Beijing China); page 4.

To determine whether there is an effect on the regulation of the immune response after a body is subjected to qi, an experiment was made using mice specimen.

After receiving the emitted qi from well-trained qigong masters, experiments on the body indicate that qi energy can significantly enhance the phagocytic function of the peritoneal

THE NATURE OF THE ENERGY BODY

macrophages and the activity of acid phosphatase, suggesting that the qi could activate peritoneal macrophages forming part of the immune system.

4. *Effects of Qigong on Psychosomatic and Other Emotionally Rooted Disorders* by Richard R. Pavek (U.S.A.); page 150.

Shen, a specific form of qigong, was found to have a beneficial effect on suspected emotionally-rooted disorders particularly involving menstrual and pre-menstrual distress, migraine, irritable bowel syndrome, eating disorders, chronic low back syndrome (both pre-surgery and post-surgery), and other emotional disorders such as anxiety, depression, blocked grief, and sleep disorders.

5. *A Study of the Effects of the Emitted Qi on the L-1210 Cells of Leukemia in Mice* by Zhao Xiuzhen and Feng Lida (China Immunology Research Center, Beijing, China); page 6.

The mice of the experimental group received 10 to 14 minutes of emitted qi once a day for a period of 10 days, while in the control group, no treatment was given. A statistical difference was discerned ($P < 0.01$) with regard to the number of L-1210 cells still existing (using a light microscope); thereby, suggesting that the number of L-1210 cells could be remarkably reduced in the mice after receiving the emitted qi.

6. *Qigong in Australia – An Effective Weapon Against Stress* by Jack Lim (Qigong School of Australia); page 155.

Qigong is found to be an effective means for combatting stress whose physical symptoms appear as increased heartbeat, physical exhaustion and insomnia, peptic ulcers, hypertension, and heart disease. All 400 subjects presented in the survey reported marked improvement in their condition. They were from various fields of occupations, e.g., doctors, business executives, lawyers, computer specialists, artists, housewives, students, and retirees.

7. *Effects of the Emitted Qi on Healing of Experimental Fracture* by Jia Lin and Jia Jinding (National Research Institute of Sports Science, Beijing, China); page 13.

The comparative biological effects of the emitted qi for the healing of bone fractures in rabbits demonstrated that the amount and density of callus formation were better in the emitted qi group than in the control group. Similar results were also obtained for therapeutic effects on ultratrauma in overstrained muscles.

It is suspected that the mechanism involved by the emitted qi is characterized by a form of electromagnetic field resulting in a high bioactivity in the treatment of bones and muscles.

CHAPTER THREE

Elementary Pranic Healing

When the body is worn out and the blood is exhausted (of its life energy) is it still possible to achieve good results?

No, because there is no more life energy left .... vitality and life energy are considered the foundation of life .... and how then can a disease be cured when there is no life energy left within the body?

– The Yellow Emperor's
Classic of Internal Medicine
(Huang Ti Nei Ching Su Wen)

And Jesus said, ...someone has touched me, for I know that power (life energy) has gone out of me.... she (the woman) said in the presence of all the people for what purpose she had touched him (Jesus), and how she was healed immediately.

– Luke 8:45-47

Two Basic Principles in Pranic Healing	49
Hand and Finger Chakras	53
Increasing One's Energy Level by Connecting the Tongue to the Palate	54
Seven Basic Techniques in Elementary Pranic Healing	54
Sensitizing the Hands	56
Scanning	60
Procedure for Scanning the Outer Aura	60
Procedure for Scanning the Health Aura	61
Procedure for Scanning the Inner Aura	61
Interpreting Results from Scanning the Inner Aura	63
Bioplasmic Waste Disposal Unit	65

Disintegrating the Diseased Energy	67
Sweeping	67
Localized Sweeping	69
General Sweeping	71
Avoiding Diseased Energy Contamination: Washing the Hands	74
Increasing the Receptivity of the Patient	74
Energizing with Prana: Hand Chakras Technique	75
Stabilizing the Projected Prana	83
Releasing the Projected Pranic Energy	85
Suggested Practice Schedule	85
When a Healer Should Not Heal	86
Five Things to Avoid in Pranic Healing	87
Steps in Healing	89
Can you Heal Without Scanning?	91
Critical Factors in Healing	92
Insulating Garments	93
Treatments for Simple Cases	
1. Headache/ Migraine	93
2. Eyestrain or Tired Eyes	94
3. Sore Eyes	95
4. Earache	96
5. Nose Bleeding	97
6. Toothache	98
7. Sore Throat or Laryngitis	98
8. Cold with Cough and Stuffy Nose	99
9. Fever	101
10. Hiccup	105
11. Stomach Pain and Gas Pain	105
12. Poor Appetite	106
13. Diarrhea	107
14. Constipation	108
15. Parasitic Worms	109
16. Dysmenorrhea	109
17. Irregular Menstruation or Absence of Menstruation	111
18. Muscle Pain and Sprain	111
19. Low Back Pain	111
20. Difficulty in Raising the Arm (Frozen Shoulder)	113
21. Stiff Neck	114
22. Minor Arthritis or Rheumatism	115
23. Muscle Cramps	116
24. Minor Burns	116

25. Contusion and Concussion	117
26. Cuts and Inflamed Wounds	118
27. Sunburn	118
28. Eczema and Other Minor Skin Allergies	119
29. Boils	120
30. Insect and Bug Bites	120
31. Pimples	121
32. Insomnia	122
33. General Weakness	123
34. Relieving Tiredness	124
What To Do If You Are Not Sure (For Simple Ailments)	124
How Frequent Should Healing Be Done?	124
Wholistic or Integrated Approach in Healing	126
How Do You Will or Intend?	127

TWO BASIC PRINCIPLES IN PRANIC HEALING

In Pranic Healing, there are two basic principles: the *cleansing* and *energizing* of the patient's energy body with prana or life energy. *It is by cleansing or removing the diseased energy from the affected chakra and the diseased organ, and energizing them (the affected chakra and organ) with sufficient prana or life energy that healing is accomplished.* These two basic principles are the very foundation of pranic healing.

These basic principles of cleansing and energizing are also clearly manifested in the body. The body is cleansed by exhaling used-up air or carbon dioxide and is energized by inhaling fresh air or oxygen. The physical body cleanses itself through its eliminative system, and is energized by taking the proper food. The healer, therefore, must give equal emphasis on cleansing as well as energizing.

Cleansing is necessary to remove the devitalized diseased energy in the whole body or in the affected part or parts and to remove blockages in the energy channels. The health rays are cleansed, combed, and strengthened.

It must be noted that the affected part should be thoroughly cleansed before and/or after energizing is done. For more severe cases, the entire energy body has to be cleansed. Very often, after initial cleansing, the patient should be partially energized to facilitate further cleansing. This is like sweeping first a very dirty floor and then adding soap and water or cleansing chemical to clean and remove the stubborn dirt. The whole process may be repeated until the energy body is normalized. Without cleansing, the patient may suffer a *radical reaction*. This reaction refers to the drastic steps the body takes in order to correct and normalize its condition. It is usually painful and uncomfortable, and may appear as an *initial worsening condition*. However, the body gradually improves after experiencing a radical reaction. But this reaction is quite unnecessary and can be avoided if proper cleansing is applied.

One such case is that of a patient who suffered from chronic abdominal pain, loose bowel movement and vomiting due to an emotional factor. There was pranic congestion around her abdominal area. Energizing with prana was applied without cleansing the affected part. Although she was relieved, the pain, loose bowel movement and vomiting recurred and intensified within 20-30 minutes. These were radical reactions or steps taken by the whole physical body to cleanse and remove the congested diseased energy from itself in order to normalize its condition. Three hours later, cleansing and energizing with prana were applied on her abdominal area and she was completely relieved.

In several instances, the same patient was treated for the same complaint. In this case, the patient was relieved within a few minutes just by cleansing or removing the diseased energy from the

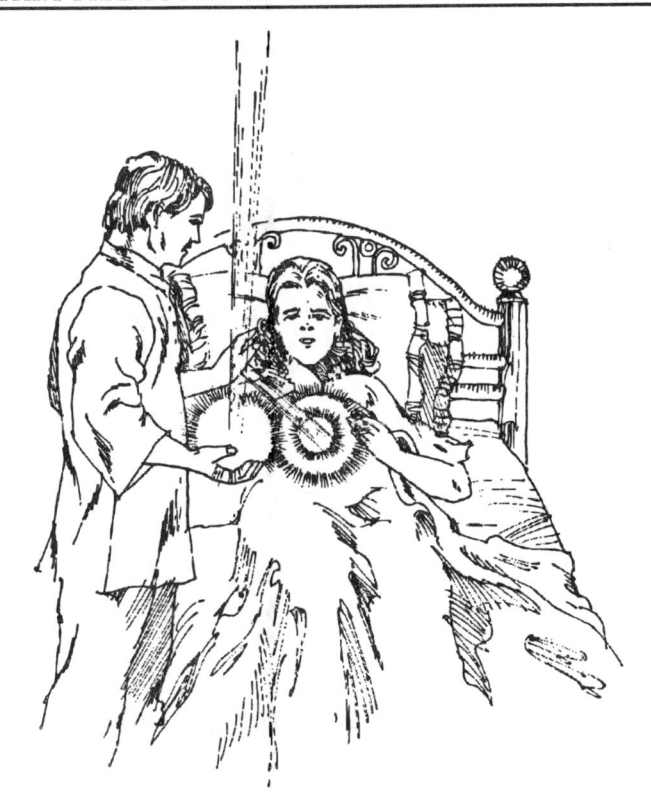

Fig. 3-1 *Pranic healing is accomplished by removing the diseased energy and by energizing the affected parts with prana or life energy.*

affected part. Energizing was not applied since the patient was relieved immediately. There was no radical reaction.

Cleansing is necessary in order to facilitate the absorption of prana or ki by the affected part. Energizing without first cleansing the part to be treated is just like pouring fresh coffee to a cup that is already filled with stale coffee; or trying to replace dirty water in a sponge by pouring clean water on top of it This approach is slow and quite wasteful. Fresh prana cannot flow easily into the affected part since the affected part is filled with diseased

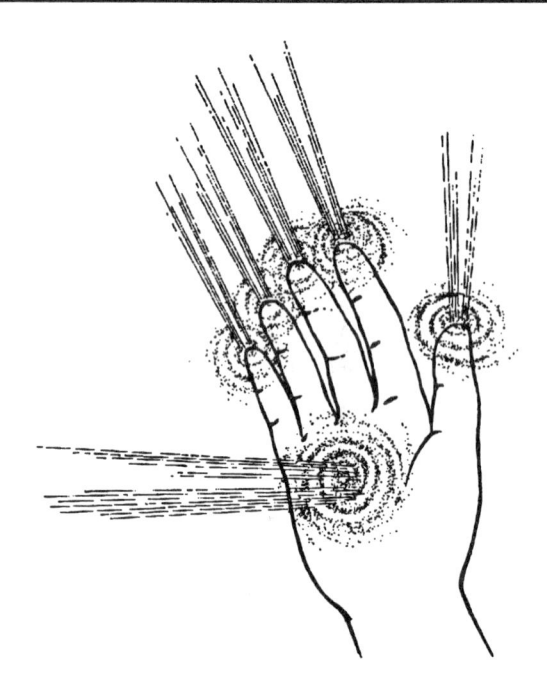

Fig. 3-2 *Hand and finger chakras (energy centers)*

energy and the energy channels are blocked. The projected fresh prana is not also fully absorbed by the treated part; therefore, it is very possible that the ailment would recur immediately or within a short period of time.

There are several reasons why cleansing should be done before energizing:

1. Absorption of prana or ki is facilitated.

2. Healing takes a shorter time and less prana is required to heal the patient.

3. The possibility of a radical reaction is reduced or eliminated.

4. The risk of damaging the finer energy channels or meridians is also reduced.

In simple cases, cleansing the energy body and/or the affected part is usually sufficient to heal the patient. In other cases, the part that has diseased energy is so depleted that the healer has to facilitate the healing process by energizing with prana.

HAND AND FINGER CHAKRAS

There are two very important chakras located at the center of each palm. These chakras are called the *left-hand chakra* and the *right-hand chakra*. They are usually about one inch in diameter. Some pranic healers have hand chakras as big as two inches or more in diameter. Although the hand chakras are considered as minor chakras, they have very important functions in pranic healing. It is through the hand chakras that prana is absorbed from the surroundings and projected to the patient. Both the right- and left-hand chakras are capable of absorbing and projecting prana or ki. But for right-handed persons, it is easier to absorb through the left-hand chakra and project through the right-hand chakra and vice-versa for left-handed persons.

There is a mini chakra in each finger. These chakras are also capable of absorbing and projecting prana. The hand chakras project less concentrated or gentler prana while the finger chakras project more intense or stronger prana. Energizing infants, the elderly, and very weak patients is done slowly and gently through the hand chakras.

By stimulating or activating the hand chakras, the hands become sensitized, thereby developing the ability to feel subtler matter and to scan the different auras. It is through scanning that the healer can locate the diseased areas in the energy body.

INCREASING ONE'S ENERGY LEVEL BY CONNECTING THE TONGUE TO THE PALATE

One's pranic energy level can be increased temporarily and easily by simply bringing the tip of the tongue up to the palate (Connecting the tongue to the palate). This has the effect of improving the connection between the back energy channels and the front energy channels, thereby improving and increasing pranic energy circulation. This manifests as the inner aura expanding in size. For example, when the light switch is on, there is light. There is connection. If the light switch is off, there is no light. In the same manner, when the tongue is connected to the palate, there is increased flow of pranic energy. When the tongue is not connected to the palate, there is decreased circulation of energy.

Connecting the tongue to the palate enables a healer to have more energy and makes healing more effective. *Therefore, when sensitizing, scanning, sweeping and energizing, the tongue should be connected to the palate.* This technique can be used also for reading, studying, meditating or other activities that require considerable energy.

SEVEN BASIC TECHNIQUES IN ELEMENTARY PRANIC HEALING

There are seven basic techniques that are followed in the practice of elementary pranic healing:

1. Sensitizing the hands

2. Scanning the inner aura

3. Sweeping (cleansing): general and localized

ELEMENTARY PRANIC HEALING

Connected   Disconnected

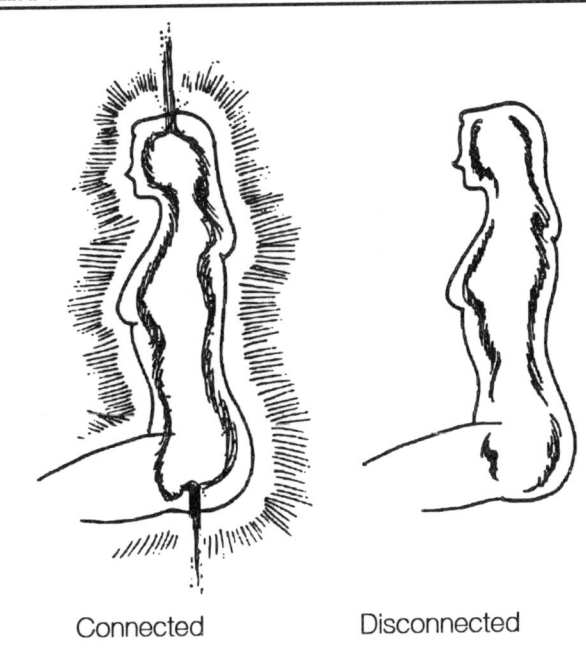

Fig. 3-3 *Connecting the tongue to the palate*

    4. Increasing the receptivity of the patient

    5. Energizing with prana: hand chakras technique

        a. Drawing in prana
        b. Projecting prana

    6. Stabilizing the projected prana

    7. Releasing the projected pranic energy

All the techniques in this chapter have been tried and tested. Most of you will be able to produce positive results in just a few sessions by following properly the instructions. It is very important to maintain an open mind and be persevering. Practice

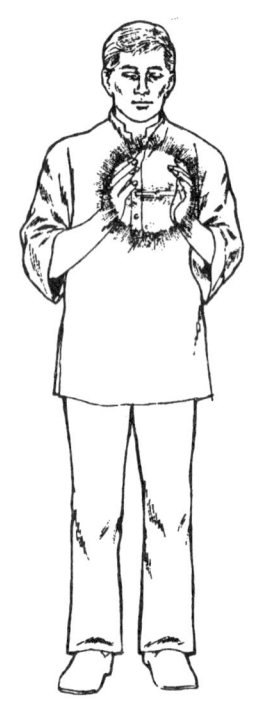

Fig. 3-4 *Sensitizing the hands: Place your hands three inches away from each other. Concentrate on the center of your palms for about 10 minutes. Inhale and exhale slowly. Many of you may feel a warm tingling sensation or pulsation.*

immediately what you have read and try them out for at least four sessions.

SENSITIZING THE HANDS

Since it takes considerable time to develop the auric sight, you should at least try to sensitize your hands in order to feel the energy field or the inner aura. This will enable you to determine which areas of the patient's energy body are depleted or congested.

ELEMENTARY PRANIC HEALING

Physical Exercises to Facilitate Sensitizing of the Hands

To make sensitizing easier, please do a set of exercises that will clean and open up the meridians of the spine, the shoulders, the hands and fingers:

1. Spine Exercise : Raise your arms forward. Twist your spine to the right and to the left. Do this exercise 10 times.

2. Hip Exercise : Rotate your hips clockwise 10 times, then counterclockwise 10 times.

3. Neck Exercise : Rotate your neck to the right in a clockwise motion. Do this 10 times. Then rotate your neck to the left in a counterclockwise motion. Do this 10 times. This exercise should not be done by a person with an occlusion in the carotid arteries.

4. Shoulder Exercise : Rotate your arms in a forward motion 10 times. Then rotate them in a backward motion 10 times.

5. Elbow and Fist Exercise : Bend your elbows close to your body and clench your fists. Then move your arms forward and open your fists. Do this exercise 10 times.

6. Wrist Exercise : Rotate the wrists to the right 10 times in a clockwise motion. Then rotate them to the left 10 times in a counterclockwise motion.

1. Spine Exercise
2. Hip Exercise
3. Neck Exercise
4. Shoulder Exercise
5. Elbow and Fist Exercise
6. Wrist Exercise

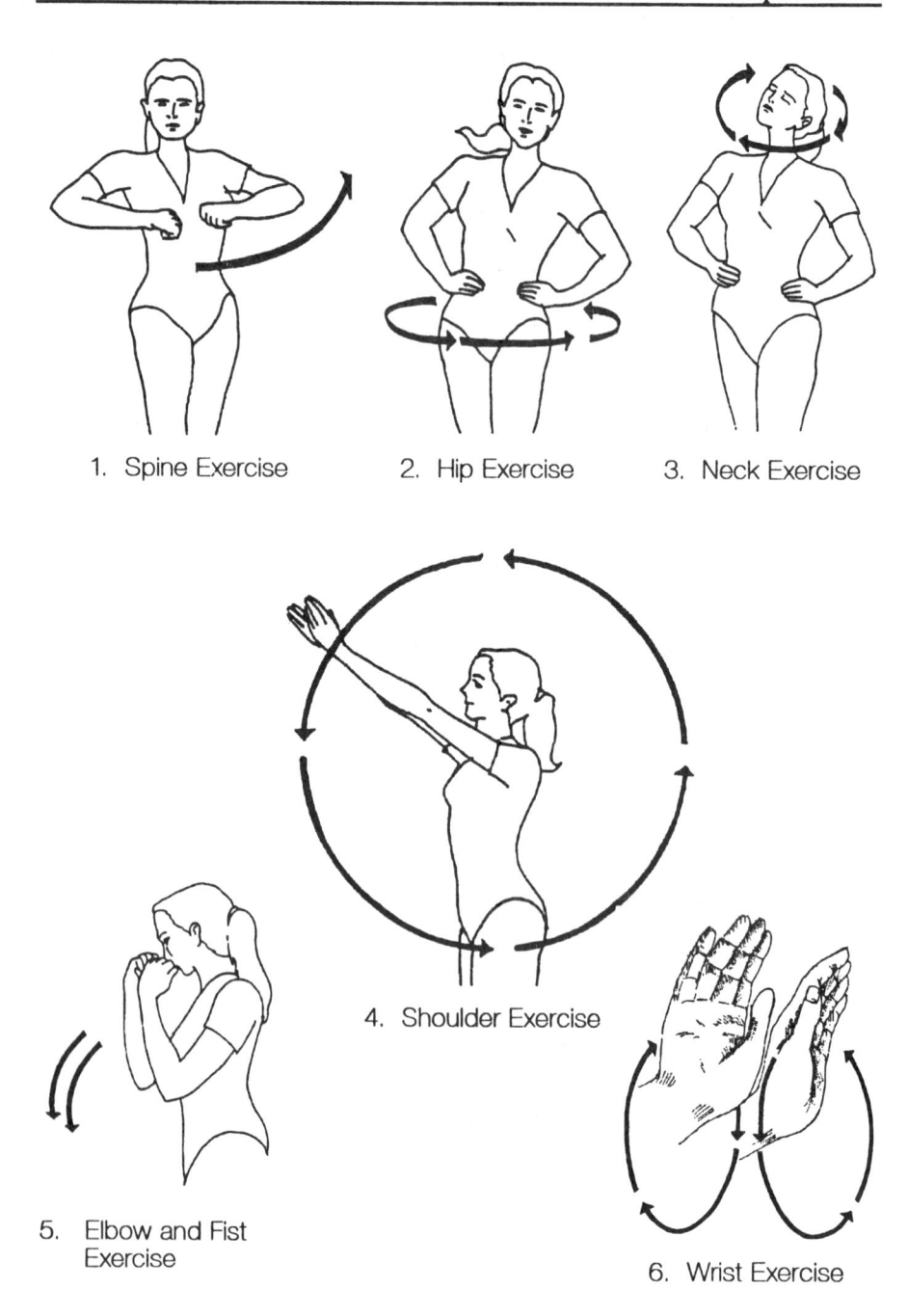

Fig 3-5 *Physical exercises to facilitate sensitizing of the hands*

ELEMENTARY PRANIC HEALING

Procedure:

1. Connect your tongue to your palate.

2. Press the center of your palms with your thumbs. This is to facilitate concentration on the center of the palms.

3. Put your hands about three inches apart parallel to each other with the armpits slightly open.

4. Be aware of the centers of your palms and the tips of the fingers. Inhale and exhale slowly. Move your hands slightly back and forth. The movement has to be done very slowly. Do this for about five minutes. By being aware of the centers of the palms and the tips of the fingers, the hand and finger chakras are activated, thereby sensitizing the hands or enabling the hands to feel subtle energy or matter.

   Eighty to ninety percent of you will be able to feel a tingling sensation, heat, pressure or rhythmic pulsation between the palms on the first try. It is important to feel the pressure or the rhythmic pulsation.

5. Proceed immediately to scanning after sensitizing your hands.

6. Practice sensitizing your hands for about a month. In general, your hands should be more or less permanently sensitized after a month of practice.

7. Do not be discouraged if you do not feel anything on the first try. Continue your practice; it is likely that you will be able to feel these subtle sensations on the fourth session. It is very important to keep an open mind and concentrate properly.

SCANNING

In scanning, it is helpful but not really necessary to first learn how to feel the size and shape of the outer and health auras before scanning the inner aura. This is to make the hands more sensitive since both the outer and health auras are subtler than the inner aura, and also to prove to yourself the existence of the outer and health auras. In healing, we are primarily interested in scanning the inner aura. It is in scanning the inner aura that the troubled spots can be located.

When scanning with your hands, always concentrate on the centers of your palms. It is by concentrating on the centers of your palms that the hand chakras remain or are further activated, thus making the hands sensitive to subtle energy or matter. Without doing this, you will have difficulty in scanning.

Procedure for Scanning the Outer Aura

1. Stand about four meters away from your subject with your palms facing the subject and your arms slightly outstretched.

2. Slowly walk towards the subject, simultaneously trying to feel with your sensitized hands the subject's outer aura. Concentrate on the centers of your palms when scanning.

3. Stop when you feel heat, a tingling sensation or a slight pressure. You are now feeling the outer aura. Try feeling the size and shape of the outer aura, its width from head to waist, waist to feet, and from front to back. In most cases, it will feel like an inverted egg, the top being wider than the bottom.

4. It is very important that you gradually learn to feel the aura in terms of pressure in order to be more accurate in determining the width of the outer, health, and inner auras.

5. The outer aura is usually about one meter in radius but in some cases it may be more than two meters wide. Some hyperactive children have outer auras as big as three meters.

Procedure for Scanning the Health Aura

1. After determining the size and shape of the outer aura, gradually move forward a little, still retaining the earlier position.

2. Stop when you feel the subtle sensations again. These sensations may be slightly more intense. You are now feeling the health aura. Feel the size and shape of the health aura.

The health aura is usually about two feet in width. When a person is sick, his health rays droop and are entangled, and his health aura decreases in size. Sometimes the health aura may decrease to twelve inches or less. The health aura of a very healthy and energetic person may be as big as one meter or more. It usually feels like a tapering cylinder, bigger at the top and smaller at the bottom.

Procedure for Scanning the Inner Aura

1. Proceed to feel the inner aura with one or both hands. Move your hands slowly and slightly back and forth. The inner aura is usually about five inches in thickness. Concentrate on the centers of your palms when scanning in order that the hand chakras may remain or be

further activated, thereby making the hands sensitive to subtle energy or matter.

2. Scan the subject from head to foot and from front to back. Scan the left part and right part of the body. For example, scan the left and right ears or scan the right and left lungs. When the inner aura of the right and left parts of the body are scanned, they should have about the same thickness. If one part is bigger or smaller than the other, then there is something wrong with it. When, for instance, the ears of a patient were scanned and the inner aura of the left ear was found to be about five inches thick while that of the right ear was only about two inches, it turned out, after questioning the patient, that the right ear had been partially deaf for the past 17 years.

Pranic congestion   Pranic depletion

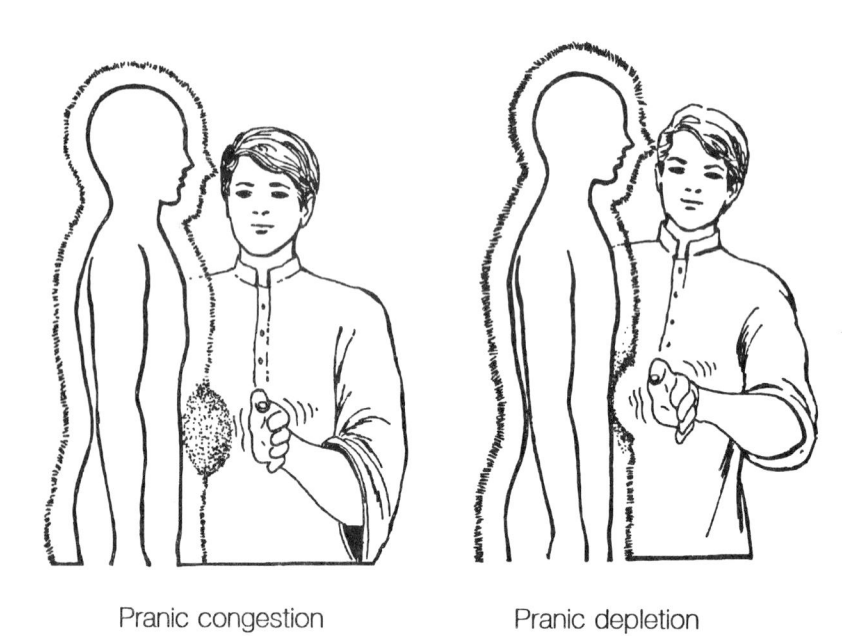

Fig. 3-6 *Scanning the inner aura*

3. Special attention should be given to the major chakras, the vital organs, and the spine. In many cases, a portion of the spine is usually either congested or depleted even if the patient does not complain about back problems.

4. The chin should be raised to accurately scan the throat area. The inner aura of the chin tends to interfere or camouflage the actual condition of the throat.

5. Scanning of the lungs should be done at the back and at the sides rather than the front in order to get accurate results. The nipples have two mini chakras that tend to interfere in the proper scanning of the lungs. A more advanced technique is to scan the lungs at the front, at the back and at the sides by using two fingers, instead of the entire hand.

6. Special attention should be given to the solar plexus since many diseases of emotional origin negatively affect the solar plexus chakra.

Interpreting Results from Scanning the Inner Aura

1. In scanning your patient, you will notice that there are hollows or protrusions in some areas of the patient's inner aura. A hollow in an area is caused by *pranic depletion*. The affected part is depleted of prana or there is insufficient prana in the affected area. The surrounding fine meridians are partially or severely blocked preventing fresh prana from other parts to flow freely and vitalize the affected part. In pranic depletion, the affected chakra is depleted and filled with dirty diseased energy. Usually, it is partially underactivated.

2. When the area protrudes, it means there is *pranic congestion*. Too much prana and bioplasmic matter on the affected area causes the surrounding fine meridians to be partially or severely blocked. The excess prana and bioplasmic matter cannot flow out freely. This congested prana becomes devitalized and diseased after a certain period of time since fresh prana cannot flow in freely or its inflow is greatly reduced, and the devitalized matter cannot flow out freely or its outflow is greatly reduced. In pranic congestion, the affected chakra is congested and filled with diseased energy. Usually, it is partially overactivated.

3. An affected part may have pranic congestion and pranic depletion simultaneously. It means that a portion of the affected part is hollow and another portion is protruding. For instance, a liver is congested or protruding on the left portion and is hollow or depleted on the right portion. Another example is that a portion of the left heart is congested or protruding and a portion of the right heart is severely depleted.

4. The smaller the inner aura, the more severe is the pranic depletion. The bigger the protrusion of the inner aura, the more congested is the affected part. The smaller or bigger is the inner aura of the diseased part, the more severe is the sickness.

5. An area may have a *temporary pranic surplus* in which case there is nothing wrong. For instance, a person who has been sitting down for a long time, when scanned, may have a big protrusion of the inner aura around the buttocks area. Since the surrounding meridians are not blocked, the condition normalizes after a short period of time.

6. An area may have a *temporary pranic reduction* in which case there is also nothing wrong with it. An altercation that has just occurred is likely to cause a temporary pranic reduction around the solar plexus area. After a few hours of rest, the condition will normalize. But habitual altercation or anger may cause pranic depletion around the solar plexus area which results in abdominal ailment and possibly heart disease.

7. The physical condition of the patient should be observed carefully and the patient should be thoroughly questioned or interviewed before jumping to any conclusion.

8. As stated earlier, diseases manifest first on the energy body before manifesting on the visible physical body. There are cases in which there is pranic depletion or pranic congestion in the inner aura of an affected part, although medical findings would show a negative result or normality of the affected part. In this case, the disease has not yet manifested on the visible physical body. *Therefore, pranic healing should be applied before the disease can manifest physically.*

BIOPLASMIC WASTE DISPOSAL UNIT

The diseased energy has to be disposed properly so that the energy of the room will remain clean and in order to avoid contaminating yourself and the other patients from this dirty energy. The diseased energy, when removed from the patient's body, is still connected to the patient by energy or etheric threads. The Hawaiian shamans (healers) or kahunas call the energy thread as invisible aka thread. In esoteric parlance, this is called etheric thread. Unless the diseased energy is disposed properly, there is the possibility that it may go back to the patient.

To make a bioplasmic waste disposal unit, simply put about a liter of water into a bowl and add a handful of salt into the water. It has been clairvoyantly observed that water is capable of absorbing dirty energy and salt breaks down the dirty energy. *(The word "disposal unit" will be used to replace the term "bioplasmic waste disposal unit" from here onwards.)*

After every sweeping or cleansing, you should flick your hands toward the disposal unit.

You can perform this simple experiment:

Get two bowls of water and put salt in one bowl. Do not put salt in the other one. Scan the two bowls before and after flicking the dirty energy to each bowl. The dirty energy can be obtained from sweeping your patients. Leave the bowls for about two hours and note the difference. The diseased energy in the bowl of water with salt will have dissipated, which means you can hardly feel the diseased energy, while that on the other bowl with water without salt is still intact.

Some healers use water, sand, water with tobacco, meat and other organic matters as disposal units. Some American Indian shamans use twigs. The twigs are placed in the mouth of the shaman and the diseased energy is sucked out or extracted by the use of the mouth. The twigs are used to catch the diseased energy. The diseased energy is symbolically seen by some clairvoyants as spiders or insects or some other repulsive forms. Some shamans do not place anything in their mouths. They just simply suck out the diseased energy and "dry vomit" it out. For beginners, there is the danger of literally swallowing the diseased energy. It is safer to use sweeping.

DISINTEGRATING THE DISEASED ENERGY

If there is no water and salt preparation available, you can use the following methods:

1. Will or intend the diseased energy to disintegrate when you flick your hand.

2. Visualize green or orange fire beside you and throw the dirty energy into it. Make sure that you put off the fire to avoid unnecessary risk. It is real in the invisible world. What manifests in the invisible world can and often does inevitably manifest in the physical world. Therefore, failing to extinguish the fire may create unpredictable problems for you.

SWEEPING

Sweeping is generally a cleansing technique. It can also be used for energizing and distributing excess prana. When cleansing is done on the whole energy body, it is called *general sweeping*. Cleansing which is done on specific parts of the body is called *localized sweeping*.

The hands are used in sweeping. There are two hand positions: *cupped-hand position* and *spread-finger position*. These two hand positions are used alternately. The cupped-hand position is more effective in *removing the diseased energy* while the spread-finger position is more effective in *combing* and *disentangling the health rays*. General sweeping has been called aura cleansing or combing by some esoteric students.

Sweeping produces the following results:

1. It removes congested and diseased energy. Blocked

meridians or energy channels are cleansed and unclogged. This allows prana from other parts of the body to flow to the affected part, facilitating the healing process.

2. Expelling of toxins, wastes, germs, and dirty energy is greatly facilitated by disentangling and partially strengthening the health rays. The health rays are further strengthened by energizing the whole body with prana.

3. By disentangling and strengthening the health rays, the health aura which acts as a protective shield is normalized. This increases one's resistance against infection.

4. Sweeping automatically *seals holes in the outer aura* through which prana leaks out. Without sealing the holes in the outer aura, the healing process is very slow even if the patient is energized with prana because prana would just simply leak out. This is one of the contributing factors why sometimes there is regression or the disease comes back in a few minutes or hours after the patient has been healed.

5. Absorption of prana by the patient is greatly facilitated after sweeping or cleansing.

6. Sweeping is also used to distribute excess prana in a treated area to other parts of the body after it has been energized to prevent possible congestion.

7. Sweeping is used to energize by directing excess prana from the surrounding areas of the body or from a chakra or chakras to the affected part that is low in prana. For instance, a mild form of arthritis of the fingers was cured in minutes just by cleansing the

fingers and sweeping or directing the excess prana from the hand chakra to the affected fingers.

8. Radical reaction is reduced or avoided by simply sweeping the patient thoroughly.

Sweeping is a very important pranic healing technique and is very easy to learn. It cleanses, strengthens, and greatly facilitates the healing process. Many simple illnesses can be healed just by sweeping.

Localized Sweeping

1. Place your hand or hands above the affected area. Concentrate on your hand and on the affected part, then slowly sweep away the diseased energy. This is just like cleaning a dirty object with your hand.

2. Apply localized sweeping five times on the affected part, then flick your hand forcefully to throw away the diseased energy to the disposal unit. This process should be repeated until the patient is partially or completely relieved.

3. For simple ailments, localized sweeping should be done 30 to 50 times. In many cases, the patient may feel partial or complete relief. This is very useful especially in treating dysmenorrhea, stomach pains, loose bowel movement, headache and others.

4. The sweeping movements can be done in any direction: vertically, horizontally, diagonally or in L-shape.

5. For more severe ailments, the number of localized sweeping should be increased. For cyst, apply localized sweeping about 100 times or more; for acute hepatitis,

70   Chapter Three

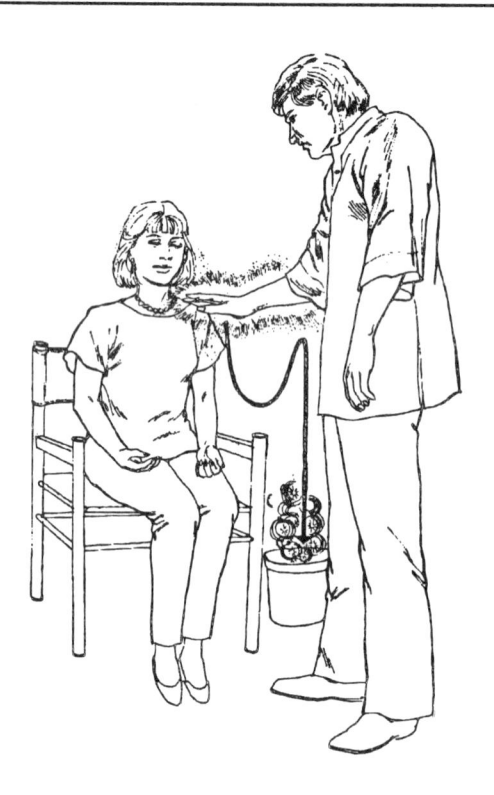

Fig. 3-7 *Localized Sweeping: The rate of healing is increased by cleansing or removing the diseased energy from the affected part. Many minor ailments can be partially or completely relieved by applying localized sweeping about 30-50 times on the affected area.*

about 200 times or more, since the affected part is very inflamed; for tumor or cancer, about 300 to 500 times because the affected part is extremely congested. In some cases, the relief from pain is very substantial. For infants and small children, the number of localized sweeping is reduced.

6. For experienced and proficient pranic healers, the number of sweeping is also greatly reduced.

Sweeping is very easy and can be learned almost immediately by most people. Sometimes in localized sweeping, the diseased energy is transferred from the affected part to another part of the body. For instance, one practitioner was sweeping away the congested energy at the back of the head of a patient when a part of it was transferred to the neck and shoulder areas. This caused the pain at the back of the head to partially move to the neck and shoulder areas. Should you encounter a similar situation, just simply apply localized sweeping on the newly affected area.

General Sweeping

General sweeping is done with a series of downward sweeping movements only. In downward sweeping, you start from the head down to the feet. Upward sweeping movements are not used in cleansing but are used only to reawaken patients who may have fallen asleep or may have become slightly drowsy. In upward sweeping, you start from the feet up to the head.

Procedure:

1. Cup your hands and place them six inches above the head of the patient. Do not touch the patient unnecessarily. Maintain a distance of about two inches between the patient's body and your hands.

2. With your hands still cupped, sweep your hands slowly downward from the head to the foot following line No. 1 as shown in the illustration (Fig. 3-8). Raise your hands slightly and flick them strongly downward to throw away the dirty diseased energy. This is very important to avoid recontaminating the patient with the diseased energy, and also to avoid contaminating your-

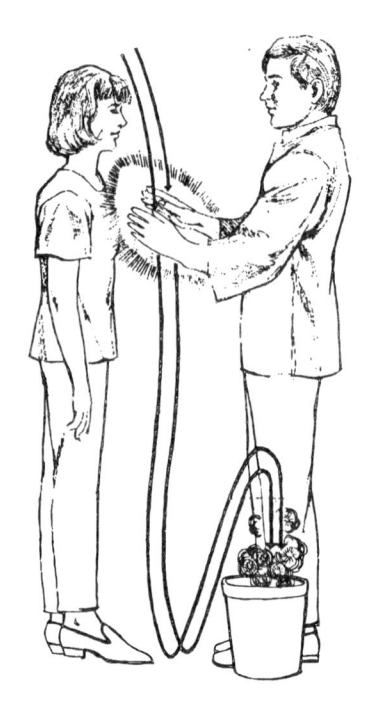

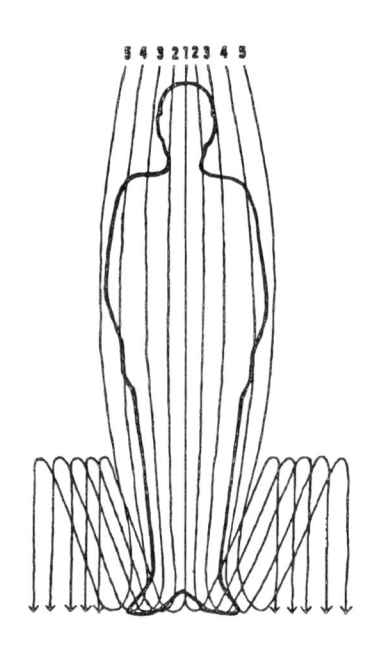

Fig. 3-8 *General Sweeping: By cleansing or removing the diseased energy, circulation of life energy or prana is enhanced, thereby increasing the rate of healing. General sweeping can be done with the patient standing, sitting or lying down. This technique is very effective in treating fever.*

self. This would manifest not only as pain in your fingers, hands, and palms but may result in the weakening of your body and/or illness similar to that of the patient.

3. Repeat the process in procedure no. 2 with spread-finger position instead of the cupped-hand position. This is called combing and is used to disentangle and strengthen the health rays.

ELEMENTARY PRANIC HEALING

4. Repeat the whole process in procedure nos. 2 and 3 on lines 2, 3, 4, and 5 as shown in the illustration.

5. Apply downward sweeping on the back of the patient by following the procedure in nos. 2, 3, and 4.

6. It is very important to concentrate and have the intention to remove the diseased energy. Without this, the sweeping process becomes less effective and more time-consuming. It is the intention or the application of the will, with the aid of the hands, that the diseased energy is thoroughly and quickly removed.

   With regular practice, you can apply sweeping with great ease and with minimum effort.

7. After the downward sweeping, some patients may become sleepy. You may apply a few upward sweeping to reawaken or make the patient more alert. Since upward sweeping is not a cleansing technique, there is no need to flick your hands after doing it. It should be applied only after the patient has been relatively cleansed.

Warning: Applying upward sweeping before downward sweeping may result in the diseased energy going to or getting stuck in the head area. This may have negative physical effects.

How many times should general sweeping and localized sweeping be applied on a patient? The answer is as many times as required. There is no fixed number of times.

AVOIDING DISEASED ENERGY CONTAMINATION: WASHING THE HANDS

Before healing, after sweeping, and after energizing — wash thoroughly with water or water with salt both hands up to the elbows. This is to wash away some of the diseased energy left on the hands of the healer and also to reduce the possibility of contaminating oneself or absorbing the diseased energy into one's system. Otherwise, this may manifest as pain in the fingers, hands, arms or manifestation of the patient's symptoms in the healer's body. Washing is also necessary to prevent diseased energy contamination of your next patient. You may also use 70 percent ethyl or isopropyl alcohol; this has a disintegrating effect on the diseased energy.

When treating patients with contagious diseases, the hands should preferably be washed with germicidal soap to reduce the possibility of infecting yourself and the next patient.

INCREASING THE RECEPTIVITY OF THE PATIENT

Healing will be a lot easier if the patient is relaxed and receptive or does not offer strong resistance. If the patient is relaxed, his body can absorb more pranic energy. The projected prana can be rejected for the following reasons: first, if he has a strong bias against this type of healing; second, if he dislikes the healer; and third, if he does not want to get well.

It is, therefore, advisable to establish rapport with the patient to reduce resistance. Rapport can be established by smiling at the patient - greeting and treating him in a kind, courteous manner. If he does not know anything about pranic healing, then the healer should explain briefly and clearly the nature of pranic healing.

ELEMENTARY PRANIC HEALING

If there is strong resistance on the part of the patient, request him to assume the receptive pose during the treatment. Request the patient to turn his palms upward and to bend his head slightly downward. Ask him to close his eyes. This is to reduce his resistance and, therefore, make the healing a lot easier.

To further increase the receptivity of a skeptical patient, instruct him to mentally repeat several times during the treatment the following affirmation: "I willingly, fully and gratefully accept all the healing energy... in full faith, so be it!" Or, when the patient is being energized, you may request him to visualize his body and the affected part being filled with light or pranic energy, or that he is inhaling light or pranic energy into his body and the affected part. This will greatly facilitate the rate of assimilation of pranic energy.

ENERGIZING WITH PRANA: HAND CHAKRAS TECHNIQUE

When projecting prana to the patient's energy body, one should simultaneously draw in air prana or air vitality globules from the surroundings. This would prevent draining or exhausting oneself and becoming susceptible to infection and diseases.

There are many ways of drawing in prana and projecting prana; one of the safest and easiest ways is through the hand chakras. One of the hand chakras is used to draw in air prana and the other to project prana or life energy to the patient. Both left and right hand chakras can either predominantly draw in or project prana. The hand chakra is alternately drawing in and projecting prana at a rapid rate. Whether it predominantly draws in prana or predominantly projects prana is a matter of intention or will. You can use the right-hand chakra to project prana and the left-hand chakra to draw in prana or vice-versa. This is a matter of personal preference. With the right-handed, it is easier to draw in

a/b.) Press the center of your palms with your thumb for a few seconds to facilitate your concentration.

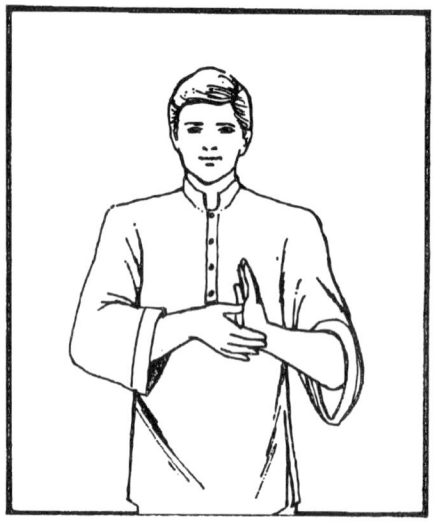

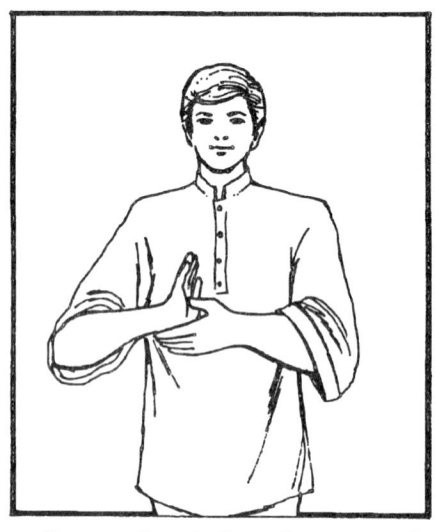

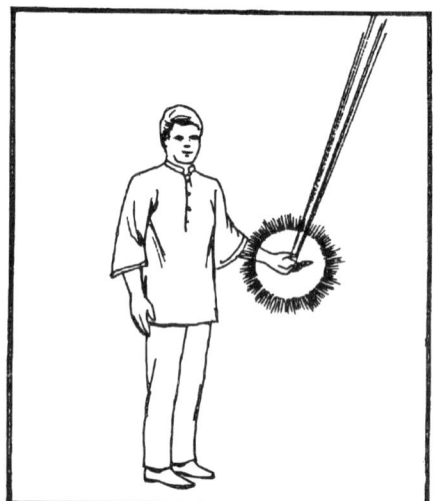

c.) Concentrate on the center of your palm that will be used for drawing in pranic energy for about 15 seconds.

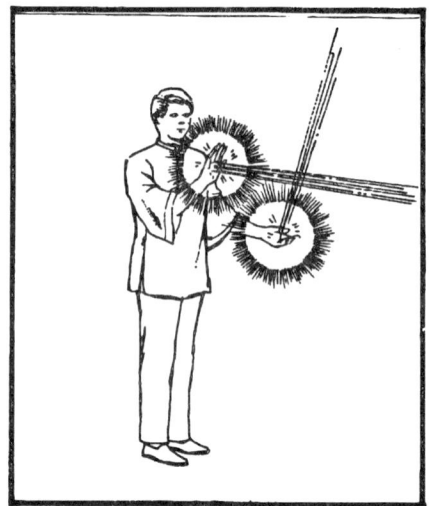

d.) Simultaneously concentrate on the center of each palm. Many of you will feel some sort of energy or current after several minutes.

Fig. 3-9 *Energizing with prana: hand chakras technique. To energize, place the projecting hand near the affected part and concentrate simultaneously on the center of each palm.*

ELEMENTARY PRANIC HEALING 77

localized sweeping   energizing

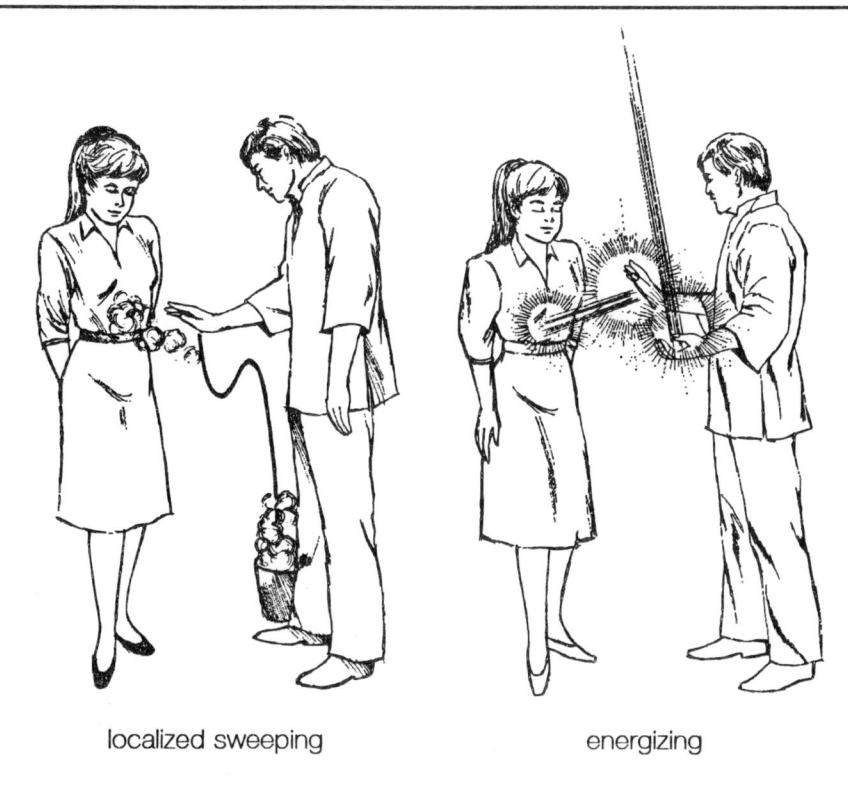

Fig. 3-10 *How to treat minor ailments: Just apply localized sweeping about 30 times or more, and energize the affected part.*

prana using the left-hand chakra and project prana with the right-hand chakra, and vice-versa for the left-handed persons.

Prana is drawn in through one of the hand chakras and projected through the other hand chakra. Attention or concentration should be focused on the hand chakras (on the centers of the palms) and on the part to be treated, with more emphasis on the hand chakras. Focusing too much on the part being treated than on the two hand chakras is a common mistake done by beginners. This would tend to reduce the flow of prana coming in and going out.

Procedure:

1. Press the center of each palm with your thumbs to facilitate your concentration.

2. The drawing-in hand should be turned upward while the projecting hand should be turned downward or outward. The reason behind this is because we have been conditioned to receive with the hand turned upward and to give with the hand turned downward or outward. When a child asks for something from the parent, the parent gives with the hand turned downward while the child receives with the hand turned upward.

3. Concentrate or focus your attention on the center of your palm that will be used for drawing in pranic energy for about 10 to 15 seconds. This is to partially activate the hand chakra, thereby enhancing its ability to draw in pranic energy. If you intend to draw in pranic energy through your left hand, then concentrate on its center.

4. Place the other hand near the affected part and concentrate simultaneously on the center of both hands. If you intend to project with your right hand chakra, place your right hand near the affected part. Maintain a distance of about three to four inches away from the patient. Continue concentrating or focusing your attention on the centers of your palms until the patient is sufficiently energized. For simple cases, this may take about 5-15 minutes for beginners.

5. There should be an initial expectation or intention to draw in prana from one hand chakra and to project prana through the other hand chakra. Once the initial intention or expectation has been formed, there is no need to further consciously expect or will to project.

The position of the hands, the initial expectation, and the concentration on the centers of the palms will cause prana to be drawn in automatically through one of the hand chakras and projected out through the other hand chakra.

6. Some healers commit the mistake of concentrating too much on the projecting hand and not enough on the receiving hand. As a result, they are not able to project enough pranic energy because they are not drawing enough of it. Also, they tend to become easily exhausted since they are using their own pranic energy instead of that from the surroundings. Therefore, the healer should concentrate more on the receiving hand than on the projecting hand in order to avoid being depleted.

7. When energizing or projecting prana, you must gently will or form an initial intention, directing the projected prana to go to the affected chakra and then to the affected part. It is critically important that the projected prana be directed to the affected part. This will produce a much faster rate of relief and healing. Just energizing the affected chakra without willing or directing the pranic energy to go to the affected part will result in a slower distribution of prana or life energy from the treated chakra to the affected part, thereby producing a slower rate of relief and healing.

8. The left and right armpits should be slightly open to allow easier flow of prana from one hand chakra to the other hand chakra. This is important.

9. If you feel a slight pain or discomfort on your hand while energizing, flick your hand. When energizing, the hand should be flicked regularly to throw away the diseased energy.

10. Energizing should be continued until the treated part is sufficiently energized. The affected part has enough prana if you feel a slight repulsion coming from the treated area or if you feel a gradual cessation of the flow of prana from your palm to the treated area. The flow of prana may feel like a warm moving current or just a plain subtle moving current. The feeling of slight repulsion or cessation of flow is due to the equalization of the pranic energy level between your hand and the treated area. For beginners, energizing with prana may take 5-15 minutes for simple cases, and about 30 minutes or more for more severe cases.

11. Cross-check whether the treated area is sufficiently energized by simply rescanning the inner aura of the treated part. If it is not, then energize further until the treated part has sufficient prana.

12. If the treated part is overenergized to a high degree, apply distributive sweeping to prevent possible pranic congestion. This is done by sweeping the excess prana with your hand to the surrounding areas. Cross-check the result by scanning. If the treated part is overenergized to a slight degree by only three inches, then just leave it as is.

13. Prana or ki may also be projected through the fingers or finger chakras other than the hand chakra. The prana coming out from the finger chakras is more intense. If the projected prana is too intense, the patient may feel pain and a boring or penetrating sensation which is quite unnecessary. It would be better to master energizing through the hand chakras before trying to energize through the finger chakras.

ELEMENTARY PRANIC HEALING

In energizing, visualization is helpful but not necessary. You may or may not imagine white light going to the treated part or chakra. In advanced pranic healing, color pranic energy or colored light is used to facilitate the rate of healing. Just relax and concentrate calmly on the hand chakras. The result will automatically follow. The technique is simple, easy, and quite effective. Try it and judge for yourself.

If the healer prefers to visualize, he can visualize the projected pranic energy as a "white light", not "colored light." Elementary and intermediate pranic healers should preferably avoid using color pranic energy when healing since its improper use may cause adverse effects on the patient. This should be done preferably by advanced pranic healers only.

In drawing in prana, there are several possible positions: "reaching for the sky" pose, "egyptian" pose, and "casual" pose. In the "reaching for the sky" pose, raise the receiving arm and turn the palm upward. The act of raising the arm upward is similar to unbending a water hose. There is a meridian or energy channel in the armpit area which is connected to the left hand chakra and the right hand chakra. The unbending of this meridian allows prana to flow with minimum resistance. The act of concentrating on the receiving hand chakra is like turning on the water pump. When you concentrate on the receiving hand, its chakra is activated and draws in a lot of prana.

In the "egyptian" pose, bend the elbow of the receiving hand until it is almost parallel to the ground. The arm is moved slightly away from the body to make a small opening in your armpit area. This has the effect of unbending the meridians in the armpit area. The palm is turned upward. This conditions the mind to receive prana.

In the "casual" pose, let your receiving arm hang loosely and casually. The arm is moved slightly away from the body to allow a

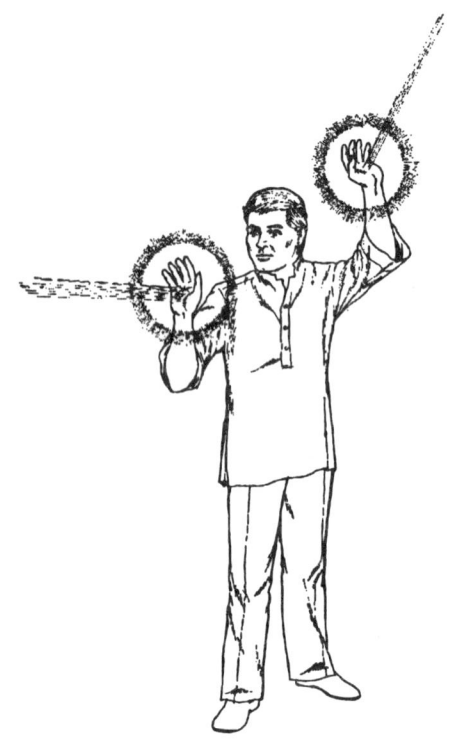

Fig. 3-11 *Energizing: Reaching for the sky pose*

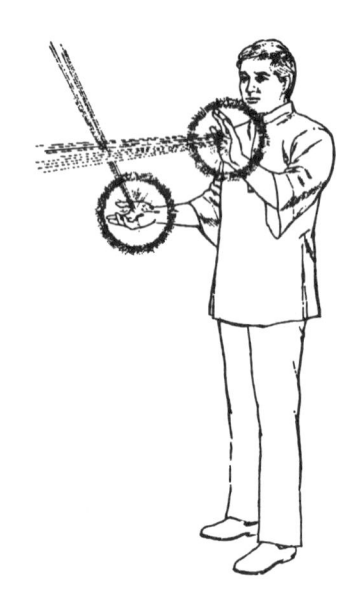

Fig. 3-12 *Energizing: Egyptian pose (standing position)*

small opening in the armpit area. The palm is in a casual position and is not raised upward. The casual position requires more concentration for beginners since the upward position of the palm which conditions the mind to receive prana is not used.

The author usually uses the "egyptian" pose because it is more comfortable and does not look too strange. This reduces the resistance from the patient. It is quite possible for a patient to partially and unintentionally block most of the prana projected to him by the healer if he finds the healer too strange or if he strongly rejects and disbelieves this form of healing. That is why it is better to establish rapport with the patient to make healing faster and easier.

ELEMENTARY PRANIC HEALING

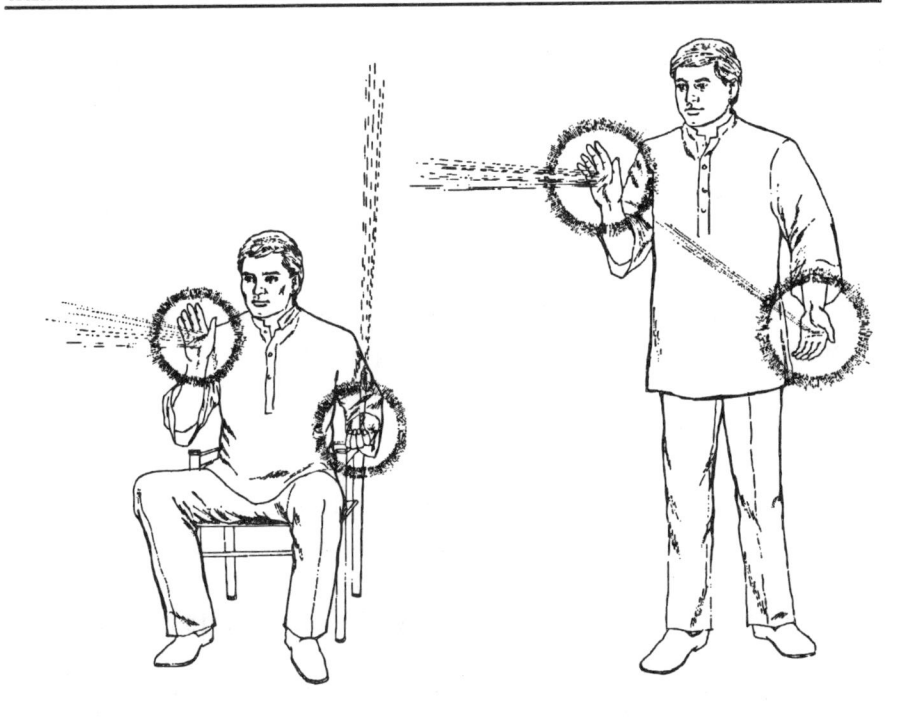

Fig. 3-13 *Energizing: Egyptian pose (sitting position)*

Fig. 3-14 *Energizing: Casual pose*

STABILIZING THE PROJECTED PRANA

One of the potential problems in pranic healing is the instability of the projected prana. The projected prana tends to gradually leak out causing the possible recurrence of the illness. This potential problem can be handled by thoroughly cleansing or sweeping the part to be treated and by stabilizing the projected prana.

The projected prana can be stabilized in two ways:

1. After energizing, "paint" the treated part with light blue

for three to four seconds. If you are not good in visualizing, simply say, "light blue, light blue, light blue" while "painting" the treated part.

2. Will or mentally instruct the projected prana to remain or stabilize.

You can perform this experiment to prove to yourself the validity of these principles and techniques:

Procedure:

1. Using the hand chakras technique, project "white" prana on top of a table for about one minute and simultaneously visualize and form it into a ball without willing it to remain. This is the first pranic ball.

2. Project, visualize and form a blue pranic ball for about one minute without willing it to remain. This is the second pranic ball.

3. Project and form a white pranic ball for about one minute and will or mentally instruct the pranic ball to remain for an hour. This is the third pranic ball. Make sure the locations of these balls are properly marked.

4. Scan the three pranic balls to make sure they are properly formed.

5. Wait for about 20 minutes and scan the three pranic balls again. You may find that the first pranic ball is already gone or greatly reduced in size while the second and third pranic balls are still quite intact.

Do try this experiment immediately. It is simple and easy to perform.

RELEASING THE PROJECTED PRANIC ENERGY

A healer will notice that it is relatively easier to be detached when healing strangers than when healing one's own children, relatives or close friends. This is due to the tendency of the healer to be "overconcerned" or too anxious with the result because of the emotional attachment to the patient. Clairvoyantly, this attachment is seen as an etheric or energy cord (cord of light) linking the healer to the patient. Because of this cord, there is a tendency that the projected prana may return to the healer; therefore, the patient may get well slowly instead of rapidly. To avoid this, the healer should visualize himself cutting the etheric cord or "cord of light" with an imaginary pair of scissors or knife.

Also, it is better not to think about the patient immediately after the treatment because the etheric link might be re-established. Furthermore, if the patient is very depleted, there is a possibility for the healer to unknowingly continue energizing the patient even long after the treatment, which in the long run, will cause the healer to be depleted. Should this happen, the healer must calmly visualize himself cutting the etheric cord again.

Under normal circumstances, when the healer is calm and detached (but not indifferent to the patient), the projected pranic energy is released and the etheric cord is automatically cut.

SUGGESTED PRACTICE SCHEDULE

1. Sensitizing the hands - 5-10 minutes per day
2. Scanning - 5-10 minutes per day
3. General and localized sweeping - 10 minutes per day
4. Energizing with prana - 10 minutes per day

The above schedule should be followed for about three to five weeks to prepare you in case there is a sudden need to heal somebody like your own child or others of simple cases such as fever, loose bowel movement, gas pain, muscle pain, insect and bug bites, etc.

Preferably, these techniques should be applied on actual patients. If this is not possible, then practice on a friend or a relative.

If you are one of those few who are not able to sensitize your hands on the first session, just proceed to sweeping and energizing with prana. Continue the practice of sensitizing your hands. In general, you should be able to accomplish this in three to four sessions.

It is advisable and preferable to learn to heal simple cases first (at least 30 cases) before proceeding on your own to treat more difficult or severe ones. This is necessary in order to gain experience and confidence.

WHEN A HEALER SHOULD NOT HEAL

1. A healer should not heal when he is sick or suffering from general weakness. This is to avoid the transference of diseased energy to the patient.

2. A healer should not also heal when he is feeling very angry or irritated because the projected pranic energy will be contaminated with anger and other negative emotions. This may cause the patient to become worse.

ELEMENTARY PRANIC HEALING

FIVE THINGS TO AVOID IN PRANIC HEALING

1. Do not apply too intense and too much prana on infants, very young children, the very weak and elderly patients. With infants and very young children, their chakras (energy centers) are still small and not quite strong. With very weak and elderly patients, their chakras are weak. Applying too much prana or too intense energizing on these patients will result in a choking effect on their chakras. This is similar to the choking reaction of a very thirsty person who drinks too much water in too short a time. Infants and children should be energized gently and gradually and only for a shorter period of time for their chakras, being quite small, can easily be overenergized and congested. The ability of the very weak and old patients to assimilate prana is very slow. Therefore, this types of patients should be energized gently, gradually, and for a longer period of time since their bodies are quite depleted. They should be allowed to rest and assimilate prana for about 15-20 minutes before energizing them again.

   If the solar plexus chakra (energy center) is suddenly overenergized, resulting in the choking effect on the chakra, the patient may suddenly become pale and may have difficulty breathing. Should this happen, apply localized sweeping immediately on the solar plexus area. The patient will be relieved immediately. Although this type of case is rare, it is presented in order to show what to do in case something like this happens.

   Treating infants, children and elderly patients is just like shaking hands with infants, children and very old people; your grip tends to be gentle; whereas, when shaking hands with adults and younger people, your grip tends to be firmer and stronger.

2. Do not energize the eyes directly. The eyes, being delicate, will be easily congested with prana if energized directly and may be damaged in the long run. The eyes are energized through the back of the head (back head chakra), the area between the eyebrows (ajna chakra), and the temples (temple minor chakra). In case the eyes are sufficiently energized, the excess prana would just flow to other parts of the body.

3. Do not directly and intensely energize the heart for a long time. It is quite sensitive and delicate. Too much prana and too intense energizing may cause severe pranic congestion of the heart. The heart should be energized through the back of the spine near the heart area. In energizing the heart through the back, prana flows not only to the heart but to other parts of the body. This reduces the possibility of pranic congestion of the heart. If the heart is energized through the front, the flow of prana is localized around the heart area, thereby increasing the possibility of pranic congestion.

4. Do not energize the meng mein chakra of infants, small children, and older people. This may activate the meng mein chakra and cause the infant, small child or elderly patient to have hypertension, which may thus affect the brain. In the case of a pregnant woman, this chakra should not also be treated since it may cause adverse effects on the unborn child. This chakra should be treated only by advanced or experienced pranic healers.

5. Do not energize the spleen chakra of infants or children because they may faint as a result of pranic congestion. Should this happen, just apply general sweeping several times to remove the excess pranic energy. The spleen chakra of a patient with hypertension or a history of hypertension should not also be energized because the

the patient's condition might become worse. However, this chakra is used to treat patients who are very weak or very depleted. It is important that the spleen chakra should be treated only by advanced or experienced pranic healers.

Pranic healing is quite safe as long as you follow properly the given guidelines and instructions.

STEPS IN HEALING

1. Smile and establish rapport with the patient to enhance his receptivity. Observe and interview him.

2. Scan the affected parts, the vital organs, major chakras, and the spine.

3. Instruct him to assume the receptive pose.

4. Apply general sweeping.

5. Do localized sweeping on the affected areas.

6. Rescan the affected parts. In case of pranic congestion, scan to determine whether the congestion has been significantly reduced or not. For pranic depletion, scan to determine if the inner aura of the affected part has become a little bigger or has partially normalized.

7. For simple cases, sweeping or cleansing is sometimes sufficient to heal the patient.

8. Before energizing, make the patient receptive in order to facilitate the absorption and assimilation of the projected pranic energy.

9. Energize the affected parts with prana.

10. Get feedback from your patient. If there is some pain left, ask for the exact spots and rescan those areas. Do more sweeping and energizing.

11. If the part is highly overenergized, do distributive sweeping to prevent possible pranic congestion.

12. Rescan the treated area to determine whether the affected area has been sufficiently decongested or energized. Thoroughness is the key to dramatic healing or very fast healing.

13. In pranic congestion, cleansing is emphasized. In pranic depletion, energizing is emphasized.

14. Stabilize the projected prana. This is very important.

15. Release the projected pranic energy by visualizing the etheric cord or cord of light linking you and the patient being cut by an imaginary pair of scissors or knife.

16. Instruct your patient not to wash the part that has just been treated for about 12 hours; otherwise, the symptoms may recur. Water absorbs some of the pranic energy that has been projected to the affected part.

Patients suffering from severe ailments or general weakness should not take a bath for about 24 hours after pranic treatment. This is to enable the body to gradually absorb and assimilate the pranic energy that has been projected.

For beginners, it would be better if scanning is done before questioning the patient. This is to improve their accuracy in scanning. Scanning, like decision-making or other human faculties, can be influenced by suggestion. You should watch out for this possible flaw in scanning the patient and try to recheck your findings.

For simple localized illnesses, general sweeping may be omitted. For infectious diseases, general sweeping should preferably be applied, even if the ailment is just a simple case of eye infection or cold because the whole body is more or less affected; the outer aura usually has holes. The rate of healing is much faster when general sweeping is applied on these cases.

CAN YOU HEAL WITHOUT SCANNING?

If your ability to scan is quite limited, you still can heal without scanning. For simple cases, just ask the patient what part hurts or is causing discomfort. Then apply localized sweeping and energizing. For severe types of ailments, just follow the steps or instructions in the book. For certain severe ailments, there are patterns that can be followed. For instance, patients suffering from heart ailments usually have imbalanced or malfunctioning heart and solar plexus chakras. Therefore, cleansing and energizing these two chakras would greatly improve the condition of the patient. The heart should be energized through the back heart chakra.

Although you can heal without scanning, you would be much more accurate and effective if you use scanning. Sometimes, some of the malfunctioning chakras are located far away from the painful or ailing part.

CRITICAL FACTORS IN HEALING

1. The patient must be scanned and rescanned thoroughly and accurately. Correct pranic diagnosis will lead to correct treatment. Proper rescanning will give correct feedback as to the effectiveness of the initial treatment.

2. The patient's energy body must be thoroughly cleansed to increase the rate of healing and to avoid radical reaction.

3. The patient must be energized sufficiently with prana. Insufficient energizing would produce only slight improvement or a slow rate of healing.

4. Stabilize the projected prana to prevent it from escaping or leaking out. Many new healers become overconfident and commit the serious mistake of not stabilizing the projected prana when their patients tell them how their conditions have greatly improved. As a result, some patients experience recurrence of symptoms or ailments after about 30 minutes or a few hours. Therefore, always stabilize the projected prana after energizing.

5. When the healer is calm and detached, the projected energy is released and the etheric cord linking the healer and patient is automatically cut. However, if the healer is anxious or attached to the result, he should use the visualization technique in cutting the etheric cord in order to prevent the projected pranic energy from going back to him.

ELEMENTARY PRANIC HEALING

INSULATING GARMENTS

Materials such as silk, rubber, and leather goods tend to act as partial insulators to prana. Patients should be requested not to wear silk since it makes projection of prana on them difficult. Leather or rubber shoes and leather belts should preferably be removed to make general sweeping more effective. Some healers prefer to remove their shoes when healing in order to absorb more ground prana.

TREATMENTS FOR SIMPLE CASES

1. Headache / Migraine

    a. Scan the crown, forehead and ajna chakras, the back of the head, the entire head and the neck. Headaches could be caused by pranic depletion or congestion on these parts. The eyes, the temple and solar plexus chakras should also be scanned.

    b. Apply localized sweeping and energizing on the crown, forehead and ajna chakras, the back of the head, and the affected head area. If the cause is due to pranic congestion, localized sweeping is usually sufficient to remove the pain. Or just ask the patient what part is aching and apply localized sweeping and energizing alternately on the affected part until the patient is relieved.

    c. If the headache is due to eyestrain, apply the treatment for "eyestrain or tired eyes."

    d. If the patient has a migraine, or if the headache is due to some emotional problems or stress, apply localized sweeping thoroughly and energizing on the front and

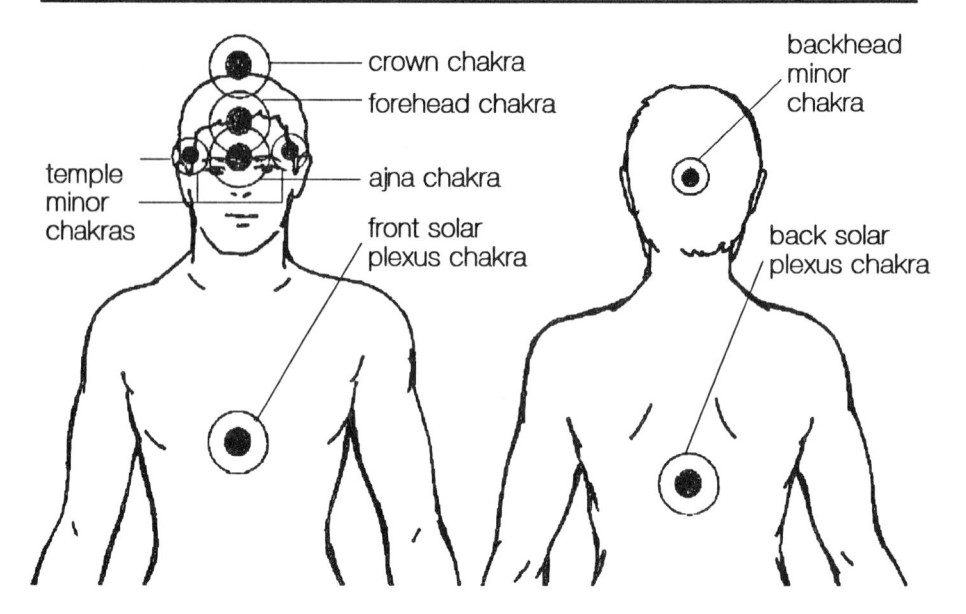

Fig. 3-15 *Pranic treatment for headache and migraine*

back solar plexus chakras first before treating the head area. The emphasis should be on localized sweeping. The front and back solar plexus chakras may require 100 to 200 sweepings each. Repeat the treatment several times a week for as long as necessary. Remember to always get feedback from the patient and always rescan the treated area to determine whether the treatment has been done properly.

e. Stabilize the projected pranic energy.

2. Eyestrain or Tired Eyes

a. Scan the eyes, ajna, temple and back head chakras. These are usually depleted; occasionally, some of them may be congested.

ELEMENTARY PRANIC HEALING

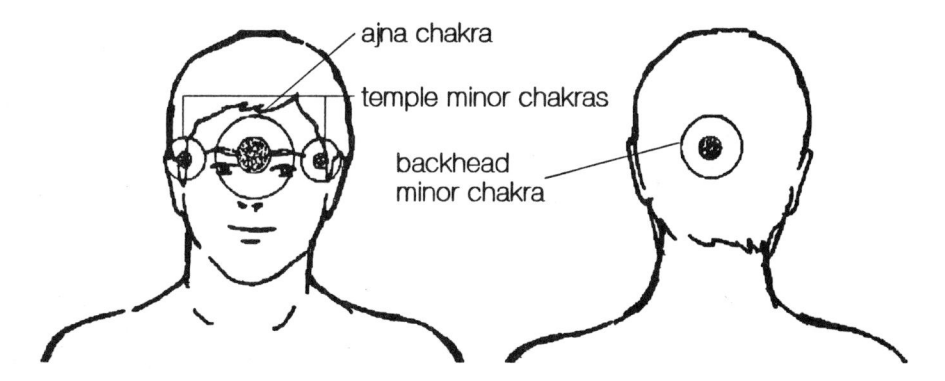

Fig. 3-16 *Pranic treatment for eyestrain or tired eyes*

    b. Apply localized sweeping thoroughly on the eyes. Rescan to determine whether the inner aura of the eyes has increased in size. If it has, it means cleansing has been successful.

    c. Apply localized sweeping and energizing on the ajna, back head, and temple minor chakras. Energizing is done more on the ajna and back head chakras, less on the temple minor chakras. When energizing, you may visualize white light or pranic energy going inside the eyes. Do not energize the eyes directly since they may be damaged in the long run.

    d. Stabilize the projected pranic energy.

3. Sore Eyes

    a. Apply general sweeping two or three times.

    b. Then apply the same treatment for "eyestrain or tired eyes." Be sure to clean the eyes thoroughly.

96   Chapter Three

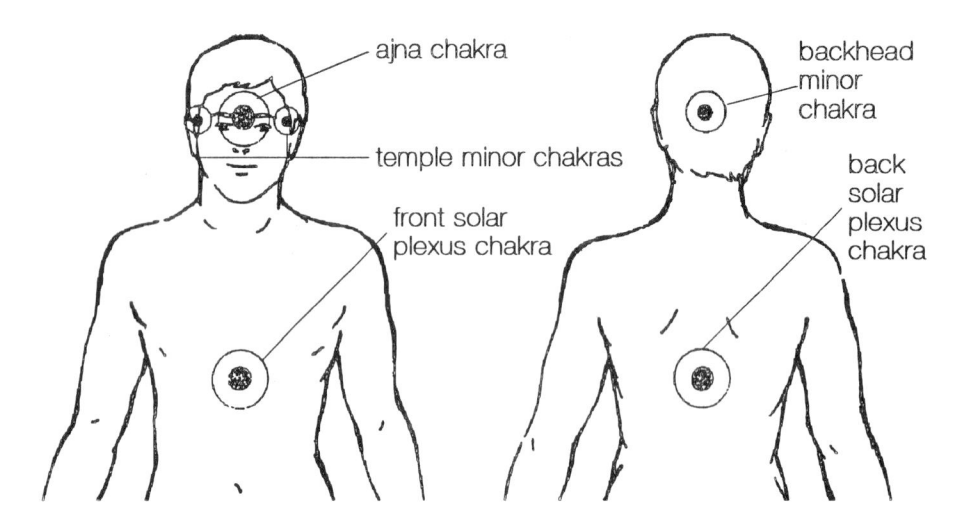

Fig. 3-17 *Pranic treatment for sore eyes*

   c. Apply localized sweeping and energizing on the front and back solar plexus chakras. This is to energize and strengthen the whole physical body.

   d. Repeat the treatment two or three times a day for as long as necessary.

   e. In severe cases, clean and energize gently the spleen chakra. Observe the patient. In rare cases, he may get congested and may faint. Do not highly energize the spleen chakra if the patient has hypertension.

   f. Stabilize the projected pranic energy.

4. **Earache**

   a. Apply localized sweeping and energizing thoroughly on the affected ear and the jaw minor chakras.

   b. If the patient has a stuffy nose, apply localized sweeping

ELEMENTARY PRANIC HEALING

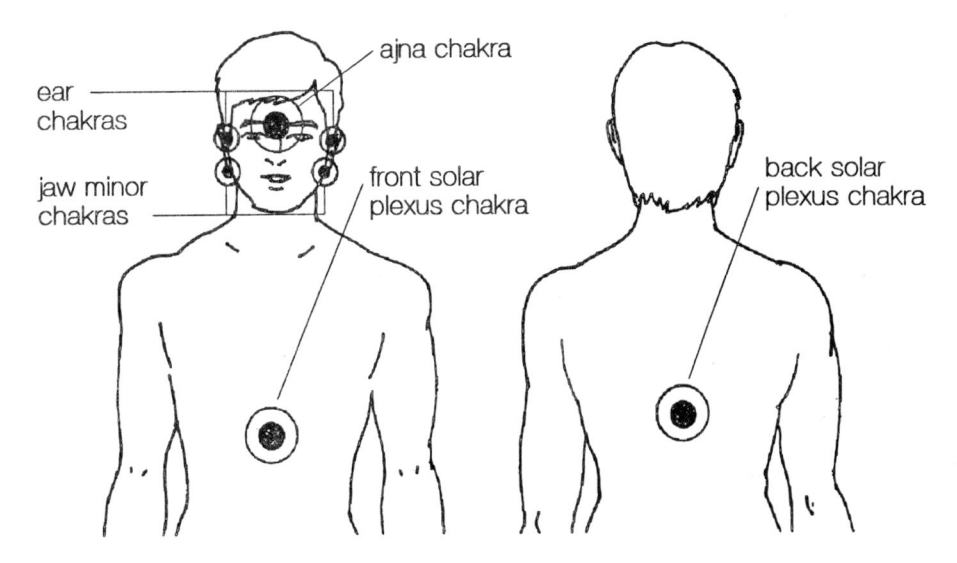

Fig. 3-18 *Pranic treatment for earache*

and energizing on the ajna chakra.

c. Apply localized sweeping and energizing on the front and back solar plexus chakras to energize and strengthen the whole physical body.

d. Repeat the treatment two to three times a day for as long as necessary. If symptoms persist, consult a medical doctor.

e. Stabilize the projected pranic energy.

5. Nose Bleeding

a. Clean and energize the ajna chakra.

b. Stabilize the projected pranic energy. In many cases, the healing is instantaneous.

ajna chakra

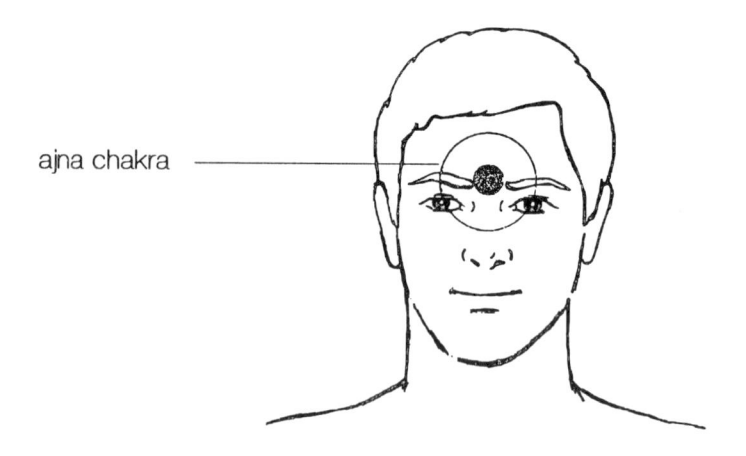

Fig. 3-19 *Pranic treatment for nose bleeding*

6. Toothache

    a. Scan the affected part. There is usually pranic depletion on the painful area.

    b. Clean the affected area by applying localized sweeping thoroughly.

    c. Energize the affected part with the fingers instead of the palm until the patient is substantially relieved. The projected pranic energy from the fingers is more penetrating than that of the palm.

    d. Stabilize the projected pranic energy.

    e. Instruct the patient to see a dentist as soon as possible.

ELEMENTARY PRANIC HEALING

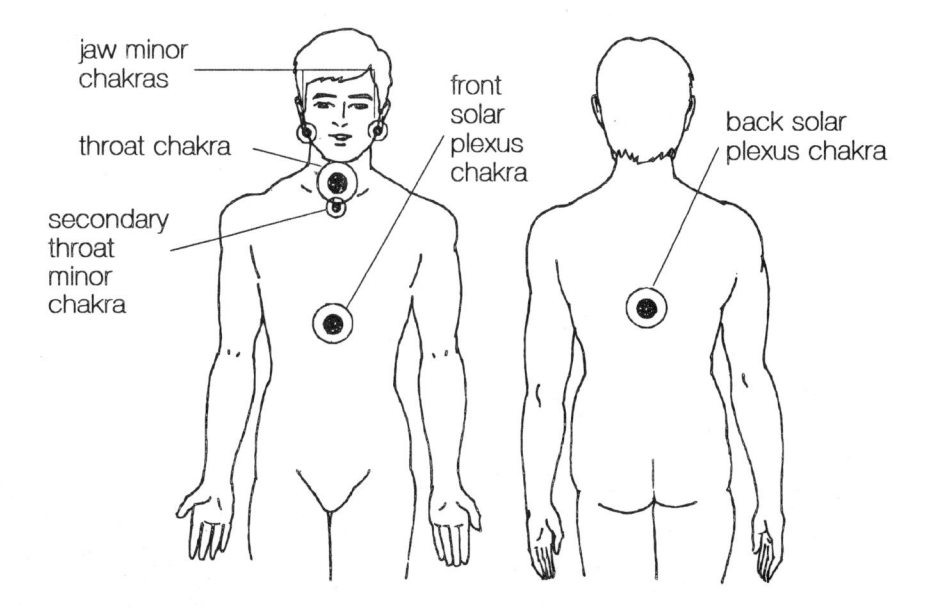

Fig. 3-20 *Pranic treatment for sore throat or laryngitis*

7. Sore Throat or Laryngitis

    a. Apply general sweeping three times.

    b. Apply localized sweeping and energizing on the throat, secondary throat (the hollow soft portion of the throat) and jaw minor chakras (the lower portion behind the ears).

    c. Apply localized sweeping and energizing on the front and back solar plexus chakras. This is to energize and strengthen the whole physical body.

    d. Stabilize the projected pranic energy.

    e. Repeat the treatment several times a day for as long as necessary.

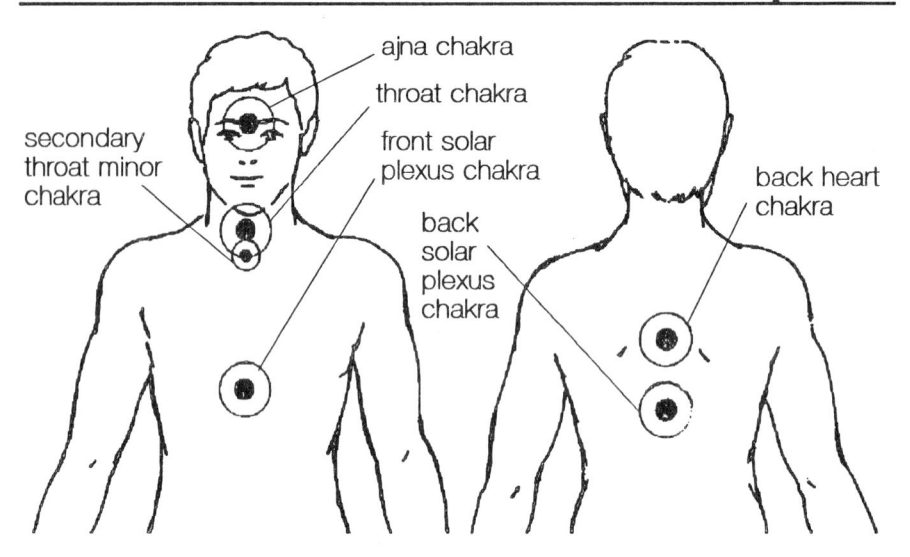

Fig. 3-21 *Pranic treatment for cold with cough and stuffy nose*

8. Cold with Cough and Stuffy Nose

a. Scan the ajna, throat, secondary throat (the hollow soft lower portion of the throat) and back heart chakras, the lungs (front, side, and back), and the front and back solar plexus chakras. These areas may be congested and/or depleted.

b. Since the whole body has been affected to a certain degree, apply general sweeping three times to clean the whole body.

c. If the patient has a stuffy nose, apply localized sweeping and energizing on the ajna chakra.

d. If the patient has a cough, apply thorough sweeping and energizing on the throat and secondary throat chakras.

e. If the lungs are partially affected, apply localized sweeping on the lungs and the back heart chakra. Energize the lungs through the back heart chakra.

f. Apply localized sweeping and energizing on the front and back solar plexus chakras. This is to energize and strengthen the whole physical body.

g. Stabilize the projected pranic energy.

h. Rescan the treated areas and get feedback from the patient. If the treatment has been done properly, the patient should be greatly relieved.

i. The patient may be given another treatment after four hours to reinforce the earlier treatment.

j. Instruct the patient to rest and not to eat too much. Eating too much consumes a lot of prana which is needed for the rapid healing of the body.

9. Fever

The treatment for fever is divided into three parts: bringing down the fever; increasing the pranic energy level of the body and strengthening its defense mechanism by energizing the bones in the arms and legs; and treating the cause or the affected part.

Fevers are usually caused by respiratory or gastrointestinal infections. Tonsillitis is also a common cause of fever in children.

a. Scan the whole body, especially the chakras and organs connected to the respiratory and gastrointestinal systems. Patients with fever are usually depleted, their inner auras being small (about two inches or less), and the solar plexus chakra congested.

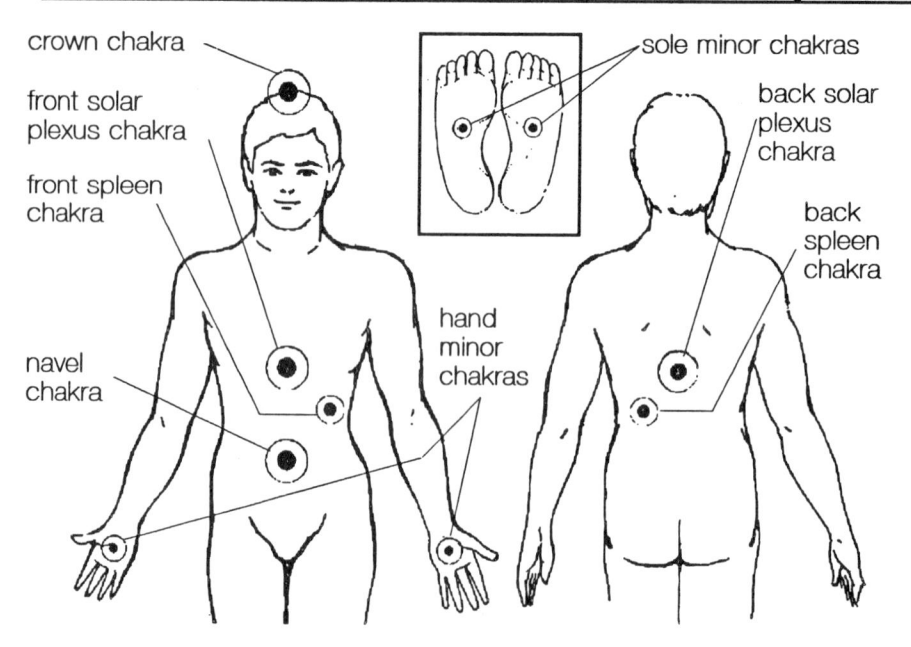

Fig. 3-22 *Pranic treatment for fever*

b. Interview the patient and ask him about the symptoms of his ailment.

c. Clean the whole body thoroughly by applying general sweeping three to five times.

d. Apply localized sweeping on the front and back solar plexus chakras for about 50 to 100 times, then energize the front solar plexus chakra. Stabilize the projected pranic energy. Energizing the solar plexus chakra without thorough cleansing may cause the fever to become worse. This is a radical reaction.

Steps c and d are very important in rapidly bringing down the fever. The emphasis is on cleansing. Thorough cleansing of the entire body and the solar plexus chakra is very important. Although the body is depleted, it is filled with red-hot pranic energy and the solar plexus chakra is usually congested with muddy, red-hot pranic energy. In general, the fever can be brought down rapidly by removing the congested, dirty red energy from the solar plexus chakra.

e. In many cases, applying general sweeping several times and localized sweeping thoroughly on the front and back solar plexus chakras is sufficient to bring down the temperature.

f. Apply localized sweeping and energizing on the navel chakra, the hand and sole minor chakras. You may visualize the pranic energy or white light going inside the bones of the hands and legs in order to strengthen the defense mechanism of the body. This is also to partially activate the hand and sole minor chakras, thereby increasing their capacity to absorb air and ground prana. This will gradually and steadily energize the whole body, providing it with sufficient prana or life energy to fight the infection.

Do not stabilize the projected pranic energy on the sole and hand minor chakras since this would partially inhibit them.

g. Do not energize directly the basic chakra because if it is overenergized, the fever might go up. It is no longer necessary to energize the basic chakra because when the sole chakras are energized, the basic chakra is automatically energized without being overenergized.

h. Apply localized sweeping and energizing thoroughly on the crown chakra.

i. Fever which is accompanied by vomiting, loose bowel movement, and abdominal pain is usually associated with gastrointestinal infections. Apply localized sweeping thoroughly on the front and back solar plexus chakras, stomach, navel chakra, small intestine and large intestine. Energize the solar plexus and navel chakras slowly and gently. The emphasis should be on thorough cleansing. Energizing without thorough cleansing may cause a radical reaction and worsening of the symptoms.

j. Fever which is accompanied by stuffy nose, cough and/or difficulty in breathing is usually associated with respiratory infections. Apply localized sweeping and energizing on the ajna, throat, secondary throat, jaw minor and back heart chakras, and the lungs. Then stabilize the projected pranic energy.

In case of severe infection, clean and energize gently the front and back spleen chakras to improve the immune and defense system of the body. Observe the patient. In rare cases, he may get congested and may faint. Do not highly energize the spleen chakra if the patient has hypertension.

When this technique is done properly, most patients will show dramatic improvement in a few hours. In rare cases, patients may experience a slight increase in temperature in the first few hours. This is partly due to the radical reaction and the intensified fight between the germs and the white blood corpuscles. The slight increase in temperature can be avoided or corrected by applying general sweeping three to five times and localized sweeping about 50 times or more on the front and back solar plexus chakras.

k. The treatment should be given two to three times a day to greatly increase the rate of healing. The patient is likely to recover in less than a day or two.

l. With infants and small children, just apply general sweeping thoroughly and localized sweeping thoroughly on the front and back solar plexus chakras. This is usually sufficient to bring down the temperature in a short period of time. Treatment may be repeated several times a day if necessary.

m. If symptoms persist, instruct the patient to consult a medical doctor as well as a certified pranic healer immediately.

10. Hiccup

a. Apply localized sweeping and energizing on the front and back solar plexus chakras. Treatment should be continued until the patient is relieved.

b. If the patient is suffering from chronic or long-standing hiccup, apply localized sweeping and energizing on the navel chakra until the patient is substantially relieved.

c. Stabilize the projected pranic energy.

d. Repeat the treatment if necessary.

11. Stomach Pain and Gas Pain

a. Scan the front and back solar plexus and navel chakras and the abdominal area.

b. Apply localized sweeping thoroughly on the front and back solar plexus and navel chakras, and the abdominal area. In many cases, just applying thorough localized sweeping on the front and back solar plexus and navel chakras, and the upper and lower abdominal areas is sufficient to partially or completely relieve the patient.

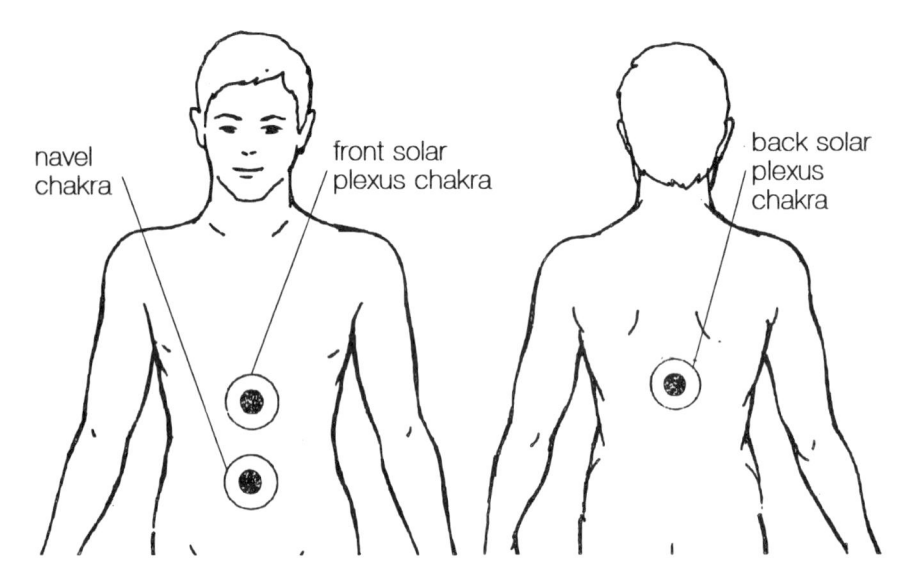

Fig. 3-23 *Pranic treatment for hiccup, stomach pain and gas pain*

    c. Energize the front and back solar plexus and navel chakras. If localized sweeping is not done thoroughly, the patient may experience radical reaction or a worsening of the condition.

    d. Stabilize the projected pranic energy.

    e. If symptoms persist, instruct the patient to consult a medical doctor immediately as well as a certified pranic healer.

12. Poor Appetite

    a. Apply localized sweeping and energizing on the front and back solar plexus, navel and basic chakras.

    b. Stabilize the projected pranic energy. Repeat the treatment if necessary.

ELEMENTARY PRANIC HEALING

front solar plexus chakra

navel chakra

back solar plexus chakra

basic chakra

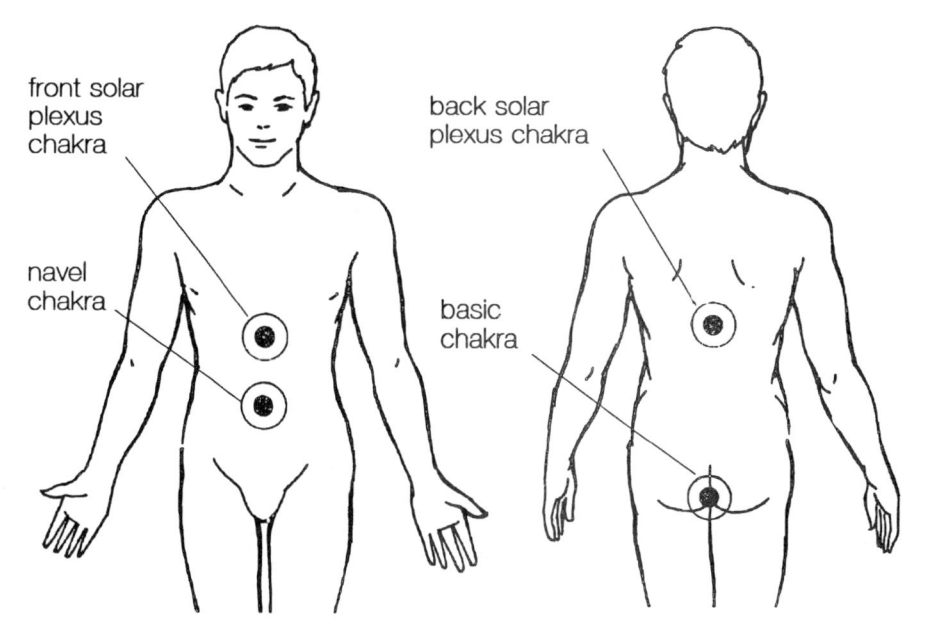

Fig. 3-24 *Pranic treatment for poor appetite, diarrhea, constipation, and parasitic worms*

13. Diarrhea

  a. Scan the front and back solar plexus and navel chakras, and the abdominal area.

  b. Apply general sweeping three times.

  c. Apply localized sweeping thoroughly on the front and back solar plexus and navel chakras, and the abdominal area. The emphasis should be more on the abdominal area. Usually, a patient can be partially or completely relieved by just applying localized sweeping thoroughly.

  d. Energize the front and back solar plexus and navel chakras. The patient should experience relief after a short period of time.

e. If the patient is quite weak but does not have fever, apply localized sweeping and energizing on the basic chakra to strengthen the body.

f. Stabilize the projected pranic energy.

g. If the pain becomes more intense and the loose bowel movement more frequent, this means that the patient has not been cleansed thoroughly. Therefore, apply more localized sweeping on the solar plexus and navel chakras, and the lower abdominal area.

h. If symptoms persist, instruct the patient to consult a medical doctor immediately, as well as a certified pranic healer.

14. Constipation

a. Scan the front and back solar plexus and navel chakras, the abdominal area, and the basic chakra.

b. Apply localized sweeping and energizing on the front and back solar plexus, navel, and basic chakras.

c. Be sure to stabilize the projected pranic energy.

d. Usually the patient will be relieved in a short period of time. For acute and chronic constipation, it may take several hours before the patient is relieved. For chronic constipation, repeat the treatment several times a week for as long as necessary. This treatment, when applied regularly, will improve and strengthen the eliminative system.

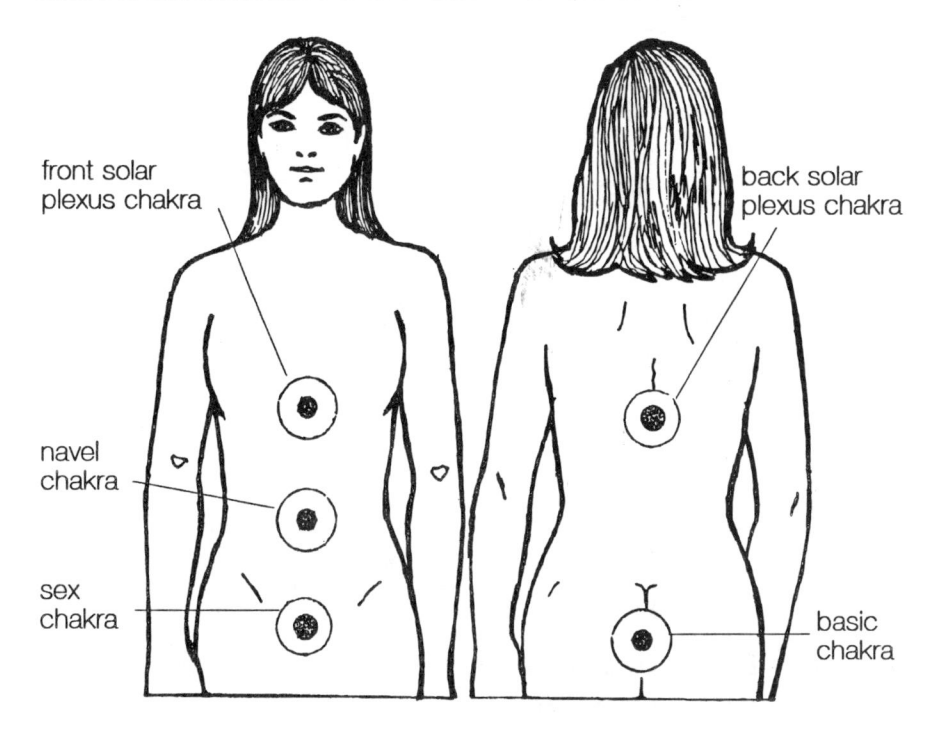

Fig. 3-25 *Pranic treatment for dysmenorrhea*

15. Parasitic Worms

    a. Apply the same treatment for "constipation" several times a week for as long as necessary. Instruct the patient to consult a medical doctor.

16. Dysmenorrhea

    a. Scan the sex and navel chakras, the lower abdominal area, and the basic chakra.

    b. Apply localized sweeping and energizing on the sex, navel, and basic chakras. The emphasis should be on applying localized sweeping thoroughly on the sex

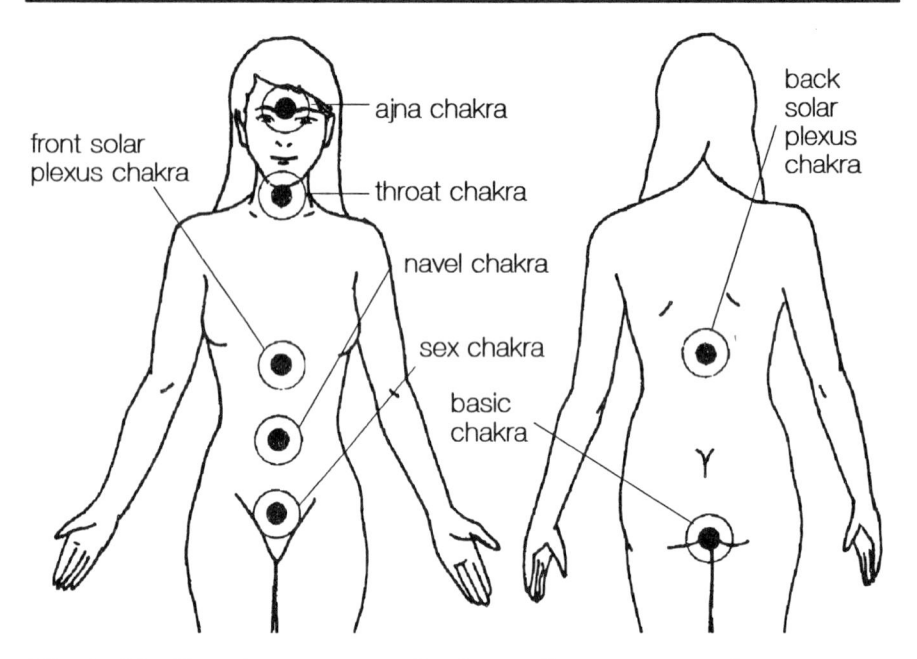

Fig. 3-26 *Pranic treatment for irregular menstruation or absence of menstruation*

chakra. In many cases, patients may experience partial or complete relief.

c. If the patient is exhausted or has fainted, then the front and back solar plexus chakras should also be cleaned and energized.

d. Stabilize the projected pranic energy.

e. Most patients will be relieved in a short time.

f. This treatment can be applied three days before menstruation to avoid dysmenorrhea.

17. Irregular Menstruation or Absence of Menstruation

    a. Use the same treatment for "dysmenorrhea."

    b. Apply localized sweeping and energizing on the ajna chakra and throat chakra.

    c. Stabilize the projected pranic energy.

    d. Repeat the treatment several times a week for as long as necessary.

18. Muscle Pain and Sprain

    a. Apply localized sweeping and energizing on the affected part. The emphasis should be on energizing. Most patients will recover partially, if not completely, in a short time.

    b. For a new sprain, energizing should be continued until there is complete relief. The patient should not overexert the treated part since it has not healed completely; otherwise, the pain will recur immediately. For faster results, use the fingers for energizing.

    c. Stabilize the projected pranic energy.

19. Low Back Pain

    a. Scan the patient thoroughly, especially the spine, the front and back solar plexus chakra and basic chakra.

    b. Apply general sweeping two to three times.

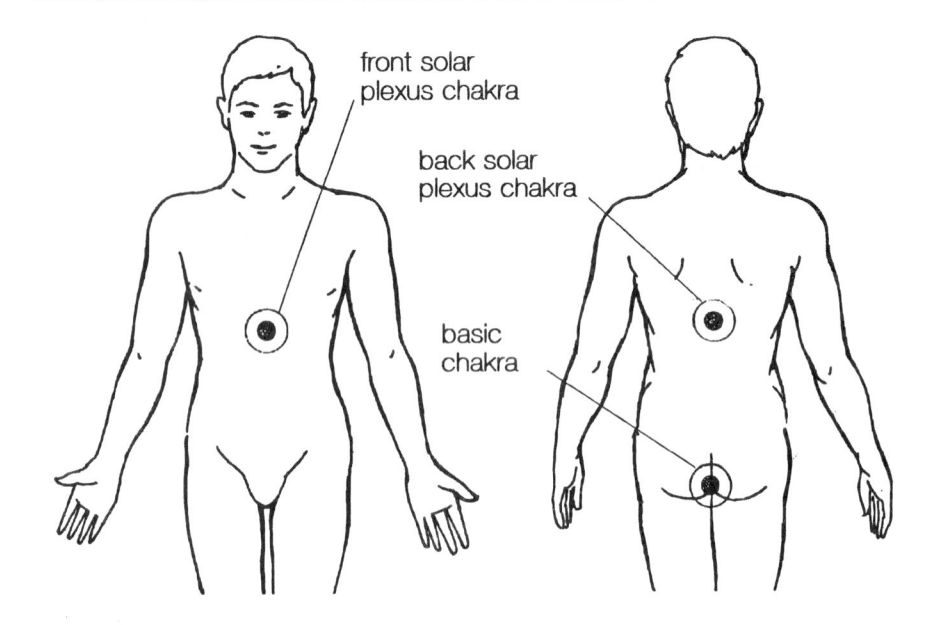

Fig. 3-27 *Pranic treatment for low back pain*

c. Apply localized sweeping 10 times or more on the entire spine.

d. Apply thorough localized sweeping and energizing on the front and back solar plexus and basic chakras. In many cases, the patient may experience partial and complete relief immediately.

e. Apply thorough localized sweeping and energizing on the affected part(s). Do not energize the meng mein chakra. The relief is usually very fast.

f. Be sure to stabilize the projected pranic energy.

g. Repeat the treatment two to three times a week for the next few weeks. This is necessary to make the healing permanent.

ELEMENTARY PRANIC HEALING

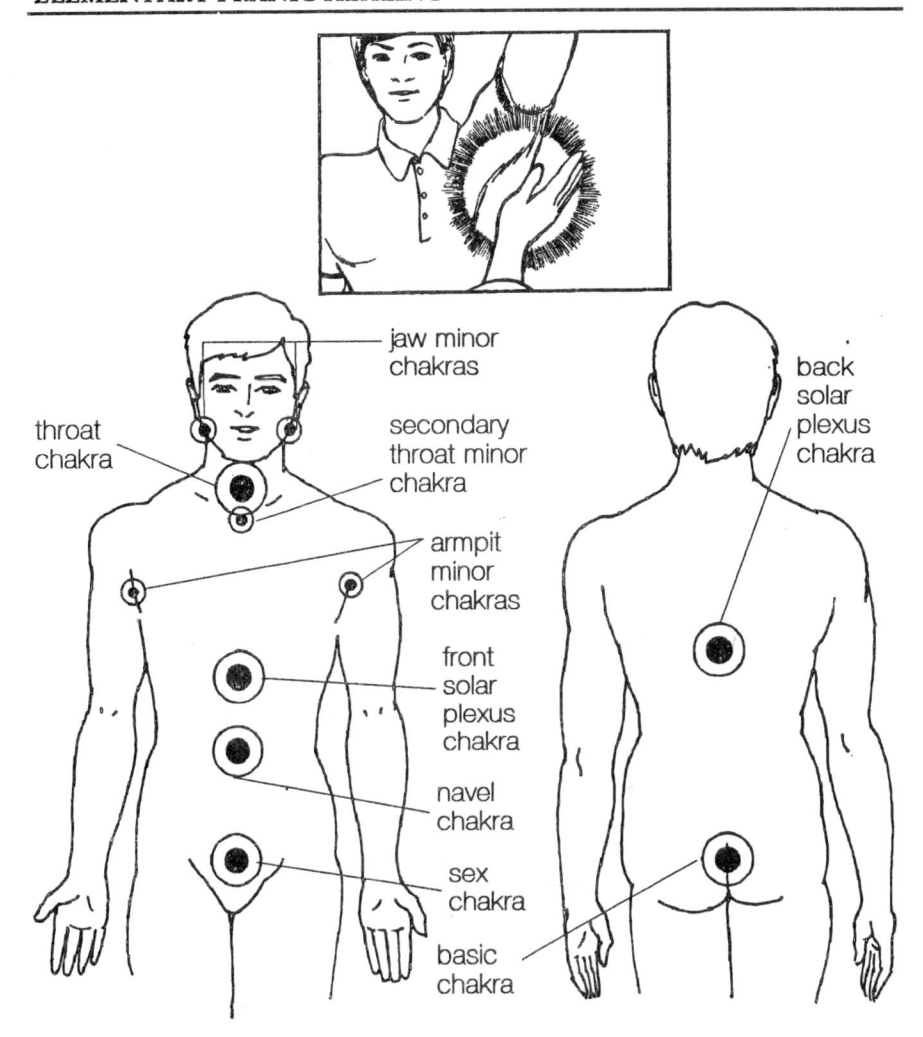

Fig. 3-28 *Pranic treatment for difficulty in raising the arm (frozen shoulders)*

20. Difficulty in Raising the Arm (Frozen Shoulder)

a. Scan the patient thoroughly. The armpit minor chakra of the affected shoulder is usually congested. In some cases, just by applying localized sweeping without energizing the armpit will cause partial or complete relief.

b. Apply general sweeping two to three times.

c. Apply thorough localized sweeping and energizing on the affected shoulder and armpit. By thoroughly cleansing and energizing the armpit area, many patients will experience dramatic improvement in just a short period of time.

d. Apply localized sweeping and energizing on the throat, secondary throat, jaw minor, front and back solar plexus, navel, sex and basic chakras. The emphasis of the treatment is on thorough cleansing and energizing of the solar plexus and basic chakras, and the neck area. The basic chakra controls and energizes the muscular and skeletal systems of the body; therefore, it is advisable to treat this chakra.

e. Be sure to stabilize the projected pranic energy.

21. Stiff Neck

a. Scan the throat, the entire neck, the shoulders, and the armpits. Scan the throat, secondary throat, jaw minor, front and back solar plexus and basic chakras.

b. Apply general sweeping three times.

c. Apply localized sweeping and energizing thoroughly on the front and back solar plexus, navel, basic, throat, secondary throat and jaw minor chakras, and the affected parts. If the treatment is done properly, the effect is quite dramatic. The emphasis of treatment is on the solar plexus chakra, basic chakra, and the neck area.

d. Be sure to stabilize the projected pranic energy.

e. Stiff neck could also be due to a heart ailment or hypertension. So, if symptoms persist, consult a medical doctor, and also a certified pranic healer.

22. Minor Arthritis or Rheumatism

a. Apply localized sweeping and energizing alternately on the affected part until there is partial or substantial relief.

b. Apply localized sweeping thoroughly on the spinal column.

c. Apply thorough localized sweeping and energizing on the front and back solar plexus chakras, liver, navel chakra, sex chakra and basic chakra. The basic chakra controls and energizes the muscular and skeletal systems of the body; therefore, it is advisable to treat this chakra.

d. Stabilize the projected pranic energy.

e. Repeat the treatment several times a week for as long as necessary.

Sometimes, arthritis could be localized in origin: for example, poor sleeping habits may cause stiff neck, or an accident on the knee may result in arthritis of the knee after several years. If this is the case, the basic chakra may not necessarily be depleted, though in many cases it is usually depleted.

After the first or several treatments, the patient may be completely relieved. This does not necessarily mean that the patient is completely healed. It may mean that the patient is partially healed and is in the process of improving. Therefore, it is necessary to give the patient several more treatments.

23. Muscle Cramps

a. Scan the affected part.

b. Apply localized sweeping and energizing alternately on the affected part until there is substantial or complete relief. The emphasis should be on energizing.

c. Apply localized sweeping and energizing on the front and back solar plexus, navel, sex and basic chakras.

d. Be sure to stabilize the projected pranic energy.

24. Minor Burns

a. If the burn is caused by hot oil or boiling water, gently wipe off the oil or water immediately.

b. Apply localized sweeping and energizing alternately on the affected part. The patient may experience substantial relief within 20 to 30 minutes. When the treatment is done properly, the affected part will only show a red mark instead of forming a blister. Repeat it several times a day until the red mark disappears.

c. If the burn is already a few hours or a few days old, apply thorough localized sweeping and energizing on the affected part and the basic chakra. The basic chakra is also treated in order to facilitate the healing process. Repeat the treatment several times a week for as long as necessary. Make sure the treated area is sufficiently energized.

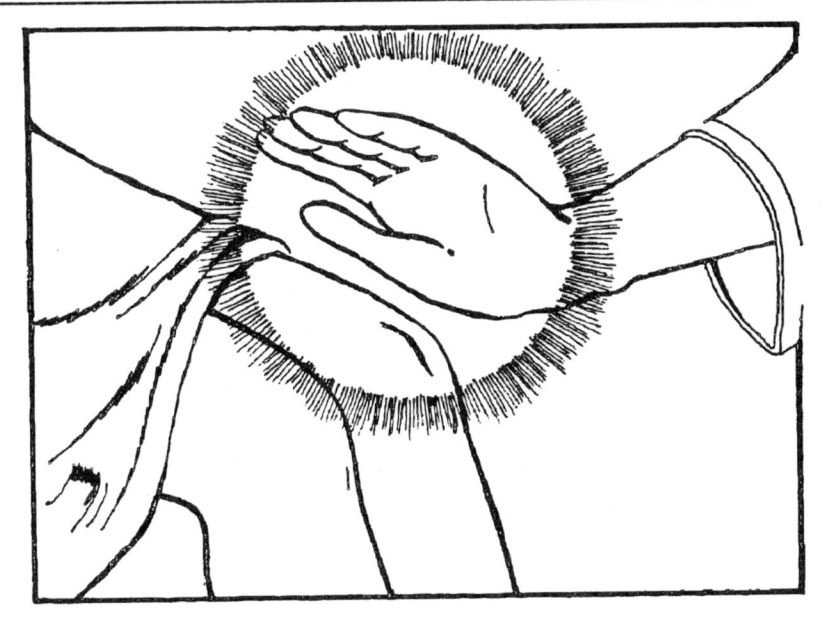

Fig. 3-29 *Pranic treatment for burns, cuts and contusions*

    d. Stabilize the projected pranic energy.

25. Contusion and Concussion

    a. Apply localized sweeping and energizing on the affected part.

    b. Repeat the treatment three or four times a day for several days.

    c. Stabilize the projected pranic energy.

    d. When the treatment is done properly and thoroughly, the rate of healing will be very fast and the treated part will not usually show any black and blue marks.

e. If the affected part is on the head area, instruct the patient to consult a medical doctor immediately, and also a certified pranic healer.

26. Cuts and Inflamed Wounds

a. For fresh wounds, apply localized sweeping immediately on the affected part and then energize thoroughly.

b. If the wound is inflamed, apply localized sweeping and energizing on the affected part. The emphasis should be on localized sweeping. Sometimes, it may even be necessary to apply as much as 50 to 100 localized sweepings.

c. To further accelerate the rate of healing, apply localized sweeping and energizing on the basic chakra.

d. Stabilize the projected pranic energy.

e. Repeat the treatment two or three times a day for as long as necessary.

27. Sunburn

a. Since the patient is suffering from congestion of solar pranic energy, apply general sweeping five times or more.

b. Apply localized sweeping thoroughly on the affected parts until the patient is substantially or completely relieved.

c. Do not energize the patient.

The effect is quite dramatic when the treatment is done properly.

ELEMENTARY PRANIC HEALING 119

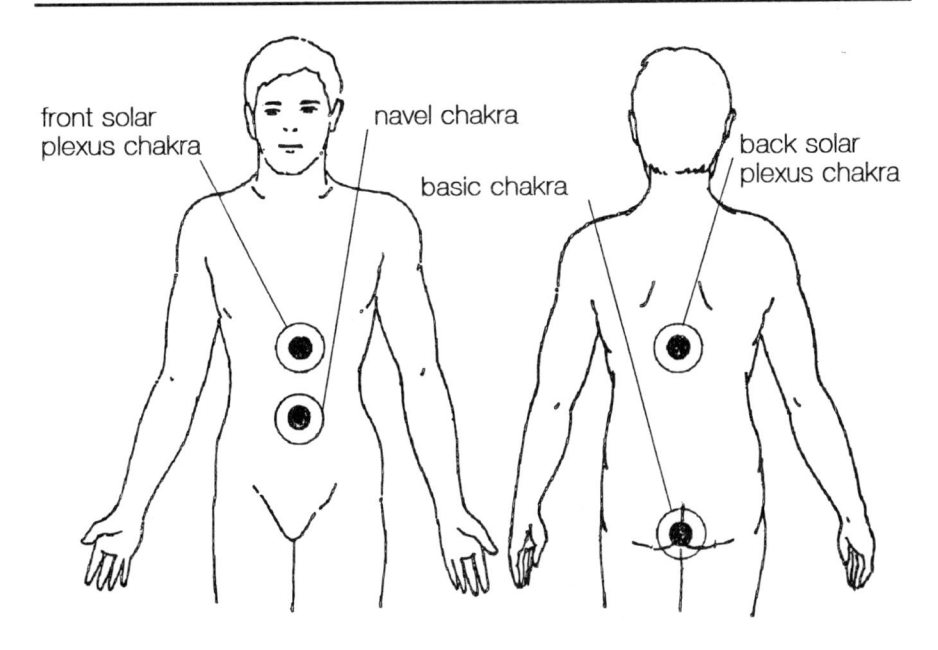

Labels on figure: front solar plexus chakra, navel chakra, basic chakra, back solar plexus chakra

Fig. 3-30 *Pranic treatment for eczema and other minor skin allergies*

28. Eczema and Other Minor Skin Allergies

a. Just apply localized sweeping thoroughly and energizing on the affected part until there is substantial relief.

b. Apply localized sweeping thoroughly on the liver (front, side and back).

c. Apply localized sweeping thoroughly and energizing on the front and back solar plexus, navel, and basic chakras. The emphasis of the treatment is on thorough cleansing of the solar plexus and basic chakras.

d. Stabilize the projected pranic energy.

e. Repeat the treatment thrice a week for as long as necessary.

29. Boils

a. Apply localized sweeping and energizing thoroughly on the affected part. The emphasis should be on localized sweeping. If this is done properly, the boil will become pinkish instead of dark red.

b. If the patient has chronic boils, apply localized sweeping thoroughly on the liver. Then apply localized sweeping thoroughly and energizing on the front and back solar plexus chakras.

c. Apply localized sweeping and energizing on the basic chakra.

d. Stabilize the projected pranic energy.

e. Repeat the treatment if necessary.

30. Insect and Bug Bites

a. Apply localized sweeping and energizing alternately on the affected part until there is substantial reduction in redness and swelling.

b. Be sure to stabilize the projected pranic energy.

c. Repeat the treatment if necessary.

ELEMENTARY PRANIC HEALING

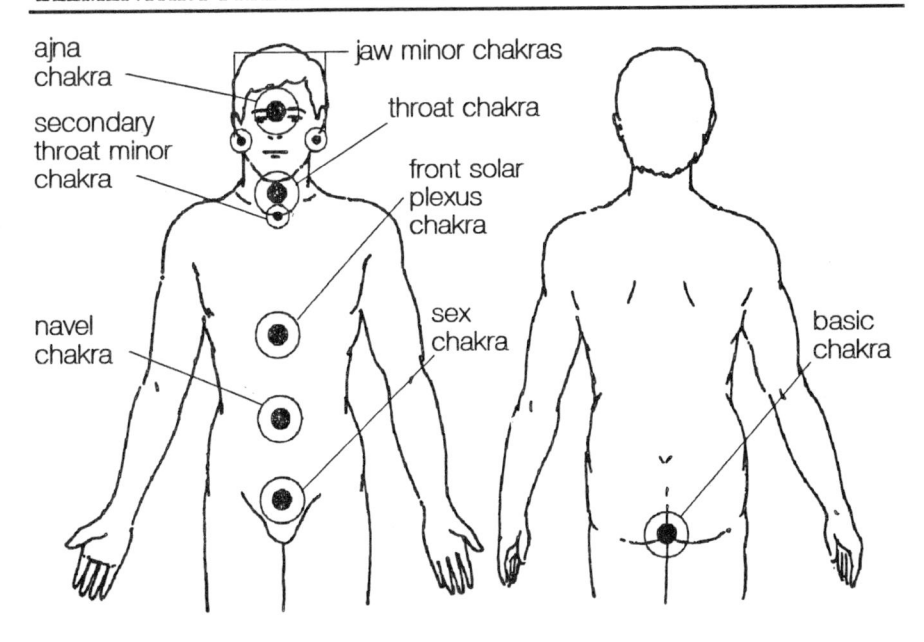

Fig. 3-31 *Pranic treatment for pimples*

31. Pimples

a. Apply thorough localized sweeping and energizing on the face. The face is depleted and the inner aura is relatively gray.

b. Scan the ajna, throat, secondary throat, jaw minor, solar plexus, navel, sex and basic chakras. Then apply localized sweeping and energizing on these chakras.

c. Stabilize the projected pranic energy.

d. The face may be treated once or twice a day while the major chakras may be treated once every two or three days.

e. The patient is expected to watch his diet and to keep his face regularly clean. Irritating the pimple should be avoided.

f. The emphasis should be on cleansing and energizing the face. Substantial improvement may occur in a few weeks' time.

32. Insomnia

The basic chakra is the center for dynamic activity. If the basic chakra is highly overactivated, it manifests as restlessness and insomnia. Overactivation of the basic chakra is usually caused by overactivation of the solar plexus chakra. By applying localized sweeping thoroughly, it is possible to normalize the front and back solar plexus chakras and the basic chakra, thereby enabling the patient to sleep deeply and easily.

a. If the patient is too excited or overenergized, apply general sweeping three to five times. Apply localized sweeping 30 to 50 times each on the front and back solar plexus chakras and basic chakra. This would be sufficient to make the patient drowsy. Apply downward sweeping only. Do not apply upward sweeping since it would tend to make the patient more alert.

b. If the patient is under stress or emotionally disturbed, apply general sweeping three to five times. Apply localized sweeping 30 to 50 times each on the crown, ajna, throat, front and back solar plexus and basic chakras. You may energize a little the treated chakras. Also, apply localized sweeping thoroughly on the meng mein chakra, and on the left and right adrenal glands which are usually congested. Apply localized sweeping and energizing on the back heart chakra to soothe the patient.

c. Stabilize the projected pranic energy.

d. Repeat the treatment thrice a week for as long as necessary.

ELEMENTARY PRANIC HEALING 123

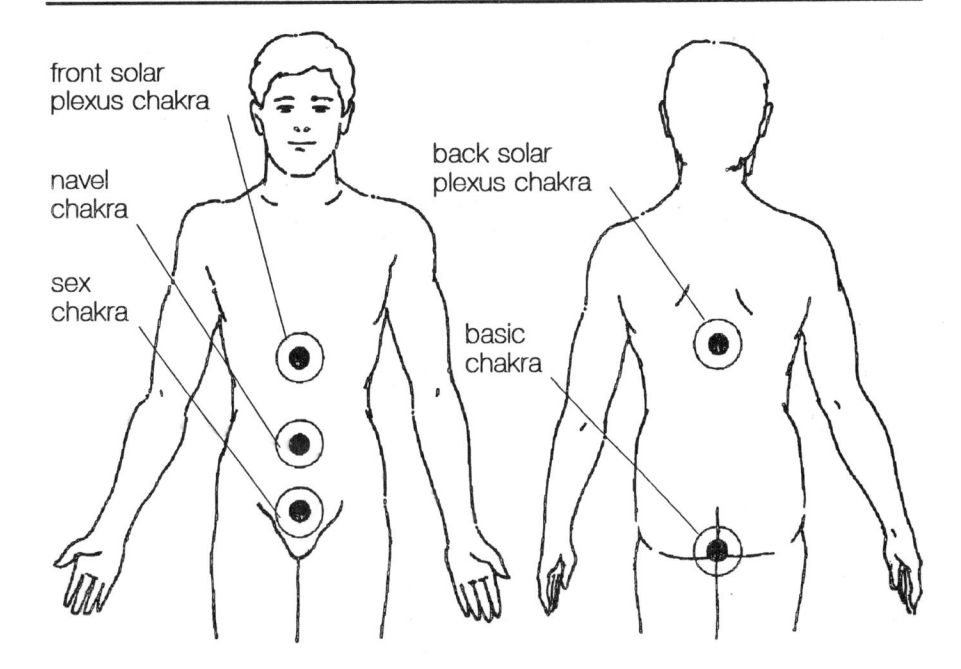

Fig. 3-32 *Pranic treatment for general weakness and for relieving tiredness*

e. If the patient is depleted, apply general sweeping several times. Apply localized sweeping and energizing on the navel and solar plexus chakras.

33. General Weakness

a. Apply general sweeping two to three times.

b. Apply localized sweeping and energizing on the basic, sex, navel, front and back solar plexus chakras.

c. Repeat the treatment three times a week for as long as necessary. This is very effective when applied regularly.

34. Relieving Tiredness

a. Apply the same treatment for general weakness. This is very helpful, especially in relieving tiredness after a hard day's work. The effect is almost instantaneous when it is done properly. This technique is used as an "energy booster" for working people.

WHAT TO DO IF YOU ARE NOT SURE
(for simple ailments)

a. Ask the patient about his complaint.

b. Apply thorough localized sweeping for about 30 to 50 times and energize the affected areas.

c. Repeat the treatment if necessary.

The author has taught many ordinary people how to heal, and they have become relatively proficient in just a few weeks' time. Pranic healing is easy. It just needs an open mind and a little perseverance.

HOW FREQUENT SHOULD HEALING BE DONE?

It depends on at least four factors:

1. *The severity and the acuteness of the ailment.* In severe cases, the rate of deterioration could be quite fast. For healing to take place, the rate of healing must be faster than the rate of deterioration. To increase the rate of healing, the frequency of the treatments has to be increased For example, in treating patients with cancer, the treatment has to be given at least once every two days. If treatment is given once every two weeks, the patient is not

likely to improve because the rate of deterioration is much faster than the rate of healing.

In emergency or critical cases, the rate of deterioration is so fast that the treatment may have to be given once every hour or once every four hours depending upon the acuteness of the case. In acute appendicitis, the treatment has to be given once every hour for the next four hours or until the condition has substantially improved. In the next few days, the treatment should be given two to three times. Not all cases of acute appendicitis can be healed by pranic healing. Some may require surgery.

2. *The rate of pranic consumption.* Tissue damage caused by burns, cuts, concussions, and acute infections consume large quantities of prana at a very fast rate. If the patient is suffering from severe infection or burn, then the affected part should be energized once every hour for the next few hours since the rate of pranic consumption is very fast. In acute pancreatitis, the patient can be treated once every four hours until he has substantially improved. Another factor is how fast the patient wants to get well. If a patient has a concussion on the arm and he wants to get well in a day or two, this would require several applications of pranic healing for the first few hours. If healing is done immediately and properly, the skin will not blacken or turn yellow and the rate of healing will be very fast - less than a day or two days at the most.

If the patient just wants a moderate rate of healing, then the treatment can be applied just once. If pranic healing is applied immediately, then the concussion will be healed within a few days.

3. *The delicateness and importance of the part being treated.* If the organ being treated is quite delicate and vital such as the head, eyes, and heart, then healing should preferably be applied at a longer interval. This is to avoid possible pranic congestion which may have serious consequences. If the part being treated is not so delicate or sensitive like the knee or the arm, then healing can be

applied once every hour for the next four hours without serious side effects or radical reactions.

4. *The age and health condition of the patient.* Patients who are very weak or old require a series of mild treatments since their ability to absorb prana is very slow.

These are factors to be considered in determining the frequency of treatments. The healer should use sound judgment or discrimination on this matter.

The author usually prefers to treat a patient at an interval of once every two to three days in most cases. In critical cases or if the patient wants a very fast rate of healing, pranic treatment is applied once every hour for the next few hours on the first day and once or twice a day for the next few days. The healer should observe or monitor the patient closely for possible radical reactions which could be serious.

WHOLISITIC OR INTEGRATED APPROACH IN HEALING

As stated earlier, disease can be caused by internal or external factors or a combination of both. Obviously, the health condition of a person depends upon the well-being of the visible physical body, the energy body, and the psychological health of the patient. Although many of the simple and serious diseases can be healed by pranic healing, it is better to reinforce the healing process by taking herbs or medicinal drugs. If the visible physical body and energy body are treated simultaneously, obviously the rate of healing would be much faster and more effective than orthodox medicine alone or pranic healing alone. An acupuncturist uses acupuncture to treat the energy body and herbs to heal the visible body by strengthening the affected organs. Although the author heals by using pranic healing only and has obtained amazing results, he also encourages his patients to consult medical doctors, take medicines, and undergo surgery, if this is necessary. The ancient famous Chinese doctor Hua To was noted not only for his skills in acupuncture and herbs but also for his surgical skills.

Although pranic healing alone can do a lot of fantastic things, it has its limitations. Proper diet and physical exercise are sometimes necessary. At times, the intake of herbs or medicinal drugs, change in lifestyle, emotional therapy or surgery is required. It is important to maintain one's objectivity and to have a proper perspective of what the other types of healing can do. Fanaticism and going to the extremes should be avoided. Just as it is foolish for some doctors trained in orthodox medicine to ignore or sometimes ridicule paranormal healing, it is equally foolish for some paranormal healers to ignore what modern medicine is capable of doing and what it has done to cure and alleviate the suffering of man from diseases.

HOW DO YOU WILL OR INTEND?

You do not have to tense your muscles or exert extraordinary effort when you "will" or "intend." You do not even have to visualize or close your eyes. When you perform with understanding, expectation, and concentration, you are already willing! The degree of concentration required is not extraordinary. The degree of concentration used in reading a book is sufficient to perform pranic healing. The author does not expect you to believe or disbelieve what he has written. What he expects from you is an open, inquiring mind with a strong interest to experiment and verify the validity of the principles and techniques suggested in this book.

The preliminary work with Kirlian photography so far seems to indicate that psychic healing involves a transfer of energy from the bioplasmic body of the healer to the bioplasmic body of his patient.

– S. Ostrander and L. Schroeder,
Psychic Discoveries Behind the Iron Curtain

A more scientific method .... first withdraws the congested and diseased matter, and then replaces it by healthier nerve ether (life energy), thus gradually stimulating the sluggish current into activity.

– C. W. Leadbeater,
The Chakras

CHAPTER FOUR

Intermediate Pranic Healing

> *Man lives only as long as he has life energy in his body. If he lacks life energy, he dies. Therefore, we should practice pranayama (the art of controlling life energy or prana through breathing).*
>
> — *Hatha Yoga Pradipika*
> Ancient Textbook On Yoga

> *... by rhythmic breathing and controlled thought, you are enabled to absorb a considerable amount of prana (life energy), and are also able to pass it into the body of another person, stimulating weakened parts and organs and imparting health and driving out diseased conditions.*
>
> — *Yogi Ramacharaka*
> The Science of Psychic Healing

Drawing in Prana through Pranic Breathing	131
How to Draw in Ground Prana, Air Prana and Tree Prana	135
Sensitizing the Hands and the Fingers through Pranic Breathing	139
Scanning with the Fingers	139
Sweeping with Pranic Breathing	141
Energizing with Pranic Breathing	142
Energizing: Distributive Sweeping Technique	145
Disposing Diseased Energy	146
Utilizing Ground Prana in Healing	146
Suggested Practice Schedule	147

Chapter Four

Rotation of the Chakras 147
Other Healing Techniques 150
Energizing Objects 152
Treatments for Simple and Serious Cases
    1. Strengthening the Body's Defense System
       by Increasing its Life Energy Level 154
    2. Measles, German Measles
       and Chicken Pox 155
    3. Mumps and Tonsillitis 157
    4. Gum Bleeding 158
    5. Pyorrhea 158
    6. Fainting 159
    7. Nearsightedness, Farsightedness
       and Astigmatism 160
    8. Cross-eyes and Walleyes 161
    9. Chronic or Acute Glaucoma 161
    10. Heart Ailments 163
    11. High Cholesterol Level 166
    12. Hypertension 167
    13. Loss of Smell 168
    14. Sinusitis 169
    15. Respiratory Ailments (Pneumonia,
        Tuberculosis, Emphysema, etc.) 170
    16. Asthma 173
    17. Hepatitis 175
    18. Gastric and Duodenal Ulcers 176
    19. Hemorrhoid 177
    20. Chronic Appendicitis 178
    21. Frequent Urination 179
    22. Bedwetting 180
    23. Enlarged Prostate Gland 180
    24. Urinary Tract Infection 180
    25. Kidney and Bladder Infections 181
    26. Sexual Impotence 182
    27. Infertility 184
    28. Broken Bones 185
    29. Arthritis and Rheumatism 186
    30. Osteoarthritis 188
    31. Gout 189
    32. Rheumatoid Arthritis 190
    33. Scoliosis 192
    34. Paralysis due to Stroke 193

35. Ailments of the Endocrine Glands	194
36. Treatment for Pregnant Women Who Have Difficulty in Giving Birth	195
37. How to Hasten the Recovery of a Woman Who Has Just Given Birth	196
38. How to Prevent a Miscarriage	197
39. Pregnant Patients who have a History of Miscarriage and are Experiencing Abdominal Pain	198
40. Treating Patients Before and After Undergoing Surgery	198
41. Relieving Cancer Patients	199
42. Reducing the Rate of Aging (Old Age)	201
43. Stress or Tension	203
What To Do If You Are Not Sure (For Difficult Cases)	203
Principle of Lag Time	204
How Long Does It Take to Completely Cure a Patient?	205
Immediate Recurrence of Pain or Symptoms	205
Reasons Why Some Patients Are Not Healed	207
Personal Health Problems that a Healer May Encounter	208
Avoid Using Too Much Will in Healing	210
Rate of Vibration of the Energy Body	210
Popularizing Pranic Healing	212

DRAWING IN PRANA THROUGH PRANIC BREATHING

In Elementary Pranic Healing, you learned to draw in prana through one of the hand chakras. In Intermediate Pranic Healing, you will learn pranic breathing in order to absorb or draw in tremendous amount of prana through the whole body from the surroundings. There are many types of yogic breathing intended for different purposes. Yogic breathing that enables the practitioner to draw in a lot of prana and facilitates the projection of prana is called pranic breathing.

Pranic breathing energizes you to such an extent that your auras temporarily expand by 100 percent or more. The inner aura expands to about eight inches or more, the health aura to about four feet or more, and the outer aura to about two meters or more. When doing pranic breathing, the healer becomes more powerful. His etheric body or his energy body becomes brighter and denser. All of these can be verified through scanning.

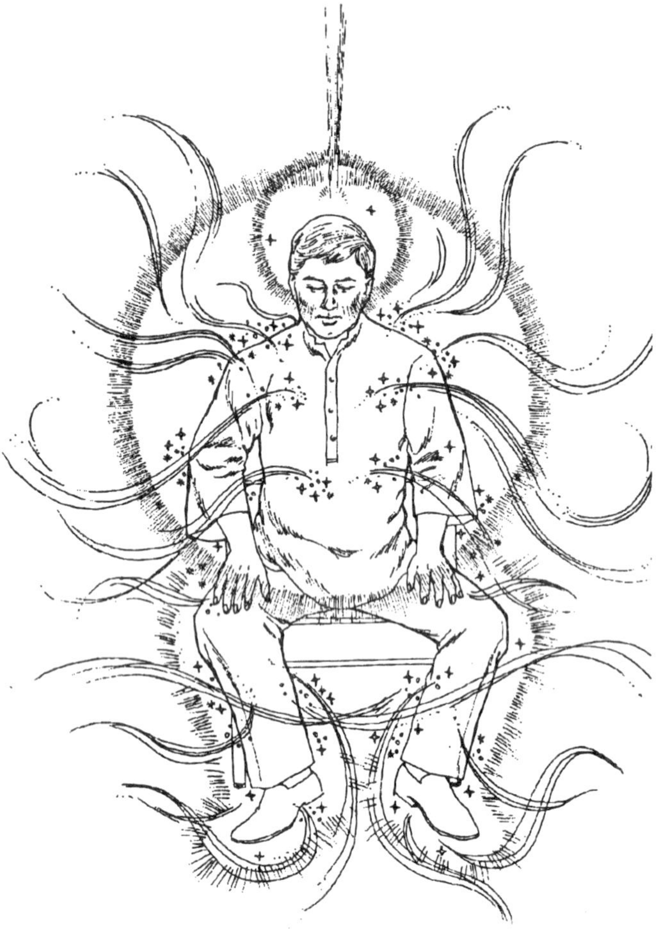

Fig. 4-1 *Pranic breathing:*
By doing pranic breathing, you are able to absorb and project tremendous amount of life energy or prana.

You can perform this simple experiment:

Ask a friend to do pranic breathing for several minutes. Scan your friend before, during and after pranic breathing. Note the changes in the size of the auras. You may even feel a rhythmic pulsation or expansion. It is important that you perform this and other experiments so that your knowledge will be based on solid foundations.

Method 1 - Deep Breathing with Empty Retention

1. Connect your tongue to your palate.
2. Do abdominal breathing.
3. Inhale slowly and retain for one count.
4. Exhale slowly. Retain your breath for one count before inhaling. This is called empty retention.

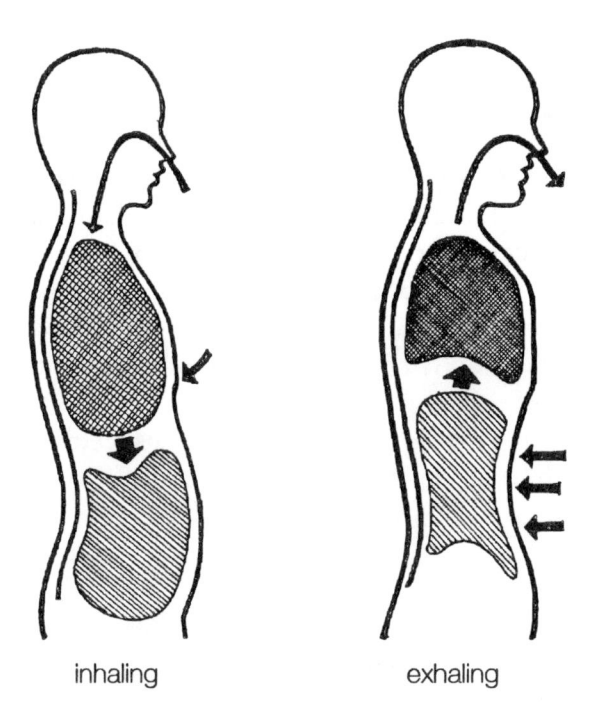

inhaling   exhaling

Fig. 4-2 *Abdominal breathing*

Method 2 - 7-1-7-1

1. Connect your tongue to your palate.
2. Do abdominal breathing.
3. Inhale for seven counts and retain for one count.
4. Exhale for seven counts and retain for one count.

Method 3 - 6-3-6-3

1. Connect your tongue to your palate.
2. Do abdominal breathing.
3. Inhale for six counts and retain for three counts.
4. Exhale for six counts and retain for three counts.

In doing abdominal breathing, you expand your abdomen slightly when inhaling and contract your abdomen slightly when exhaling. Do not over-expand or over-contract your abdomen. This would make breathing unnecessarily difficult.

The critical factors involved are the rhythm and the empty retention. Holding your breath after exhalation is called empty retention; and holding your breath after inhalation is called full retention. Through clairvoyant observation, it is noted that there is a tremendous amount of prana rushing into all parts of the body when inhalation is done after empty retention. This does not take place if the inhalation is not preceded by empty retention.

When drawing in prana, you may use either the pranic breathing method or the hand chakras technique or both of them simultaneously.

Doing pranic breathing before and after healing is important. Before healing patients, do five cycles of pranic breathing to increase the energy level of your etheric body, and thereby increase the healing power. After healing, wash your hands and do five

INTERMEDIATE PRANIC HEALING

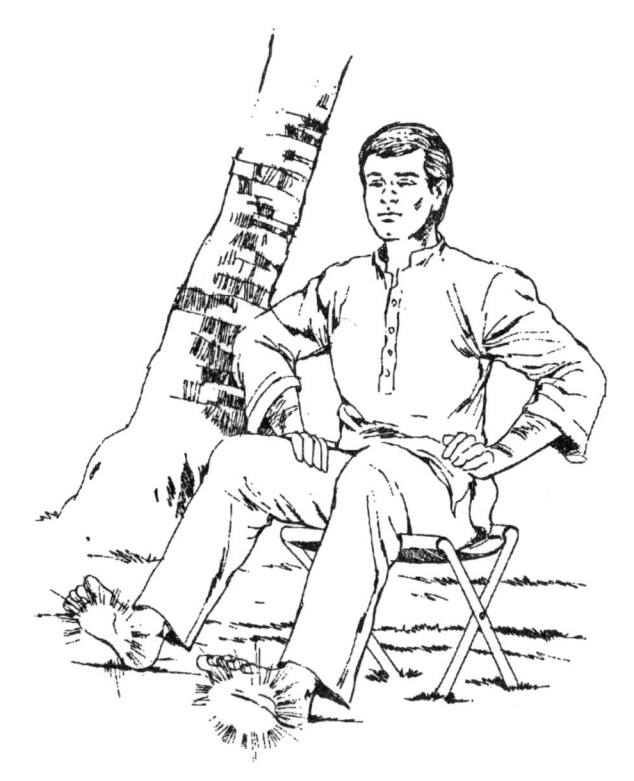

Fig. 4-3 *Drawing in ground prana*

cycles of pranic breathing to recharge your body and avoid pranic depletion. If the instructions are followed, the healer will be able to treat many patients in one day without getting depleted.

HOW TO DRAW IN GROUND PRANA, AIR PRANA AND TREE PRANA

There is a minor chakra in each foot. This chakra is called the sole chakra. By concentrating on the sole chakras and simultaneously doing pranic breathing, you can tremendously increase the amount of ground prana absorbed through the sole chakras. Concentrating on the sole chakras activates them to a certain degree. Pranic breathing greatly helps the sole chakras in drawing in ground

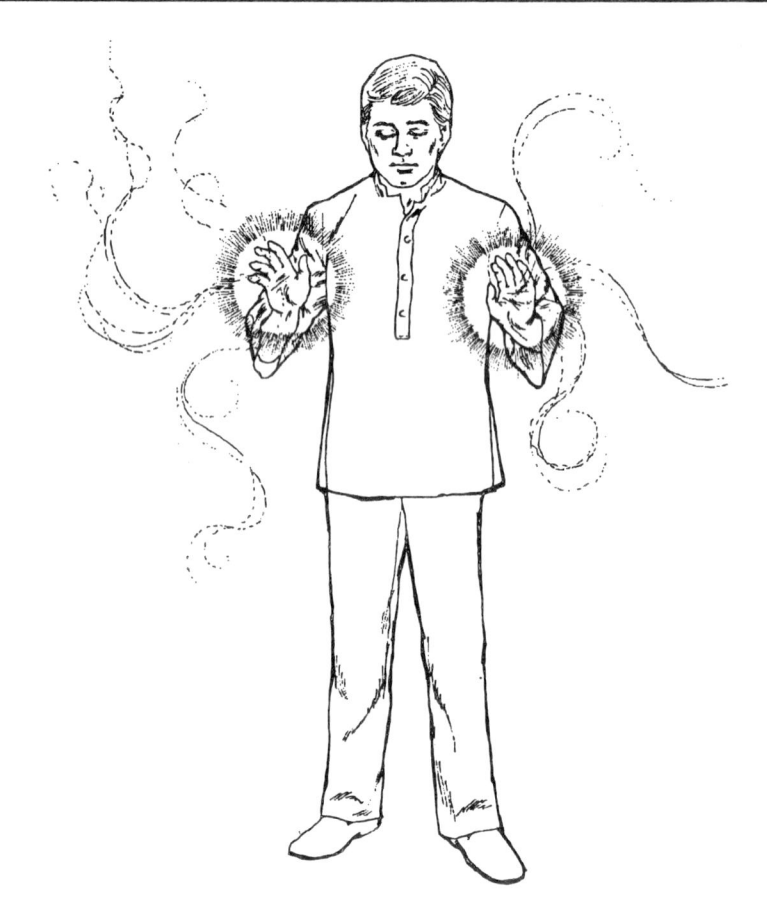

Fig. 4-4 *Drawing in air prana*

prana. Drawing in ground prana is one way of energizing yourself. Ground prana seems to be more effective in healing the visible physical body than air prana. For example, wounds and fractured bones seem to heal faster with ground prana than air prana.

This technique of drawing in ground prana or earth ki is practiced in Chinese esoteric martial art or ki kung (qigong).

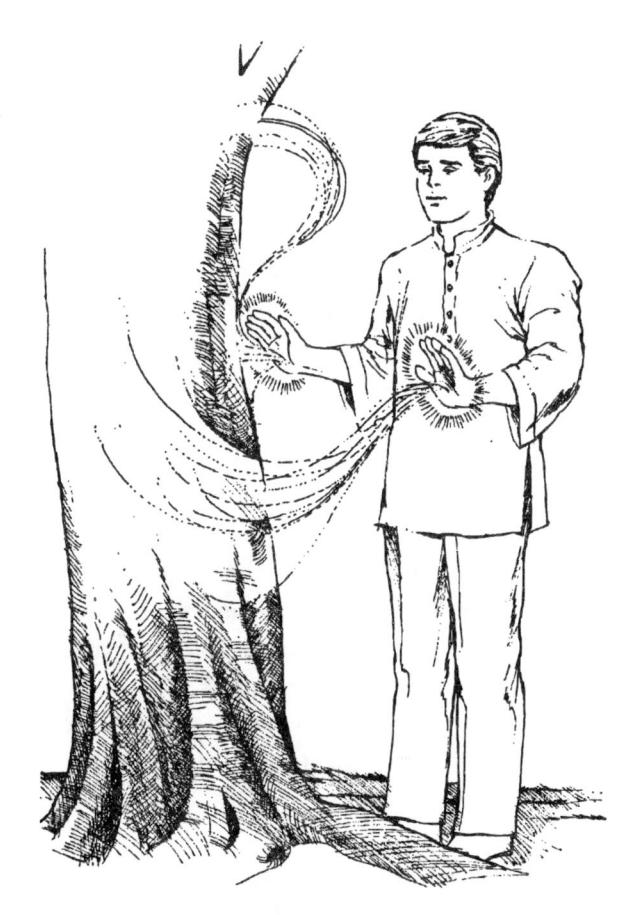

Fig. 4-5 *Drawing in tree prana*

Procedure:

1. Remove your shoes. Leather shoes and rubber shoes reduce the absorption of prana by about 30 to 50 percent.

2. Connect your tongue to your palate.

3. Press the hollow portion of your feet with your thumbs to make concentration easier.

4. Concentrate on the soles of your feet and do pranic breathing simultaneously. Do this for about 10 cycles.

Practice only in clean places. Do not practice on top of a septic tank. Otherwise, this will cause the practitioner to be severely contaminated with dirty energy. This type of ailment is difficult to heal because the dirty energy is absorb deeply into the system of the practitioner. It usually manifests as extreme difficulty in urination.

You can use the same principle to draw in air prana or tree prana through the hand chakras to energize yourself. To draw in air prana through the hands, just concentrate on the hand chakras and simultaneously do pranic breathing. To draw in tree prana through the hand chakras, choose a big healthy tree and ask mentally or verbally the permission of the tree to draw in its excess prana. Put your hands on the trunk of the tree or near it. Concentrate on the centers of your palms and simultaneously do pranic breathing. Do this for ten cycles and thank the tree for the prana. Some of you may experience numbness or a tingling sensation throughout your body.

After energizing yourself, it is advisable to circulate the prana throughout the body. Visualize yourself filled with white light or prana and circulate the prana continuously from the back to the front several times, then from the front to the back several times also.

Once esoteric principles and techniques are fully explained, they are usually very simple.

SENSITIZING THE HANDS AND THE FINGERS THROUGH PRANIC BREATHING

By now, most of you should have more or less permanently sensitized your hands. However, sometimes you may experience moments wherein the hands seem not to be able to feel or scan. This can be immediately remedied by concentrating simultaneously on the centers of your palms and the tips of your fingers while doing pranic breathing for about seven cycles. This will cause the hand chakras and finger chakras to be activated, energized and sensitized so that you can scan accurately with your palms and your fingers.

It is important to connect the tongue to the palate when sensitizing the hands and fingers and when scanning. This will facilitate the sensitizing and scanning process.

SCANNING WITH THE FINGERS

After sensitizing your hands, scan your own palm with your two fingers. Move your fingers slowly and slightly back and forth to feel the inner aura of your palm. Try to feel the thickness of your palm and the different layers of the inner aura. Practice also scanning your palm with one finger. Always concentrate on the tips of your fingers when scanning with them. This will activate or further activate the mini finger chakras, thereby sensitizing the fingers.

When scanning with your palms and fingers, always concentrate on the centers of your palms and on the tips of your fingers. This will cause the hand chakras and the finger chakras to remain activated or become more activated, increasing the sensitivity of your palms and fingers.

Being able to scan with the palms is not sufficient. You must also learn to scan with your fingers. This is required in locating or proper scanning of small troubled spots which is difficult to do with the palm. The palm may only feel the healthier surrounding areas around the small troubled spots. The small troubled spots are camouflaged by the healthier parts.

For instance, a person with eye problems usually has pranic depletion in the eyes, while the inner auras of the surrounding areas may be normal. Since the palm is quite big and the inner aura of the eyes is about two inches in diameter, it is likely that the palms may feel only the healthy areas of the eyebrows and forehead without becoming aware of the small troubled spots. This could be avoided if the fingers were used in scanning. The spinal column should also be scanned by using one or two fingers in order to locate small troubled spots.

In scanning a patient, you do not have to scan the outer and health auras. You were taught how to scan these auras in order to prove to yourself their existence. What is important is scanning the inner aura of the patient. In scanning the inner aura, it is important to feel the general energy level or the general thickness of the inner aura of the patient. The general energy level will be used as a reference point or standard in comparing the conditions of some of the major chakras and vital organs. The accuracy of scanning will be affected if that area is scanned for too long because the scanned area will become partially energized.

It is important that you should be able to feel the pressure when scanning in order to determine the thickness of the inner aura of the part being scanned. Some of you may feel pain in your hands or fingers when in contact with a diseased part. The inner aura has several layers. In scanning the inner aura, you may feel pressure at about five inches and another layer which is denser or stronger in pressure at about two or three inches away from the skin. Sometimes the inner aura of a certain part may seem normal. But when scanned further within, the next layer is rather thin which means that the part is quite depleted. In scanning the inner aura, it is important to scan not only its first layer but also its inner

INTERMEDIATE PRANIC HEALING

layers. An advanced yogi or an advanced practitioner of ki kung (the art of generating internal power) has an inner aura that is comparatively big and has many layers. Sometimes the inner aura is several meters in thickness.

Scanning is also very useful in determining whether an infant or a child has hearing or eyesight problems.

In treating serious cases, the 11 major chakras, the relevant minor chakras, all the major and vital organs, and the spine should be scanned thoroughly. It is through proper scanning and correct understanding of the nature of the ailment that the correct treatment can be determined.

SWEEPING WITH PRANIC BREATHING

General and localized sweeping are more effective when used with pranic breathing since the patient is cleansed and energized simultaneously to a substantial degree. This type of sweeping is quite effective and very often sufficient to heal simple ailments. Sweeping can be done several feet away from the patient and with fewer strokes. You do not have to bother with what hand position to use. Just follow the instructions given in elementary pranic healing on how to apply general sweeping and localized sweeping, and simultaneously do pranic breathing.

You may visualize luminous white prana sweeping and washing the patient from the crown to the feet when doing downward sweeping. Visualize the health rays being straightened. You do not have to do upward sweeping unless the patient is quite sleepy or has weak legs. When doing upward sweeping, you may visualize ground prana going up from the sole chakras to the crown chakra. This should be done after the patient has been cleansed sufficiently with downward sweeping. To apply upward general sweeping before applying downward sweeping may result in the transference of diseased energy to the head and brain areas. This may result in serious harm to the patient.

You may or may not visualize when you do sweeping, but with some healers sweeping is more effective when it is accompanied by visualization. What is important is the intention to clean and energize the patient's energy body.

In sweeping, special attention should be placed on the back energy channel or the governor meridian which interpenetrates the spine, and the front energy channel or functional meridian which is opposite to the spine. Except for the spleen chakra, almost all the major chakras are directly located along these two channels or nadis. Cleansing or applying localized sweeping on these two channels would clean the major chakras located along these two meridians, resulting in a much faster rate of healing. You must remember that all the major and vital organs are energized and controlled by the major chakras.

When applying localized sweeping, visualize the fingers and the hands penetrating into the diseased part and the grayish diseased energy being removed.

ENERGIZING WITH PRANIC BREATHING

Prana is drawn in by using pranic breathing and is projected through one or both of the hand chakras.

1. Do pranic breathing slowly for about three to five cycles and simultaneously calm and still your mind.

2. Continue doing pranic breathing and simultaneously put your hand or hands near the part to be treated. Concentrate on the center of your palm or palms.

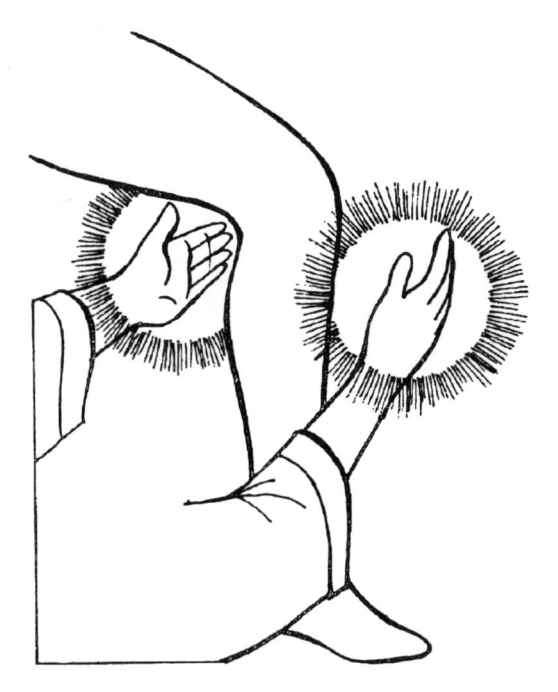

Fig. 4-6 *Parallel double energizing*

3. Will or direct the projected pranic energy to the affected chakra and then to the affected part. This is important. In many cases, it will produce rapid relief since the affected part or organ will be quickly provided with sufficient pranic energy. The attention should be focused primarily on the hand chakra or chakras and on directing the pranic energy, less on the breathing.

4. Stop energizing when you intuitively sense the patient has enough prana or life energy. Rescan the patient to determine whether he is sufficiently energized. In elementary pranic healing, you were instructed to stop energizing when you feel a slight repulsion or a cessation of flow of energy. As you become more advanced in healing, this guideline is no longer valid because your pranic energy level becomes much higher compared to

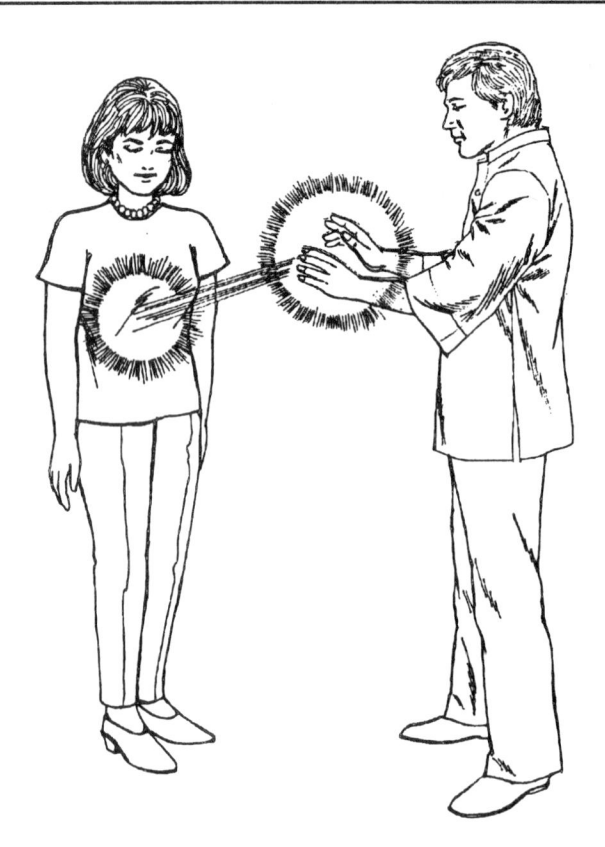

Fig. 4-7 *Non-parallel double energizing*

that of the patient. Equalizing your pranic energy level with the affected part of the patient may result in pranic congestion on the part being treated.

5. If the patient has severe infection, burns, or cuts, then the treatment has to be repeated after half an hour or after an hour. These types of cases consume pranic energy at a very fast rate; therefore, the treatments have to be repeated more frequently.

Energizing should be done simultaneously with pranic breathing. It is preferable to do pranic breathing for three to five cycles before you start energizing and to continue doing pranic breathing for three cycles after you have stopped energizing. This is to prevent possible general pranic depletion on the part of the healer.

There are two types of double energizing, or energizing with two hands: parallel double energizing and non-parallel double energizing. In parallel double energizing, simply place your hands facing and parallel to each other with the affected part in between them. In non-parallel double energizing, the hands are directed to the affected part but are not parallel to each other. In parallel double energizing, an intense energy field is created causing the hand to rhythmically expand and contract. Tingling sensation is felt not only in the affected part but also in other parts of the body. At times, the patient may even feel a slight electric shock. Double energizing is usually used in cases that require tremendous amount of prana. Cleansing must be done before double energizing. Double energizing can also be used to quickly relieve simple ailments or illnesses which have been mentioned in elementary pranic healing.

ENERGIZING: DISTRIBUTIVE SWEEPING TECHNIQUE

Energizing with the use of distributive sweeping technique simply means the use of sweeping to redistribute excess prana from other parts of the body to the ailing part.

1. Clean the ailing part by applying localized sweeping.

2. Sweep the excess prana with the use of your hand from the surrounding parts and chakras to the treated part.

This type of energizing is quite effective in healing simple ailments but not the more serious ones since they require tremendous amount of prana.

DISPOSING DISEASED ENERGY

There are times when it is inconvenient or impossible to throw away the diseased energy into a disposal unit. Should this happen, just simply will the diseased energy to disintegrate when you flick it away. This technique is applicable only for the more proficient healers.

For beginners, you can try to heal in open spaces and throw the diseased energy deep into the ground. It is a common practice among shamans to dispose of objects filled with diseased energy by burning them, exposing them to the air for a prolonged period of time or burying them under the ground.

UTILIZING GROUND PRANA IN HEALING

There is greater concentration of prana just above the ground than in the air. The density of prana just above the ground is about four or five times greater than the prana contained in the air. This concentration of ground prana can be used for healing.

Ask your patient to lie down on the ground. A cotton blanket or mat made of natural material may be used to lie down on. Avoid using leather, rubber, synthetic foam, mat or blanket for this purpose. They tend to act as insulators which hinder the free flow of ground prana into the body.

Apply general sweeping and localized sweeping several times. Let the patient rest and gradually absorb the ground prana. The act of cleansing causes a sort of partial "pranic vacuum" that results in the rushing of ground prana into the energy body of the patient and into the treated part. Energy tends to flow from a level of greater intensity to lower intensity or from a level of greater concentration to lower concentration. Once the patient is cleansed, energizing with ground prana occurs automatically and gradually. The healer should preferably energize the patient after sweeping to shorten the time required to substantially energize the affected part.

This is also the reason why some shaman healers go to the extent of burying the patient in the ground so that he can absorb more ground prana. If one is not feeling too well, one can take a swim in the sea for about 10-15 minutes to cleanse the energy body; after that he may bury his body in the sand to gradually absorb ground prana.

SUGGESTED PRACTICE SCHEDULE

1. Sensitizing the hands and the fingers through pranic breathing - three minutes
2. Scanning with two fingers - three minutes
3. Pranic breathing with drawing in of air prana through the hand chakras - three minutes
4. Energizing with pranic breathing - three minutes

Follow this schedule for about three to five weeks. You should also try to treat many difficult cases. If you follow consistently the instructions in this book, your healing skills will develop very rapidly. You will be able to do a lot of things that may be considered by others as "impossible" or "miraculous."

ROTATION OF THE CHAKRAS

Some students think a chakra rotates counterclockwise while some think it rotates clockwise. Both are partially correct and partially wrong. A chakra is rapidly rotating alternately clockwise and counterclockwise. Clockwise motion draws in pranic energy to the chakra while counterclockwise motion projects or draws out pranic energy from the chakra. Clockwise motion of the chakra is absorbing while counterclockwise motion of the chakra is projecting or expelling. When a healer draws in pranic energy through a chakra, the chakra is predominantly rotating clockwise and to a much lesser degree, rotating counterclockwise. When a healer projects pranic energy through a chakra, it is predominantly rotating counterclockwise and, to a much lesser degree, rotating clockwise. Under normal conditions, a chakra is rotating clockwise and counterclockwise in equal proportions. So the amount of pranic energy coming in and going out is about the same.

When energizing, the hand chakra is predominantly rotating counterclockwise and to a lesser degree clockwise (drawing in). This is why the energizing hand also absorbs diseased energy and has to be flicked regularly to throw away the diseased energy. It is better to clean before energizing not only to reduce the possibility of radical reaction but also to minimize the quantity of diseased energy that will be absorbed by the healer when energizing. This is why the author does not recommend healers to energize with the use of their eyes or with a major chakra because the eyes are very delicate and difficult to clean while a major chakra controls a vital organ or several organs. It is possible for the corresponding organ or organs to fully absorb the diseased energy which is harmful to the healer.

Under normal conditions, a chakra draws in and projects pranic energy alternately at a rapid rate. The amount of pranic energy drawn in and projected are more or less equal. The chakra rotates clockwise at 180 degrees and counterclockwise at 180 degrees in the opposite direction alternately at a rapid rate. When the hand chakra predominantly projects, the counterclockwise motion is 360 degrees and the clockwise motion is only 180 degrees. When the hand chakra rotates counterclockwise, it projects pranic energy and stops for a split second, then rotates in clockwise motion and draws in pranic energy and stops for a split second. The entire process is repeated. The pranic energy projected is not continuous and neither is the pranic energy drawn in. It only appears as continuous because the chakra is moving rapidly and alternately clockwise and counterclockwise, thereby giving an appearance of continuous projection of pranic energy or continuous drawing in of pranic energy. The difference in the intensity of pranic energy projected depends on the rate of rotation of the chakras. The faster it rotates, the more intense is the projected pranic energy and the slower it rotates, the less intense is the pranic energy projected. When a hand chakra is predominantly absorbing, it makes a 360-degree clockwise rotation and a 180-degree counterclockwise rotation and vice-versa when it is predominantly projecting pranic energy. The intensity of pranic energy projected or absorbed does not involve changes in the pattern of rotation of the chakra but is dependent upon the rate of rotation of the chakra. The faster it rotates, the more intense is the projected or absorbed prana.

In India and China, there are yogis and chi kung practitioners who heal by placing the hand near the affected part, then moving it in a circular motion. If the yogi or chi kung healer wants to clean or decongest an affected part, he applies localized sweeping by moving his hand several times in a counterclockwise motion to increase the chakra's counterclockwise motion, thereby facilitating the removal of diseased energy. He then flicks his hand to throw away the diseased energy. This process is continued until the affected chakra becomes substantially clean. If the yogi wants to energize an affected chakra, he projects pranic energy and simultaneously moves his hand clockwise to make the affected chakra draw in more pranic energy by increasing the chakra's clockwise motion. The clockwise motion is for energizing while the counterclockwise is for cleansing or decongesting. The technique is simple and easy to apply.

The appearance of the chakra is dependent upon its speed of rotation. Under normal conditions, the rapid clockwise and counterclockwise rotations produce an optical effect making the chakra look like a lotus flower with many pointed petals. The pointed petals are "optically produced" by the combined motions of pranic energy moving clockwise and counterclockwise. This is why in ancient Tibetan, Chinese and Sanskrit books on yoga, the chakras are usually presented as lotus flowers with many pointed petals. When a chakra is deliberately slowed down, the actual shape and number of petals can be seen clearly. The shape of the petals of a chakra is round. This is why the petals of the chakras described by Leadbeater are round, not pointed. When the chakra is moving very rapidly, the chakra bulges out or becomes quite thick. When it is rotating at an extremely rapid rate, the chakra appears as a dazzling point of light. When a spiritual aspirant is meditating, spiritual and pranic energies are attracted to the head area. This is why advanced yogis or saints are clairvoyantly seen with a dazzling or blinding light on the head area (spiritual "halo").

OTHER HEALING TECHNIQUES

The healing techniques that were explained earlier are those often used by the author and his friends. There are many other healing techniques used by other healers, but the basic principles are the same: cleansing and energizing the affected parts.

Other healing techniques:

1. Extraction technique

    a. Primitive
    b. Elementary
    c. Advanced

2. Short circuiting - cleansing and energizing

3. Short Circuiting - redistribution of prana

Extraction Technique - Primitive

There are several types of extraction technique and the simplest is done sometimes, if not usually, by natural-born healers who have had no training in healing. These healers simply touch the affected part and involuntarily extract or absorb the pain and the diseased energy into his body without expelling it. This is because they do not really know how to expel the diseased energy and do not understand the process. Consequently, they are affected by the diseased energy but recover after a good night's sleep. This technique is definitely not advisable.

Extraction Technique – Elementary

Another type of extraction technique is absorbing the diseased matter through one of the hand chakras and expelling it through the other hand chakra. You may use either of the hand chakras for extraction and expelling. Although this is an improvement over the primitive technique, it is still not advisable because there is always the possibility that some diseased energy will remain in the healer's body. Just imagine what will happen to the healer if he extracts dirty energy from 20-50 patients a day for 250 days a year. It is quite unlikely that the healer will remain healthy for long. He might even end up with so many strange diseases. The idea of absorbing dirty, sticky, grayish diseased energy is just plainly repulsive.

Extraction Technique – Advanced

Another type of extraction technique is simply extracting the diseased energy from the affected part by an act of will. The hand is placed a few inches away from the affected part and the diseased energy is extracted by willing it to come out. No sweeping movement is done. The diseased energy is caught by the hand and flicked into the disposal unit.

Short Circuiting – Cleansing and Energizing

Short circuiting can be done either to clean and energize simultaneously an affected part or to redistribute prana from one area to another part. Short circuiting (cleansing and energizing) is done by simply placing the energizing hand at the back of the chakra to be treated and the extracting hand in front of it.

Procedure:

1. Do pranic breathing.

2. Place your energizing hand at the back of the chakra to be treated.

3. Place your extracting hand in front of the chakra. Visualize your extracting hand surrounded by a layer of bright light.

4. Energize the back of the chakra. Visualize and will the dirty energy to come out. The diseased energy should not penetrate the layer of bright light on the extracting hand. Do not absorb the dirty energy into your body!

5. Flick the dirty energy into the disposal unit.

Short Circuiting – Redistribution of Prana

One hand is used for drawing in prana from the source and the other is used for energizing the part to be treated. For example, in treating a headache, the hand that is drawing in prana is placed in front of the throat chakra and the energizing hand is placed on the affected part.

There are other healing techniques not dealt with here but the basic principles which are cleansing and energizing are the same.

ENERGIZING OBJECTS

Objects like water, food, herbs, medicine, alcohol, oil, ointment, balm, lotion, band aid, bandage and cotton can be charged with prana to facilitate the healing process. Herbs, drugs, ointment, balm, lotion and oil can be energized to increase their effectivity and potency. Rubbing alcohol can be energized to increase its disinfecting action and hasten the rate of healing. Band aid, bandage and cotton can also be energized for similar purposes. Energized water can be taken internally by the patients to facilitate the healing process. Cold water absorbs more prana while warm water absorbs much less.

The transference of pranic energy or healing energy, contained in energized oil, to the affected part or chakra is the principle behind the religious practice of anointing the sick with holy or energized oil.

There are some patients who involuntarily or willfully resist the healing process. A patient who resists can, to a certain extent, block or prevent the entry of prana into his body. In this case, energized oil can also be used as an entry point for prana. It acts as a "gate or a hole" for prana to enter the patient's body.

For healing skin diseases, energized ointment, lotion or balm can be used after the initial pranic treatment. Instead of healing the patient so many times, healing sessions can be reduced. The healing process is hastened by the use of energized ointment or medicine. Therefore, the healer will have more time to treat more serious cases.

It is quite likely that in a few decades from now, most drugs or medicines will be energized with prana to produce faster and more effective results.

Objects can be energized by using pranic breathing and the energizing technique. Energizing can also be done through physical means.

TREATMENTS FOR SIMPLE AND SERIOUS CASES

1. Strengthening the Body's Defense System by Increasing its Life Energy Level

Many ailments are due to bacterial and viral infections. The white blood cells that protect the body from infections are produced by the bones. By proper pranic treatment and by increasing the life energy level of the body, its defense system is strengthened and enhanced.

   a. Apply general sweeping three or four times.

   b. Clean and energize the sole and hand minor chakras. Simultaneously, you may visualize pranic energy or "white light" going inside the bones. This is to strengthen the bones in the arms and legs, and also to partially activate the sole and hand chakras so that they will absorb more prana, thereby increasing the life energy level of the body.

   Do not stabilize the projected pranic energy because this may partially inhibit the sole and hand minor chakras.

   c. Apply localized sweeping thoroughly on the front and back solar plexus chakras and on the liver (front, side and back). Energize the front solar plexus chakra. This is to strengthen the liver and to energize the whole body, especially the internal organs in the trunk. The liver detoxifies the blood; strengthening it also enhances the body's defense system.

   d. Clean and energize the navel chakra. This has two major effects: first, energizing and partially activating the navel chakra will energize and partially activate the spleen chakra so that it will absorb more prana and thus, increase the life energy level of the body. Second, the navel chakra is partially activated and stimulated to produce more "biosynthetic ki", and make the etheric body more powerful, thereby increasing the ability of the etheric body to absorb more prana.

e. For severe cases of infection, clean and energize gently the front and back spleen chakras. Observe the patient. In rare cases, he may get congested and may faint. Do not highly energize the spleen chakra if the patient has hypertension.

f. Apply localized sweeping and energizing on the basic chakra. Do not energize the basic chakra if the patient has a fever since the temperature may rise.

2. Measles, German Measles, and Chicken Pox

a. Apply general sweeping three or four times.

b. Apply localized sweeping thoroughly on the face, the throat, the front and back trunk. Special emphasis should be given on the affected part and the abdominal area.

c. To improve the body's defense system, apply localized sweeping on the liver and the solar plexus chakra for about 50 times each and then energize the solar plexus chakra. Stabilize the projected pranic energy.

d. Apply localized sweeping thoroughly on the upper and lower abdominal areas, navel chakra, hand and sole minor chakras. Energize the navel chakra, hand and sole minor chakras.

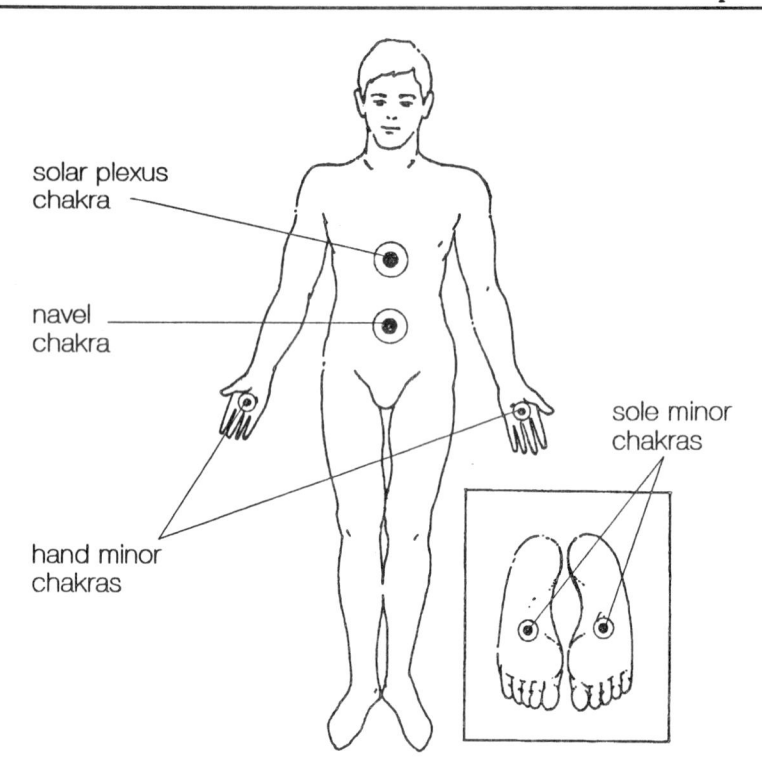

Fig. 4-8 *Pranic treatment for measles, german measles, and chicken pox*

- e. Stabilize the projected pranic energy.

- f. The emphasis of the treatment should be on the thorough cleansing of the body.

- g. Do not energize the basic chakra directly because this may increase the body's temperature. General and localized sweeping can be repeated two or three times a day.

- h. Repeat the treatment for the next several days.

INTERMEDIATE PRANIC HEALING 157

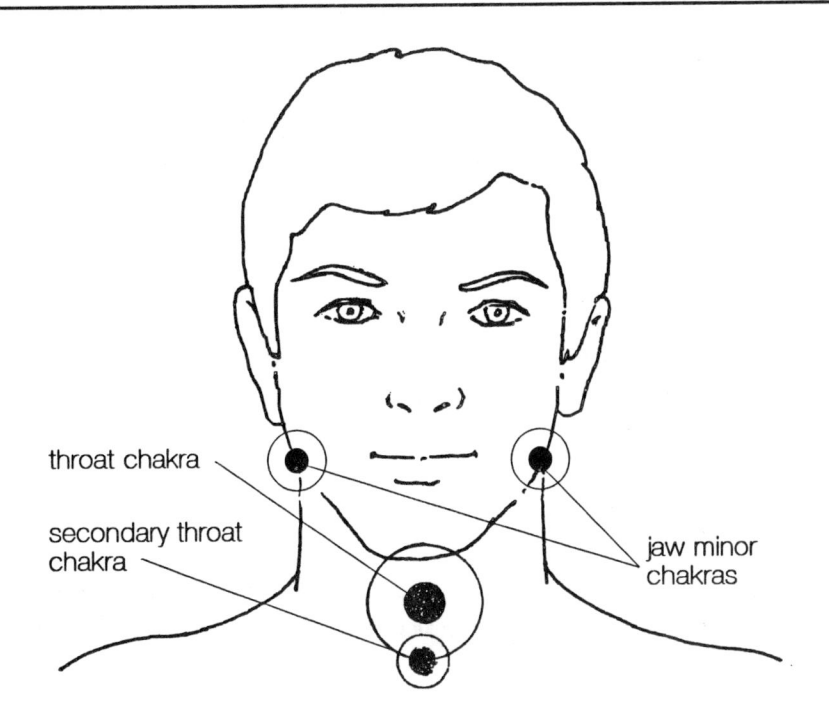

Fig. 4-9 *Pranic treatment for mumps, tonsillitis, gum bleeding, and pyorrhea*

3. Mumps and Tonsillitis

a. Apply general sweeping two or three times.

b. Apply localized sweeping thoroughly on the throat and the entire neck area.

c. Thoroughly cleanse and energize the throat and secondary throat chakras.

d. Apply localized sweeping and energizing alternately on the jaw minor chakras until the patient is substantially relieved. The jaw minor chakras are located at the lower back part of the ears. By energizing the jaw minor chakras, the entire mouth will be energized, including the parotid glands and the tonsils. Since the affected parts will consume prana at a very fast rate, the throat chakra and the jaw minor chakras should be cleansed and energized twice a day.

e. Be sure to stabilize the projected pranic energy.

f. To improve the body's defense system, apply the procedure given in "strengthening the body's defense system by increasing its life energy level".

4. Gum Bleeding

a. Apply localized sweeping and energizing thoroughly on the affected part. Repeat the treatment for as long as necessary.

b. Apply localized sweeping and energizing on the throat chakra, secondary throat, and jaw minor chakras.

c. Stabilize the projected pranic energy.

d. Repeat the treatment for as long as necessary.

5. Pyorrhea

a. Apply general sweeping two or three times.

b. Apply localized sweeping thoroughly and energizing on the affected part.

c. Apply localized sweeping and energizing on the throat chakra, secondary throat, and jaw minor chakras. Stabilize the projected pranic energy.

d. Since the rate of pranic consumption is so fast, steps b and c must be repeated two or three times a day.

e. To increase the body's defense mechanism, follow the instructions given in "strengthening the body's defense system by increasing its life energy level."

f. Instruct the patient to see a dentist immediately.

6. Fainting

a. Energize the navel chakra until the patient recovers consciousness. This increases the pranic energy level of the whole body including the head area. This approach is slower but safer.

b. Another approach is to energize the back of the head. This is faster but it may cause pranic congestion of the head due to overenergizing. This will manifest as a headache.

c. If the loss of consciousness is due to sudden emotional shock, apply localized sweeping thoroughly on the front and back solar plexus chakras and the navel chakra; then energize the navel and front solar plexus chakras.

d. If a head concussion is involved, apply localized sweeping and energizing alternately on the affected part of the head. Instruct the patient to see a medical doctor immediately.

e. Stabilize the projected pranic energy.

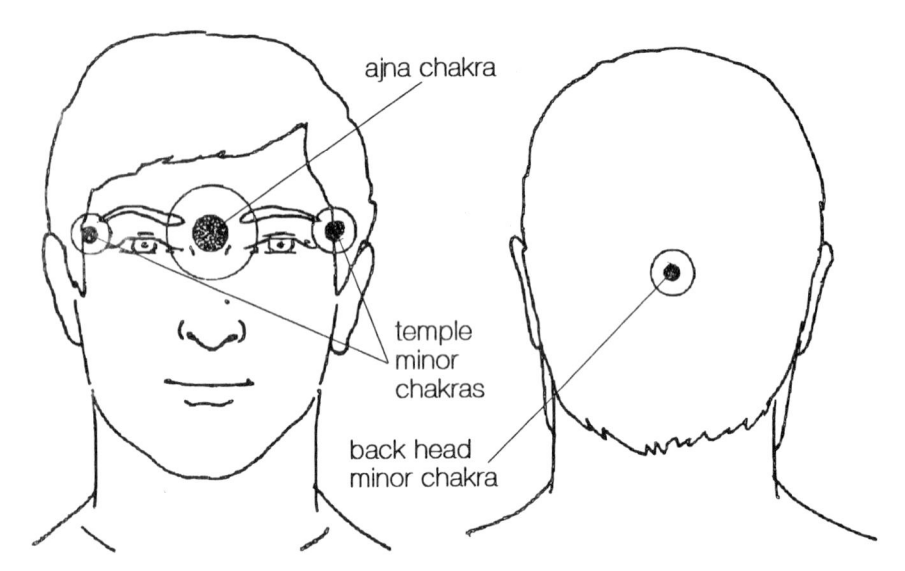

Fig. 4-10 *Pranic treatment for nearsightedness, farsightedness, astigmatism, cross-eyes, and walleyes*

7. Nearsightedness, Farsightedness and Astigmatism

The eye chakras or the eyes are usually quite depleted, the thickness ranging from less than an inch to two inches. In fewer cases, you will encounter eye ailments caused by pranic congestion.

Please take note: *The eyes should not be energized directly because they will easily be congested and their condition will become worse. The eyes are energized through the ajna, back head, and temple minor chakras.*

    a. Scan the eyes with one or two of your fingers.

    b. Apply localized sweeping thoroughly on the eyes. If localized sweeping is done properly, the inner auras of the eyes will increase slightly.

INTERMEDIATE PRANIC HEALING 161

c. Apply localized sweeping and energizing on the ajna, back head, and the temple minor chakras. When energizing, you may visualize white light or pranic energy going inside the eyes. Energize the temple minor chakras only a little.

d. Rescan the eyes and apply more localized sweeping.

e. If the patient is weak or old, apply localized sweeping and energizing on the basic, sex, navel and solar plexus chakras to strengthen the entire body and increase the rate of healing. The rate of healing does not only depend on the condition of the eyes but also on the general condition of the whole body.

f. Stabilize the projected pranic energy.

g. It is quite likely that your patient will experience a slight immediate temporary improvement. This is a good sign. The treatment should be repeated twice or thrice a week. Preferably, the patient should stop wearing eyeglasses to facilitate the healing process. Patients who suffer headaches when they do not wear eyeglasses should gradually reduce the amount of time wearing it. Complete healing may take about three to four months.

8. Cross-eyes and Walleyes

Apply the same treatment as in the preceding case.

9. Chronic or Acute Glaucoma

The eyes, eye chakras, ajna, temple minor, and back head chakras and the head are affected. Glaucoma could be aggravated or triggered by habitual stress or negative emotions. Therefore, the solar plexus chakra is also affected.

162   Chapter Four

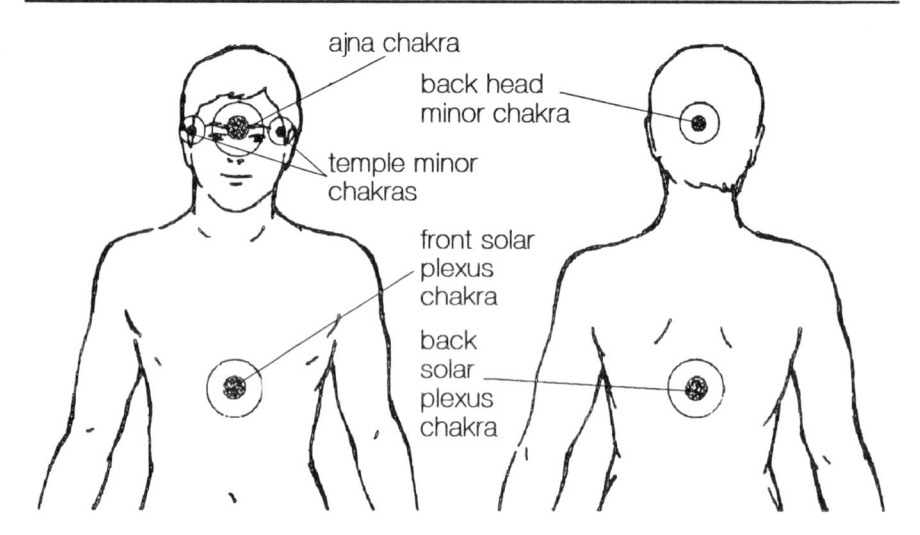

Fig. 4-11 Pranic treatment for chronic or acute glaucoma

In acute glaucoma, the patient may experience intense pain on the head and the eyes, accompanied by general weakening. He may also experience blindness for a shorter or longer period of time.

   a. Scan the eyes, eye chakras, ajna, temple, and back head chakras, the entire head area, and the front and back solar plexus chakras with one or two fingers.

   b. Apply general sweeping three times.

   c. To relieve the patient immediately of the pain or discomfort in the eyes, apply localized sweeping thoroughly on the eyes and then on the entire head area.

   d. Apply localized sweeping and energizing on the ajna, temple, and back head chakras. When energizing, you may visualize white light or pranic energy going inside the eyes.

e. Rescan the eyes. Repeat steps c and d until the patient is substantially relieved.

f. Apply localized sweeping thoroughly and energizing on the front and back solar plexus chakras. This is very important since glaucoma could be caused by habitual stress or negative emotions.

g. Stabilize the projected pranic energy.

h. If the patient has a heart ailment, then the heart should also be treated.

i. Apply the treatment thrice a week. This should be continued for several months or for as long as it is required. If the cause is emotional in origin, the patient is advised to consult a psychotherapist or a clinical psychologist. The patient should learn how to relax and meditate in order to regulate his emotions properly.

j. In acute glaucoma, the treatment may be repeated after one or two hours if he is still experiencing discomfort.

k. Instruct the patient to consult an eye specialist immediately and a certified pranic healer.

10. Heart Ailments

Heart ailments may manifest as pranic depletion or congestion, or both on the heart chakra. Although there are many types of heart ailments such as heart enlargement, partial failure of the heart muscles, rheumatic heart, and heart injury due to pacemaker malfunction, etc., the treatment is basically the same — cleansing and energizing the heart and the solar plexus chakras.

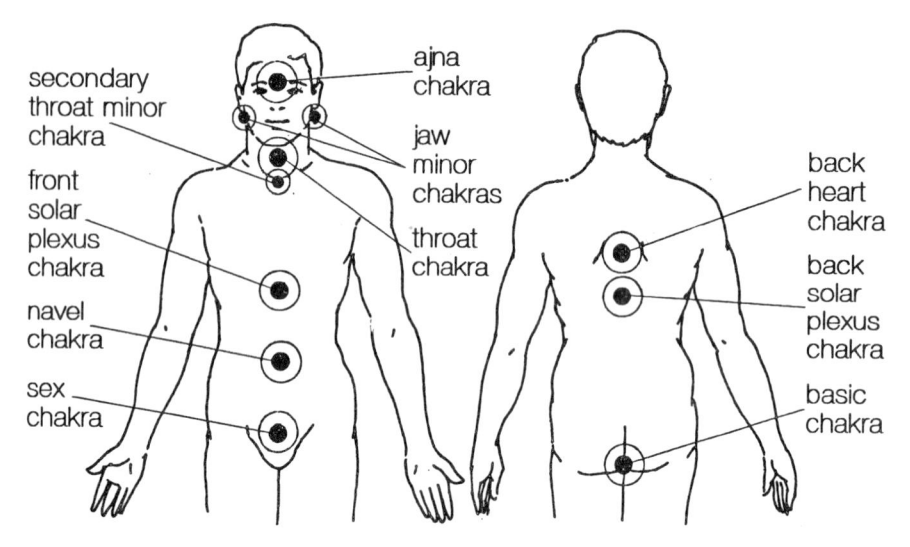

Fig. 4-12 *Pranic treatment for heart ailments*

a. Scan thoroughly the patient, especially the heart, heart chakra, front and back solar plexus, basic, throat and ajna chakras.

b. Apply general sweeping three times. General sweeping should preferably be applied first before other treatments in order to disentangle the health rays and seal off holes in the outer aura. This will definitely make healing easier.

c. Scan the heart thoroughly. Ask the patient to point out the small areas where he feels pain or discomfort. Apply localized sweeping thoroughly on the front heart chakra and on the small troubled spots with your fingers. Visualize your fingers going inside the small troubled spots and removing the diseased energy.

d. *The heart should be energized through the back heart chakra* and not through the front heart chakra. Apply localized sweeping and energizing on the back heart chakra, and you may visualize the physical heart and the front heart chakra becoming bright and clean. Get feedback from the patient to determine which spot or spots are still painful or uncomfortable. Rescan and apply more localized sweeping and energizing. If the treatment is done properly and thoroughly, the patient will experience immediate partial relief. Substantial relief may also be experienced immediately or after several hours or days. In pranic depletion of the heart, the emphasis should be on energizing, but thorough cleansing is also very important.

e. Apply localized sweeping thoroughly on the liver and the solar plexus chakra and then energize the solar plexus chakra. The emphasis should be on thorough cleansing.

f. If there is severe pranic congestion on the front heart and the front solar plexus chakras, then apply localized sweeping thoroughly. It may take about 5-10 minutes to remove thoroughly the congested diseased energy. The patient will usually be relieved immediately after the localized sweeping. Energize the heart through the back heart chakra and apply more localized sweeping. Energize the solar plexus chakra and apply more localized sweeping.

Steps c, d, e and f are very important and should be done properly.

g. Apply localized sweeping and energizing on the navel, sex and basic chakras. This will strengthen the body and further accelerate the rate of healing of the heart. The emphasis is on the basic chakra since it controls and energizes the skeletal and muscular systems. The heart is basically made up of muscles. Cleansing and energizing the basic chakra thoroughly will facilitate the recovery of the heart.

- h. In some cases, the throat chakra is affected, especially if the patient has an irregular heartbeat. Apply localized sweeping thoroughly and energizing on the throat, secondary throat and jaw minor chakras.

- i. The ajna is the master or executive chakra. Apply localized sweeping and energizing on the ajna to facilitate the proper functioning of the other chakras, thereby accelerating the healing process.

- j. Stabilize the projected pranic energy.

The treatment may last for a few minutes to about half an hour in most cases. It should be applied thrice a week. For critically ill patients, pranic treatment may be applied twice or thrice a day for the next few days. There are no fixed guidelines. You will have to use your own discretion.

It may take several weeks to about three months to heal and normalize the heart condition. The recovery period varies, depending upon the seriousness of the heart ailment, the cooperation of the patient, the frequency of pranic treatment and other relevant factors.

11. High Cholesterol Level

The cholesterol level of the body is regulated by the solar plexus chakra and the liver; therefore, they must be treated.

- a. Apply localized sweeping thoroughly on the front and back solar plexus chakras for about 50 times.

- b. Apply localized sweeping 50 times each on the liver (front, side, and back).

c. Energize the solar plexus chakra.

d. Apply localized sweeping on the front and back heart chakras, then energize the back heart chakra.

e. Apply localized sweeping and energizing on the ajna, throat, secondary throat, and jaw minor chakras.

f. Stabilize the projected pranic energy.

g. Repeat the treatment three times a week for as long as necessary.

h. Malfunctioning of the solar plexus chakra and the liver can be caused by stress and negative emotions; it is, therefore, advisable for the patient to practice relaxation and simple meditation.

12. Hypertension

Hypertension is caused by the overactivation of the meng mein chakra which is quite gray. This could be caused by several factors such as improper diet, drugs, diseased kidneys, emotional factors, and improper yogic or chi kung practices. When a person is angry, very irritated, or is under a lot of stress, the solar plexus chakra becomes overactivated. This may cause the meng mein chakra to also become overactivated, resulting in hypertension. As explained in Chapter 2, the meng mein chakra regulates the blood pressure. The basic chakra has to be treated also since it is usually gray or dirty. The solar plexus, meng mein, and basic chakras should not be highly energized since the patient may get worse.

There is too much pranic energy going up from the basic chakra to the head, thereby causing much discomfort in that area. The head, especially its back part, is quite dirty and, therefore, must be cleansed thoroughly.

a. Apply general sweeping three times or more.

b. To rapidly bring down the blood pressure, apply localized sweeping thoroughly on the front and back solar plexus and meng mein chakras for about 100 times or more each until the blood pressure has been reduced and stabilized. This can be repeated several times a day if necessary. *Please note: do not energize the meng mein chakra because the patient may become worse.* The complete treatment is given in advanced pranic healing. If the kidneys are malfunctioning, apply localized sweeping thoroughly on them.

c. Apply localized sweeping on the basic chakra since it is usually also affected.

d. Apply localized sweeping thoroughly on the crown chakra, the back of the head, and the spine to further relieved the patient.

e. Apply thorough localized sweeping and energizing on the crown, forehead and ajna chakras. Then apply more localized sweeping on the entire head area.

f. If the heart is affected then it should also be treated.

g. Stabilize the projected pranic energy.

h. Instruct the patient to see immediately a medical doctor, and also a certified pranic healer.

13. Loss of Smell

a. Apply localized sweeping and energizing on the forehead and ajna chakras, with emphasis on the latter.

b. Apply localized sweeping and energizing on the right

INTERMEDIATE PRANIC HEALING 169

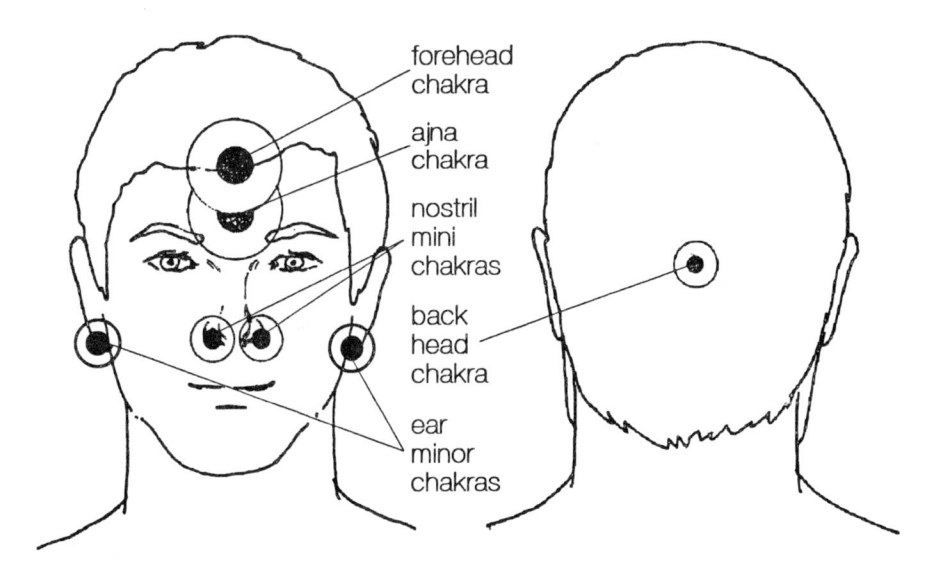

Fig. 4-13 *Pranic treatment for loss of smell*

and left nostril mini chakras. These mini chakras are located on the lower side of the nostrils.

c. Check the ear minor chakras and the back head minor chakra. If they are affected, cleanse and energize them.

d. Stabilize the projected pranic energy.

e. Repeat the treatment twice a week for as long as necessary.

14. Sinusitis

a. Apply localized sweeping thoroughly on the area above the eyebrows and the cheekbones.

b. Apply localized sweeping and energizing thoroughly on the forehead and ajna chakras, with emphasis on the ajna chakra.

c. Cleanse and energize the right and left nostril mini chakras. These mini chakras are located at the lower side of the nostrils.

d. Apply localized sweeping thoroughly and energizing on the front and back solar plexus chakras.

e. Stabilize the projected pranic energy.

f. Repeat the treatment three times a week for as long as necessary. If the patient is experiencing extreme discomfort, the treatment may be repeated twice or thrice a day.

15. Respiratory Ailments (Pneumonia, Tuberculosis, Emphysema, etc.)

There are many types of respiratory ailments but their treatments are more or less the same. There are four major chakras involved in treating the respiratory system: the ajna chakra, which controls and energizes the nose; the throat and secondary throat chakras, which control and energize the throat; the back heart chakra, which controls and energizes the lungs and the heart; and the solar plexus chakra, which controls and energizes the diaphragm.

a. Clean the entire body by applying general sweeping two to three times.

b. If the nose is affected, apply localized sweeping thoroughly and energizing on the ajna chakra.

c. If the throat, secondary throat and jaw minor chakras are affected, apply localized sweeping thoroughly and energizing on the throat and secondary throat chakras.

d. Apply localized sweeping on the lungs and cleanse them on all sides thoroughly (front, side, and back). With

INTERMEDIATE PRANIC HEALING 171

- ajna chakra
- jaw minor chakras
- throat chakra
- secondary throat minor chakra
- back heart chakra
- front solar plexus chakra
- back solar plexus chakra
- navel chakra
- sex chakra
- basic chakra

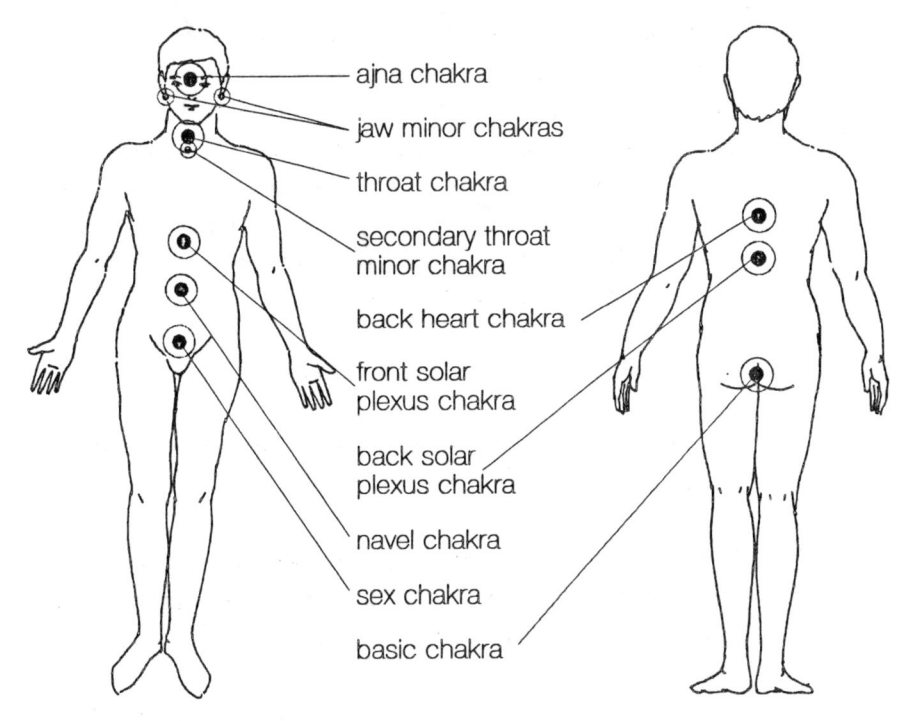

Fig. 4-14 *Pranic treatment for respiratory ailments (pneumonia, tuberculosis, emphysema, etc.)*

emphysema, apply localized sweeping 100 times or more on the front, side and back of each lung. If this is done properly, the patient may experience partial relief. Then apply localized sweeping thoroughly on the front heart and back heart chakras.

e. Energize the back heart chakra to energize the lungs and the heart. It is very important that the lungs and the back heart chakra should be sufficiently energized. If the instructions are followed thoroughly, the patient will be relieved immediately and the tightness on the chest area will be greatly reduced.

f. Apply localized sweeping and energizing thoroughly on the front and back solar plexus chakras.

g. Some patients with respiratory ailments are quite debilitated. To strengthen and increase the energy level of the body, clean and energize the front and back solar plexus, navel, sex and basic chakras. However, if the patient has a fever, do not energize the basic chakra because this may cause the body temperature to rise. Just apply localized sweeping and energizing on the hand and sole minor chakras.

h. Stabilize the projected pranic energy.

i. Apply pranic treatment twice to thrice a week until the patient fully recovers.

j. For patients suffering from tuberculosis, repeat the treatment thrice a week for about five months or more, depending upon the severity of the ailment.

k. For patients suffering from emphysema, thorough cleansing of the lungs is very important. Treatment has to be repeated twice a day for the next few days. When there is noticeable or substantial improvement, the frequency of the treatment can be reduced to once a day, then later to thrice a week for about a year or more.

l. For patients who are suffering from pneumonia, repeat the treatment three to five times a day since the rates of pranic consumption and deterioration are fast. The patient should be closely monitored for the next several days by medical doctors and by pranic healers until the condition stabilizes.

TREATMENTS FOR SIMPLE AND SERIOUS CASES   173

Diagram labels: ajna chakra; throat chakra; secondary throat minor chakra; back heart chakra; front solar plexus chakra; back solar plexus chakra; hand minor chakras; basic chakra; sole minor chakras

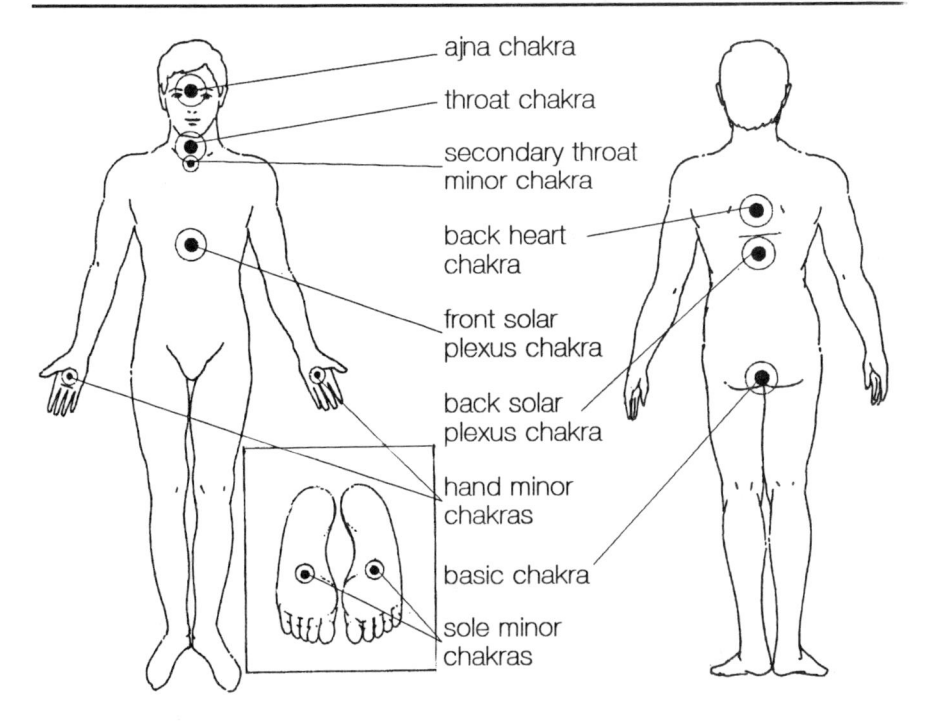

Fig. 4-15 *Pranic treatment for asthma*

16. Asthma

The treatment is divided into two parts: the first part deals with relieving the patient from asthmatic attack and greatly improving and healing the respiratory system; the second part deals with gradually removing the cause of the ailment.

   a. The outer, health and inner auras of the patient are sometimes quite gray. It is advisable to apply general sweeping two to three times.

   b. Patients suffering from asthma have depleted throat and secondary throat minor chakras. The latter is located at the lower soft portion of the throat. Apply thorough localized sweeping and energizing on the throat and secondary throat minor chakras, with emphasis on energizing.

c. Apply localized sweeping thoroughly on the lungs (front, side and back). To energize and strengthen the lungs, apply localized sweeping and energizing on the back heart chakra.

d. Apply localized sweeping on the liver (front, side and back), and the front and back solar plexus chakra. Energize the solar plexus chakra.

By treating the throat, secondary throat, back heart and solar plexus chakras, the patient will be relieved substantially. Also, treating the solar plexus chakra and the liver will gradually improve the quality of the blood produced since the liver detoxifies the blood.

e. Asthmatic patients have malfunctioning ajna and basic chakras. Clean and energize them. The basic chakra controls and energizes the bones and the quality of the blood produced.

f. To further improve the quality of the blood, the bones in the body have to be cleansed and energized. Apply localized sweeping on the entire legs. Then apply localized sweeping and energizing on the sole minor chakras, while simultaneously visualizing white light or pranic energy going inside the bones of the legs. Apply also localized sweeping on the entire arms. Then apply localized sweeping and energizing on the hand minor chakras. You may simultaneously visualize white light or pranic energy going inside the bones of the arms.

g. After energizing, be sure to always stabilize the projected pranic energy.

INTERMEDIATE PRANIC HEALING 175

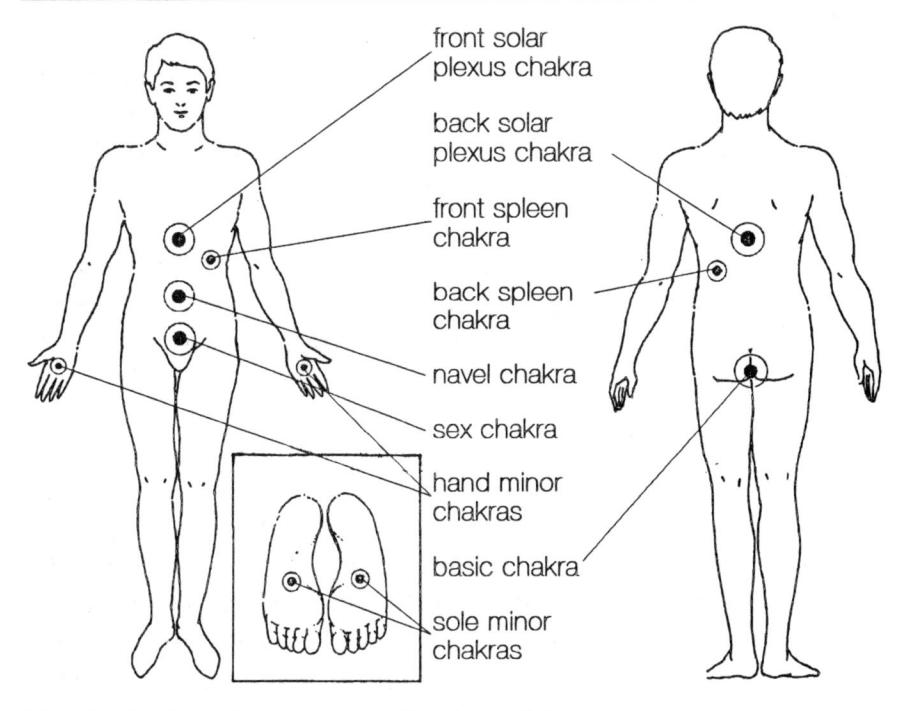

Fig. 4-16 *Pranic treatment for hepatitis*

h. Apply the entire treatment thrice a week for as long as necessary until the patient is cured. In general, the treatment may take two or three months.

17. Hepatitis

Patients with hepatitis are quite depleted and have grayish inner, health and outer auras. The inflamed liver, when seen clairvoyantly, is muddy red. The liver may be depleted and congested simultaneously. For example, the left part may be congested while the right part is depleted. The solar plexus chakra is quite depleted.

a. Apply general sweeping three to five times.

b. Apply localized sweeping thoroughly on the liver (front, side and back) about 100 times or more. Apply localized sweeping thoroughly on the front and back solar plexus chakras 50 to 100 times. Energize the front solar plexus chakra. Stabilize the projected pranic energy.

c. For severe cases of infection, clean and energize gently the front and back spleen chakras. Observe the patient. In rare cases, he may get congested and may faint. Do not highly energize the spleen chakra if the patient has hypertension.

d. To increase the energy level of the body and strengthen its defense system, clean and energize the navel, sex and basic chakras, and the sole and hand minor chakras. If the patient has a fever, just apply localized sweeping on the basic chakra; do not energize it since this may cause the temperature to rise higher. When energizing the sole and hand minor chakras, you may visualize the pranic energy or white light going inside the bones.

e. Stabilize the projected pranic energy.

f. Apply pranic treatment thrice a week for as long as necessary. This may take several months. For acute hepatitis, apply the treatment four or five times a day for the next several days. Patients with acute hepatitis should be closely monitored by medical doctors, and certified pranic healers.

18. Gastric and Duodenal Ulcers

a. Scan the front and back solar plexus chakras and the upper abdominal area.

b. Apply localized sweeping on the front and back solar

INTERMEDIATE PRANIC HEALING 177

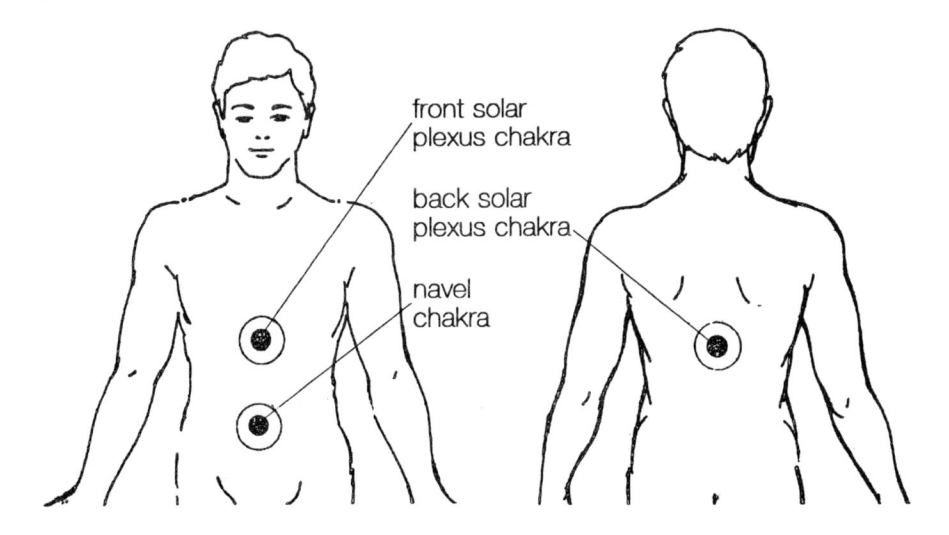

Fig. 4-17 *Pranic treatment for gastric and duodenal ulcers, hemorrhoid, and chronic appendicitis*

plexus chakras thoroughly. Then energize the front solar plexus chakra.

c. Apply localized sweeping and energizing on the affected part.

d. Apply localized sweeping and energizing on the navel chakra.

e. Be sure to stabilize the projected pranic energy.

f. Apply pranic treatment twice or thrice a week until healing is complete.

19. Hemorrhoid

Hemorrhoid manifests as pranic congestion on the anus minor chakra. The solar plexus and navel chakras are also affected. The anus minor chakra is located between the basic chakra and the anus. It is located slightly above the anus. Clairvoyantly, it is seen as muddy red.

    a. Apply localized sweeping and energizing on the anus. The emphasis is on thorough sweeping.

    b. Apply localized sweeping on the upper and lower abdominal areas.

    c. Apply localized sweeping thoroughly and energizing on the front and back solar plexus, and navel chakras. Treating the solar plexus and navel chakras is very important since the large intestine and the anus are controlled and energized by these two major chakras.

    d. Stabilize the projected pranic energy.

    e. Repeat the treatment two or three times a week for as long as necessary.

The patient may also use cold water to remove the diseased energy from the affected part. To facilitate the cleansing process, he may will or intend that the cold water is removing the diseased energy.

The patient is also expected to maintain proper hygiene.

20. Chronic Appendicitis

    a. Cleanse and energize the front and back solar plexus and navel chakras and the appendix. The patient will usually be relieved immediately.

    b. Stabilize the projected pranic energy.

    c. Repeat the treatment twice a week for as long as necessary.

INTERMEDIATE PRANIC HEALING 179

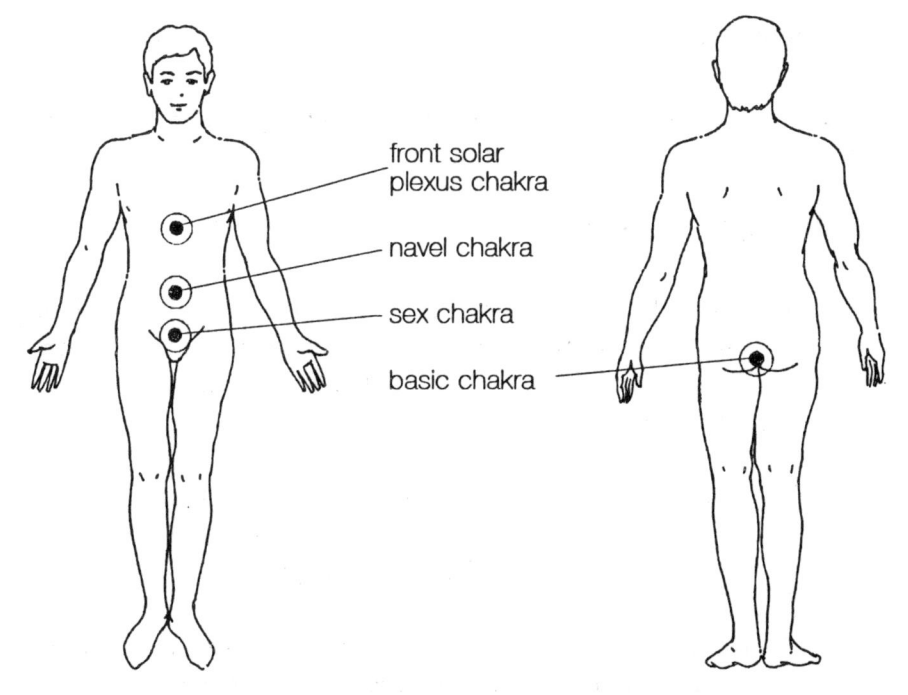

Fig. 4-18 *Pranic treatment for frequent urination, bedwetting and enlarged prostate gland*

21. Frequent Urination

a. Scan the patient thoroughly.

b. Apply localized sweeping and energizing on the sex, navel, solar plexus and basic chakras. The emphasis of the treatment should be on the sex and navel chakras.

c. Stabilize the projected pranic energy.

d. Repeat the treatment twice or thrice a week for as long as necessary.

22. Bedwetting

For grown-up children who are still bedwetting, apply the same treatment for "frequent urination."

23. Enlarged Prostate Gland

    a. Apply localized sweeping on the perineum area. This can be done by visualizing the perineum of the patient in front of you and then applying sweeping on it 30 to 50 times.

    b. Apply the same treatment for "frequent urination."

    c. Stabilize the projected pranic energy.

    d. Repeat the treatment thrice a week for as long as necessary. Instruct the patient to practice sexual abstinence during the duration of the treatment.

24. Urinary Tract Infection

    a. Apply general sweeping two to three times.

    b. Apply localized sweeping thoroughly, 100 times or more, on the sex chakra, then energize it.

    c. Apply localized sweeping and energizing on the front and back solar plexus, navel, and basic chakras.

    d. Stabilize the projected pranic energy.

    e. Usually, the patient may experience partial, if not instantaneous relief. The treatment may be repeated twice a day for the next few days.

25. Kidney and Bladder Infections

a. Apply general sweeping twice or thrice.

b. If the kidneys are infected, apply 100 sweepings or more on the affected kidney. The emphasis should be on sweeping the kidneys thoroughly. Sometimes, the ureter is also affected; therefore, it should also be cleansed thoroughly and then energize. Apply localized sweeping on the meng mein and basic chakras about 50 times each.

c. Energize the kidneys directly without passing through the meng mein chakra. The kidneys of infants and small children should be energized slightly and gently because overenergizing the kidneys may cause the blood pressure to go up.

d. After energizing the kidneys, some patients may complain of a slight headache. This may be due to the partial activation of the meng mein chakra which causes the blood pressure to go up slightly. Should this happen, apply localized sweeping 50 times or more on the meng mein chakra, and the head area until the patient is relieved.

e. If the bladder is affected, clean and energize the sex chakra.

f. Apply localized sweeping thoroughly 50 times each on the front and back solar plexus chakras. Energize a little the front solar plexus chakra. However, do not highly energize it since this may cause the meng mein chakra to be overactivated, resulting in hypertension.

g. Apply localized sweeping on the front and back spleen chakras. Energize them gently. Observe the patient. In rare cases, he may get congested and may faint. If the spleen chakra is highly energize, the meng mein chakra may become overactivated and this may lead to hypertension.

    h. Stabilize the projected pranic energy.

    i. Apply pranic treatment twice a day for the next few days until healing is complete. If the infection is acute, apply pranic treatment several times daily for the next several days.

For infants, children, pregnant women and very old patients, do not energize the meng mein chakra. Just energize the kidneys directly without passing through the meng mein chakra. Energizing or overenergizing the meng mein chakra of infants, children and very old people may cause severe high blood pressure.

The meng mein chakra and kidneys are connected to the navel chakra by a belt meridian. In some cases, the dirty diseased energy may be transferred from the kidneys to the lower abdominal area. Therefore, the patient may complain of abdominal pain instead of back pain.

26. Sexual Impotence

    a. Apply localized sweeping and energizing thoroughly on the sex, navel, and basic chakras.

    b. If the ailment is psychological in origin, apply localized sweeping and energizing thoroughly on the front and back solar plexus chakras.

    c. Apply localized sweeping on the front and back heart chakras and then energize the back heart chakra.

INTERMEDIATE PRANIC HEALING 183

- crown chakra
- back heart chakra
- front solar plexus chakra
- back solar plexus chakra
- navel chakra
- sex chakra
- basic chakra

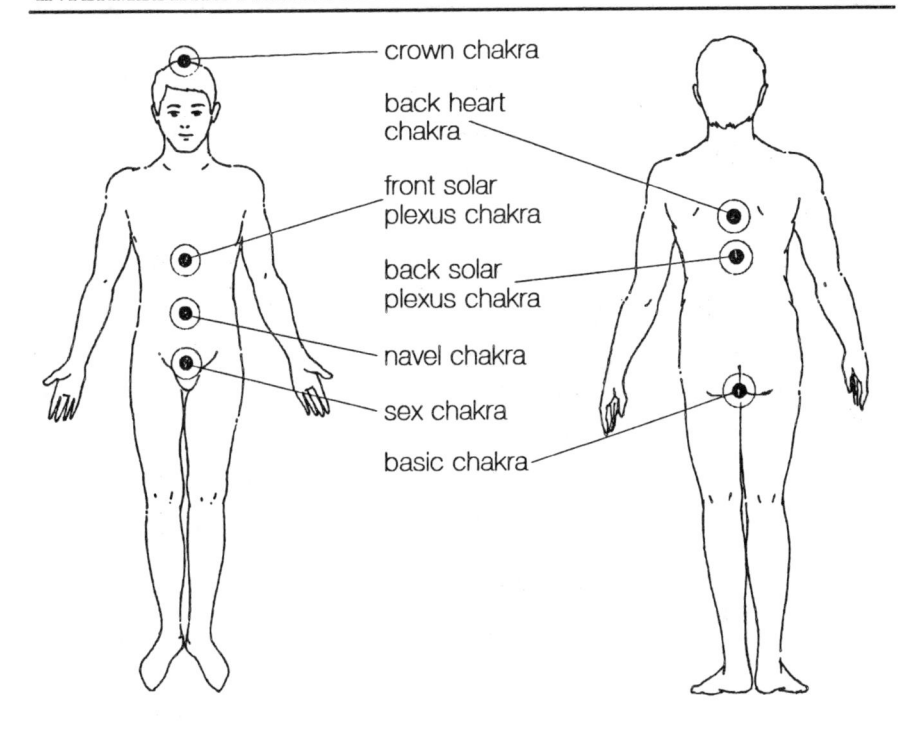

Fig. 4-19 *Pranic treatment for sexual impotence*

    d. Apply localized sweeping and energizing on the crown chakra.

    e. Stabilize the projected pranic energy.

    f. Repeat the treatment thrice a week for as long as necessary.

    g. Do not apply this treatment on patients suffering from venereal diseases or who have had a history of venereal ailment.

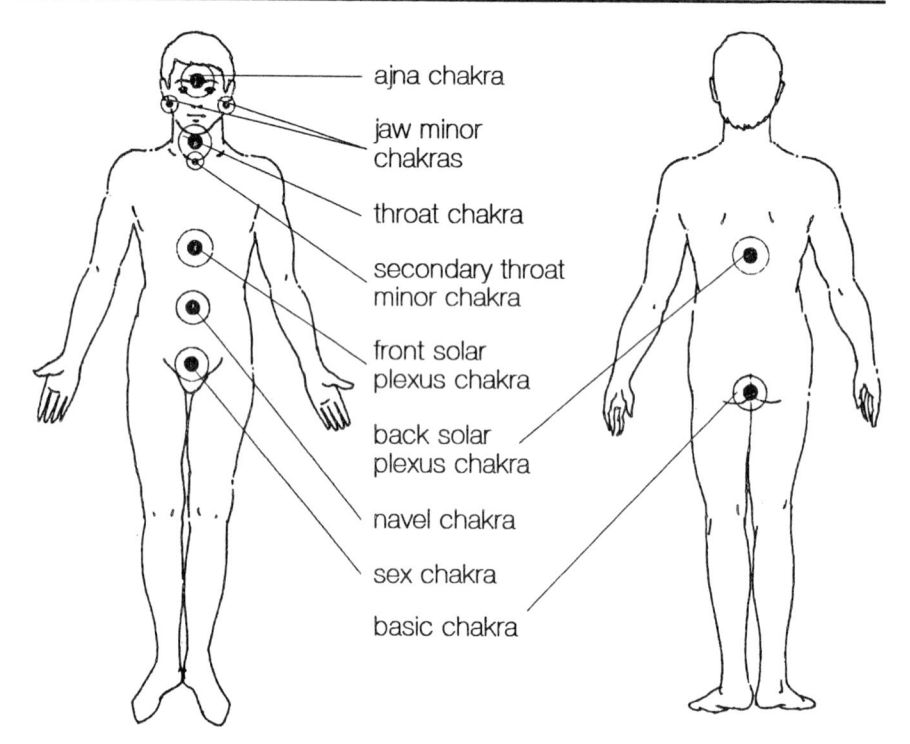

Fig. 4-20 *Pranic treatment for infertility*

27. Infertility

a. Scan the surrounding sex area, the sex, navel, basic, throat, and ajna chakras.

b. Apply localized sweeping and energizing thoroughly on the sex, navel and basic chakras. There is a minor chakra in each of the ovaries and testes; if they are affected, clean and energize them.

c. Apply localized sweeping and energizing on the front and back solar plexus chakras.

d. Apply localized sweeping and energizing on the throat, secondary throat, jaw minor and ajna chakras. Malfunctioning of any of these chakras will also cause the sex chakra to malfunction.

e. Stabilize the projected pranic energy.

f. Repeat the treatment twice or thrice a week for as long as necessary.

g. Do not apply this treatment on patients suffering from or with a history of venereal disease.

28. Broken Bones

a. Scan the affected part and the affected minor chakras. There are minor chakras on the armpits, elbows, hands, fingers, hips, knees, soles and toes.

b. Apply localized sweeping thoroughly on the injured area. Energize it thoroughly for about 20 to 30 minutes. Clean and energize the nearest minor chakras. The emphasis should be on energizing.

c. Apply localized sweeping and energizing on the hand, elbow and armpit minor chakras if the broken bone is in the arm. Apply localized sweeping on the sole, knee, and hip minor chakras if the broken bone is in the leg.

d. The healing process can be accelerated by cleansing and energizing the basic, sex, navel, and solar plexus chakras. The emphasis should be on the basic chakra because it controls and energizes the skeletal and muscular systems.

e. Stabilize the projected pranic energy.

armpit minor chakras
elbow minor chakras
front solar plexus chakra
back solar plexus chakra
navel chakra
sex chakra
basic chakra
hip minor chakras
hand minor chakras
knee minor chakras
sole minor chakras

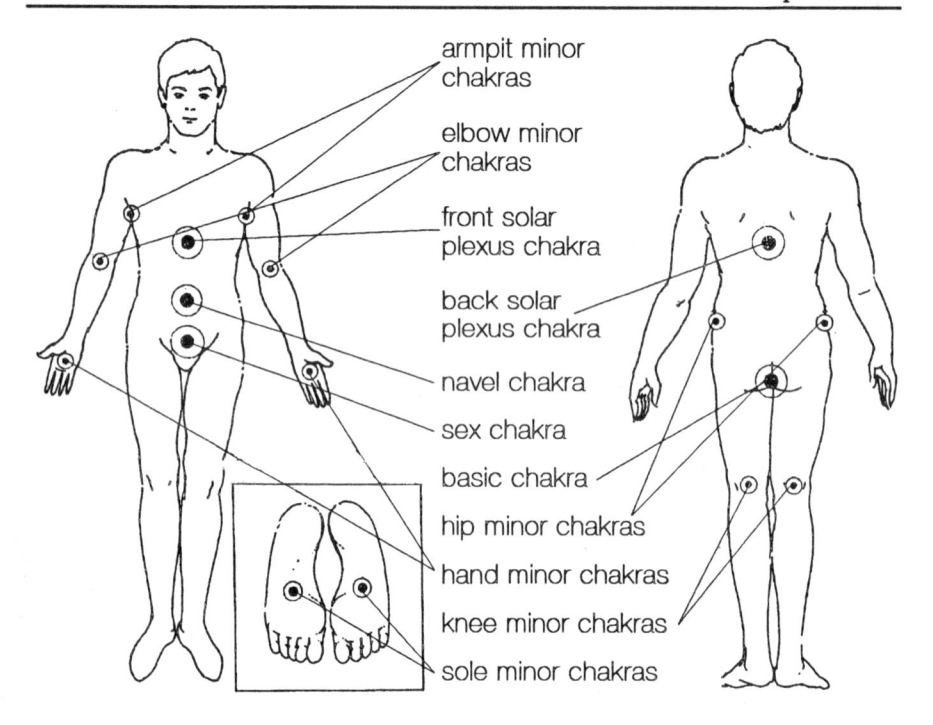

Fig. 4-21 *Pranic treatment for broken bones, arthritis and rheumatism, and osteoarthritis*

f. You may repeat the treatment once or twice a day for the first few days. The emphasis of the treatment should be on the affected part and the basic chakra

29. Arthritis and Rheumatism

In severe cases of arthritis or rheumatism, the front and back solar plexus chakras, the liver, the navel, sex and basic chakras are usually affected. They have to be cleansed and energized thoroughly. The perineum minor chakra is also affected, especially if the leg is affected. In the case of rheumatoid arthritis, the spleen chakra is also affected and has to be treated. With gout, the kidneys and the large intestine are also affected and have to be treated.

For mild arthritis or rheumatism, just apply thorough sweeping and energizing on the affected parts. Repeat the treatment several times. In some cases, patients may feel relieved almost instantaneously.

For severe cases of arthritis:

a. Apply general sweeping three times.

b. Apply thoroughly localized sweeping and energizing on the affected parts.

c. Apply localized sweeping thoroughly on the liver for about 50 times (front, side and back).

d. Apply localized sweeping thoroughly on the front and back solar plexus chakras for about 50 times. Energize the front solar plexus chakra.

e. Apply localized sweeping thoroughly on the abdominal area and navel chakra. Energize the navel chakra.

f. Apply localized sweeping thoroughly on the spine since it may be quite dirty.

g. Apply thorough localized sweeping and energizing on the sex and basic chakras. It is important that the basic chakra be energized thoroughly since it controls and energizes the skeletal and muscular systems of the body.

h. If the affected part is in the arm, the entire arm has to be cleansed. The armpit, elbow and hand minor chakras have to be cleansed and energized.

i. If the affected part is in the leg, the entire leg should be cleansed. The perineum, hip, knee and sole minor chakras have to be cleansed and energized.

j. Be sure to stabilize the projected pranic energy.

k. Repeat the treatment thrice a week for about two months or more.

30. Osteoarthritis

a. Scan the patient thoroughly.

b. Apply general sweeping two to three times.

c. Apply localized sweeping and energizing thoroughly on the affected part until there is noticeable or substantial relief.

d. If the pain is on the front knee, the cleansing and energizing have to be done not only on the front but also on the back of the knee, since the knee minor chakra is located in this area and is quite dirty.

e. If the pain is on the elbow area, the cleansing and energizing have to be done not only on the front elbow but also on the back because the elbow chakra is located in this area and is quite dirty.

f. If the affected part is on the hip, then the side of the hip should be treated since the hip minor chakra is located in this area.

g. If the affected part is on the shoulder area, the armpit has to be treated, since the armpit minor chakra is located in this area.

h. If the affected part is on the leg area, apply thorough cleansing on the entire leg. Then apply localized sweeping and energizing thoroughly on the perineum, hip,

INTERMEDIATE PRANIC HEALING 189

knee and sole minor chakras. Sometimes the pain may be experienced on the toes or on the ankles but the contributing cause may be on the hip and knee minor chakras since they may be quite dirty but not painful.

i. If the affected part is on the arm area, apply thorough cleansing on the entire arm. Then apply localized sweeping and energizing thoroughly on the armpit, elbow and hand minor chakras. Sometimes the pain may be experienced on the finger joints or on the wrist but the contributing cause may be on the armpit and elbow minor chakras, since they may be quite dirty but not painful.

j. Apply thorough localized sweeping on the spine.

k. Apply localized sweeping and energizing thoroughly on the solar plexus, navel, sex and basic chakras. These chakras are usually quite depleted. The emphasis should be on the basic chakra since it controls and energizes the skeletal and muscular systems.

l. Be sure to stabilize the projected pranic energy.

m. Repeat the treatment thrice a week for about two months or for as long as necessary.

31. Gout

a. Apply general sweeping two or three times.

b. Apply localized sweeping and energizing alternately on the affected part until it is substantially relieved. The patient may experience radical reaction or the pain may become intense if sweeping is not done sufficiently.

c. Apply localized sweeping thoroughly on the upper and

lower abdominal areas.

d. Apply thorough localized sweeping and energizing on the basic, navel and solar plexus chakras. These chakras are quite dirty and have to be strengthened. Also, by treating these chakras, the intestinal eliminative system will be improved.

e. Apply localized sweeping and energizing on the left and right kidneys to strengthen the kidneys. Do not energize the meng mein chakra.

f. If the patient experiences a slight headache after the kidneys were energized, this means that the meng mein chakra has been partially activated, thereby increasing the blood pressure. Should this happen, apply more localized sweeping on the kidneys and the meng mein chakra.

g. Stabilize the projected pranic energy.

h. Instruct the patient to watch his diet.

i. Treatment may be repeated twice a day for the next several days.

j. To minimize the possibility of recurrence, the basic, navel and solar plexus chakras have to be cleansed and energized for about two months.

32. Rheumatoid Arthritis

a. Apply general sweeping three or four times.

b. Apply localized sweeping and energizing alternately on the affected part until the patient is partially relieved. This may take about 20-30 minutes.

INTERMEDIATE PRANIC HEALING 191

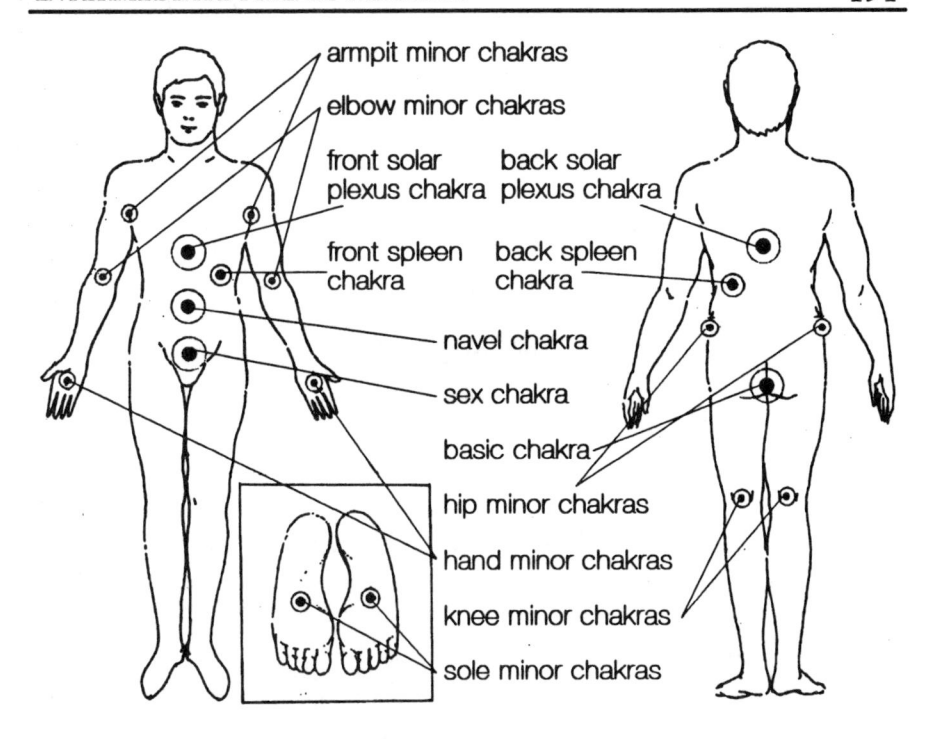

Fig. 4-22 *Pranic treatment for rheumatoid arthritis*

- c. If the affected part is in the arm, the entire arm has to be cleansed. The hand, elbow and armpit minor chakras have to be cleansed and energized.

- d. If the affected part is in the leg, the entire leg should be cleansed. The perineum, hip, knee, and sole minor chakras have to be cleansed and energized.

- e. Since the spine is usually quite dirty, apply localized sweeping thoroughly on it.

- f. From the pranic healing viewpoint, rheumatoid arthritis is caused by the malfunctioning of the basic, and solar plexus chakras, liver, and spleen chakra. The navel chakra is also partially affected. Negative emotions, in the long run, affect adversely the solar plexus chakra and the liver; it is, therefore, advisable for the patient to avoid or minimize all forms of negative emotions.

g. Apply localized sweeping thoroughly on the liver (front, side and back). Then apply localized sweeping thoroughly on the front and back solar plexus chakras. Energize thoroughly the front solar plexus chakra.

h. Apply localized sweeping and energizing thoroughly on the basic, sex, navel and spleen chakras. If the patient has hypertension or a history of hypertension, energize the spleen chakra a little to avoid causing the blood pressure to rise.

i. Stabilize the projected pranic energy.

j. The affected parts may be treated three to four times daily until the pain is substantially reduced.

k. Repeat the entire treatment thrice a week, for about two to three months or for as long as necessary.

33. Scoliosis

Patients suffering from scoliosis usually have depleted basic chakra and congested solar plexus chakra.

a. Apply general sweeping three times.

b. Apply localized sweeping thoroughly on the spine.

c. The congested solar plexus chakra is partially blocking the flow of pranic energy from the basic chakra to the spine. Apply thorough localized sweeping and energizing on the front and back solar plexus chakras.

d. Rescan the front and back solar plexus chakras and see whether they are still congested. If necessary, apply more localized sweeping.

e. Apply thorough localized sweeping and energizing on the basic chakra.

f. Apply thorough localized sweeping and energizing on the navel and sex chakras.

g. Apply also thorough localized sweeping and energizing on the affected parts.

h. Repeat treatment thrice a week for as long as necessary.

i. Instruct the patient to swim regularly if possible. Swimming has therapeutic effects on the spine.

34. Paralysis Due to Stroke

a. Scan the patient thoroughly.

b. Apply general sweeping three times.

c. Apply thorough localized sweeping and energizing on the head with emphasis on the affected part, ajna, forehead, crown and back head chakras. Localized sweeping should be done thoroughly before energizing; otherwise, the patient may experience discomfort or pain.

d. Apply localized sweeping on the spine. If the right part of the body is affected, apply localized sweeping thoroughly on the right side of the spine since it is depleted, and vice-versa if the left part is affected.

e. If the blood pressure is stable, apply localized sweeping and energizing on the basic chakra to make the body strong and to hasten the healing process. Do not energize the basic chakra if the blood pressure is high or unstable since this will aggravate the condition.

f. Apply localized sweeping thoroughly on the affected arm. Then apply localized sweeping and energizing on the armpit, elbow and hand minor chakras.

g. If the fingers are affected, then apply localized sweeping and energizing on them.

h. Also, apply localized sweeping on the affected leg. Then apply thorough localized sweeping and energizing on the hip, knee and sole minor chakras.

i. If the throat is affected, apply localized sweeping and energizing on the throat, secondary throat and jaw minor chakras.

j. Repeat the treatment thrice a week for as long as necessary.

k. It is important that the patient should have regular physical therapy.

35. Ailments of the Endocrine Glands

a. Scan the major chakras.

b. Apply general sweeping three times.

c. Apply localized sweeping and energizing on the malfunctioning chakras. The ajna chakra should be treated. Be sure to stabilize the projected pranic energy.

d. If the pancreas is affected, apply localized sweeping thoroughly on the solar plexus chakra (front and back). Then energize the back solar plexus chakra.

e. If the thyroid glands are affected, apply localized sweeping and energizing thoroughly on the throat chakra.

f. Stabilize the projected pranic energy.

g. Repeat the treatment thrice a week for as long as necessary. Instruct the patient to consult a specialist, and also a certified pranic healer.

Pregnant Women

Pregnant women should be energized slowly and gently. Overenergizing or intense and prolonged energizing should be avoided especially on the navel, sex and basic chakras. Overenergizing any of these three chakras may adversely affect the unborn child. The meng mein chakra should not be energized by elementary and intermediate pranic healers since the meng mein chakra of pregnant women are overactivated. Pregnant women are, therefore, prone to hypertension. Highly energizing the meng mein chakra of a pregnant woman may cause the blood pressure to rise or the child to be stillborn.

36. Treatment for Pregnant Women who have Difficulty in Giving Birth

a. Apply general sweeping.

b. Apply localized sweeping and energizing very gently on the navel and sex chakras to ease the labor and facilitate childbirth. This step may be repeated once every three to four hours but it has to be done gently.

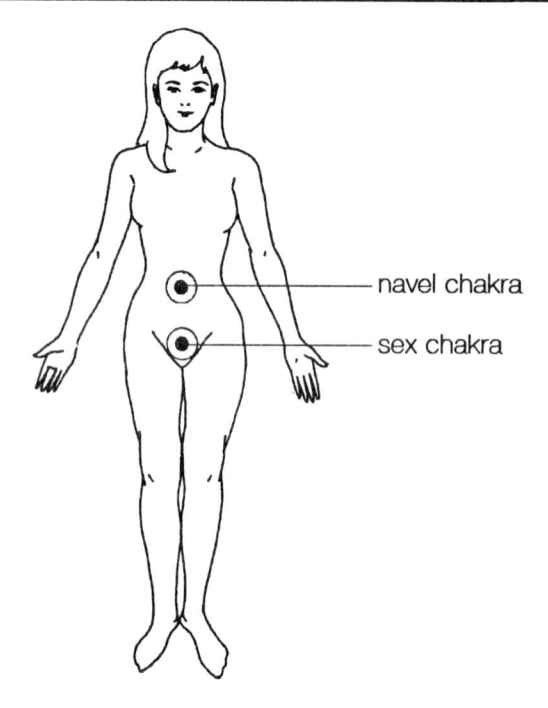

Fig. 4-23 *Pranic treatment for pregnant women who have difficulty in giving birth*

   c. If the back is painful, apply localized sweeping on the lower back for a few times. Do not energize the meng mein and basic chakras of a pregnant woman because it may affect the unborn child.

37. How to Hasten the Recovery of a Woman who has Just Given Birth

   a. Apply general sweeping three times.

   b. Apply localized sweeping and energizing on the basic, perineum, sex, navel and solar plexus chakras. Stabilize the projected pranic energy.

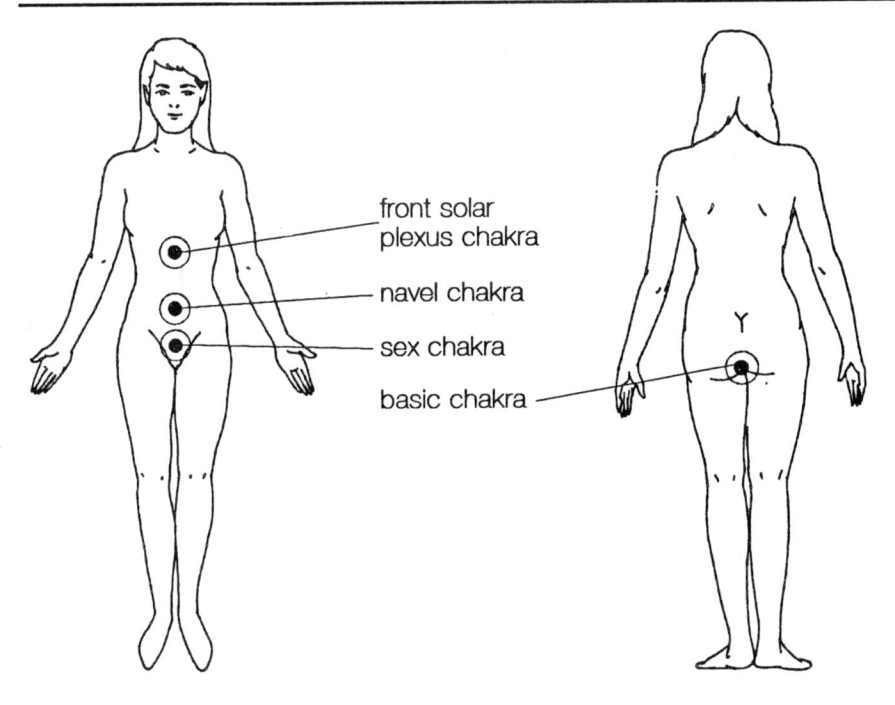

Fig. 4-24 *Pranic treatment to hasten the recovery of a woman who has just given birth*

c. Repeat the treatment twice a day for about five days. The patient should show remarkable improvement in two or three days.

38. How to Prevent a Miscarriage

Women who have had miscarriages have depleted sex, navel, and basic chakras. This treatment is applicable to patients who are not pregnant but have a history of miscarriage:

a. Apply general sweeping.

b. Apply localized sweeping and energizing on the sex, basic, navel and solar plexus chakras. Stabilize the projected pranic energy.

c. Apply localized sweeping and energizing on the throat chakra and ajna chakra.

d. Repeat the treatment twice a week for about two months.

39. Pregnant Patients Who Have a History of Miscarriage and are Experiencing Abdominal Pain

a. Scan the patient thoroughly.

b. Apply general sweeping.

c. Apply sweeping very gently on the navel, sex, and basic chakras as well as on the abdominal area.

d. Energize the navel and sex chakras very gently and slightly only.

e. Repeat the treatment several times if necessary.

40. Treating Patients Before and After Undergoing Surgery

For minor surgery:

a. Apply localized sweeping and energizing on the part that will be operated. This is to minimize or reduce bleeding.

b. Apply localized sweeping and energizing on the solar plexus, navel, sex and basic chakras. This is to strengthen the body before the operation.

c. After the surgery, apply localized sweeping and energizing on the operated area, solar plexus, navel, sex and basic chakras. This is to facilitate the healing process.

    d. Repeat the treatment.

For major surgery:

    a. Apply general sweeping several times.

    b. Apply localized sweeping and energizing on the basic, sex, navel and solar plexus chakras to strengthen the body.

    c. Apply localized sweeping and energizing on the part that will be operated and its corresponding chakra. This is to strengthen it and to minimize or reduce bleeding. Treating the nearby chakras will also be helpful.

    d. This treatment can be applied immediately before the operation or several days or weeks before.

    e. After the operation, repeat steps a, b and c for the next several days or weeks to facilitate the healing process.

41. Relieving Cancer Patients

The energy body of a cancer patient is quite dirty and depleted, but the affected part or parts are very congested. It is in these areas where there is pranic congestion that cancer cells thrive. Rapid growth of cells requires a lot of pranic energy. The objective of the treatment is to relieve the patient from the agonizing pain and to reduce the spread and growth of cancer cells by starving them of pranic energy.

    a. Apply general sweeping five times. This is to clean the energy body of the patient which is very dirty.

b. Apply localized sweeping on the affected parts 300 to 500 times. As explained earlier, the affected parts are quite congested and a few strokes of sweeping are not enough.

c. Rescan the affected parts. Apply more localized sweeping if needed.

d. Apply thorough localized sweeping about 100 times or more each on the front and back solar plexus, meng mein, and basic chakras. They are also affected and must be cleansed thoroughly. Do not energize them since, if they become overenergized, the growth rate of cancer cells will increase.

e. It is important for the healer to wash his hands regularly with water and salt while applying localized sweeping since the diseased energy is quite sticky and itchy. If this is not followed, the hands may develop arthritis of the fingers.

f. Repeat the treatment at least once a day for as long as necessary or, if possible, for the rest of the patient's life.

g. Instruct the patient to avoid meat, fish, egg, cheese and spicy foods because they can aggravate his condition. This is very important. Also, taking mega-dosage of vitamins E, C, A, B12 or royal jelly should be avoided for the same reason.

h. After cleansing the patient thoroughly, instruct him to rest under a big healthy tree or on the clean ground (make sure that there is no septic tank underneath) for about 20 minutes or more. This is to partially energize the patient. He should not try to consciously draw in pranic energy from the tree or the ground to avoid possible absorption of too much pranic energy which may aggravate his condition.

i. Sea water or salty water has very good cleansing effects. If the patient lives near the sea, you may instruct him to take a swim every day for at least 20 minutes as an alternative to pranic treatment. After swimming, the patient may rest under a shaded tree and absorb pranic energy from the surroundings. This should be done when the sun is not too hot in order to avoid pranic congestion.

j. If step i is not possible, the patient can take a bath with water and salt for about 15 to 20 minutes every day for the rest of his life, if possible. Lavender oil can be added to the water and salt bath. Lavender oil helps in cleansing and normalizing the affected chakras. The temperature of the water should be maintained at about 39-40 degrees centigrade. This is important because if the temperature is too low, the body may become weaker, and if it is too high, the cancer cells may spread faster.

All forms of anger, resentment and other negative emotions should be avoided. They can cause imbalance in the solar plexus, meng mein and basic chakras.

42. Reducing the Rate of Aging (Old Age)

You will notice that the spine of older people tend to curve downwards, their legs become weak and many or most of them tend to have arthritis. Also, they tend to fall asleep during meetings or discussions. These are due to the depletion and/or malfunctioning of the major chakras, especially the basic chakra which controls and energizes the muscular and skeletal systems, the spine, the blood, and the general vitality of a person. Therefore, the basic chakra should be treated regularly.

The following technique can be applied regularly to make older people stronger and more alert, to enable them to live a better and fuller life, and also to reduce their tendency to develop arthritis or rheumatism. It can also be applied on young or middle-aged people to reduce the rate of aging.

a. Apply general sweeping two to three times.

b. Apply localized sweeping on the liver, kidneys, the meng mein chakra and spleen chakra.

The meng mein and spleen chakras should preferably not be energized by elementary and intermediate pranic healers. If the chakras are overenergized, the patient may become severely congested or may develop high blood pressure.

c. Apply localized sweeping and energizing on the basic, sex, navel, front and back solar plexus chakras.

d. Apply localized sweeping on the front and back heart chakras. Then energize the back heart chakra.

e. Apply localized sweeping and energizing on the throat, ajna, forehead, crown and back head chakras.

f. Stabilize the projected pranic energy.

g. Repeat the treatment once or twice a week indefinitely.

h. Do not apply this treatment on patients suffering from or with a history of venereal disease or those with tumor, leukemia or hypertension. The proper treatments for these ailments are given in advanced pranic healing.

      i. Repeat the treatment for as long as necessary. This is very effective when applied properly.

43. Stress or Tension

Stress or tension manifests as malfunctioning of the solar plexus chakra. The health rays are partially affected and are clairvoyantly seen as wavy instead of straight. The outer aura is slightly grayish.

    a. Apply general sweeping three times.

    b. Apply thorough localized sweeping and energizing on the front and back solar plexus chakras, with more emphasis on localized sweeping. Rescan and apply more sweeping if they are still congested.

    c. Apply localized sweeping on the front and back heart chakras. Energize the back heart chakra.

    d. Apply localized sweeping and energizing on the crown, ajna, throat and basic chakras.

    e. Repeat the treatment thrice a week or more for as long as necessary.

    f. For more severe cases, repeat the treatment several times a day for as long as necessary.

WHAT TO DO IF YOU ARE NOT SURE (for difficult cases)

    a. Apply general sweeping several times.

    b. Apply localized sweeping and energizing on the affected parts or organs.

c. Apply localized sweeping on all the vital organs.

d. Apply localized sweeping and energizing on all the major chakras, except the spleen and meng mein chakras. Apply localized sweeping on the meng mein and spleen chakras, but do not energize them.

e. Repeat the treatment regularly.

Generally, these procedures can be used for many types of ailments, but not on patients suffering from cancer, leukemia and venereal diseases.

Instruct the patient to see a medical doctor immediately, and also a certified pranic healer.

PRINCIPLE OF LAG TIME

The principle of lag time means that the rate of healing of the energy body is much faster than that of the visible physical body. Therefore, in some cases the patient may not experience immediate relief or cure because the visible physical body heals at a slower pace than the energy body. For example, even though the heart area has been thoroughly cleansed and energized and looks quite bright, a patient may claim that he has experienced only very slight immediate relief after the pranic treatment. He may, however, experience substantial relief and improvement after a few hours or after a day or two. This delay or lag time in relief or cure is especially common in more severe cases. The degree of delay or lag time will depend on the degree of damage, the age, the physical condition and the receptivity of the patient.

HOW LONG DOES IT TAKE TO COMPLETELY CURE A PATIENT?

The length of time required to completely cure a patient depends on several factors: the frequency of treatment, the age, and physical condition of the patient, the patient's degree of receptivity, the presence of intervening or causal factors which cause the delay of or prevent healing from manifesting, the degree of damage, the nature of the ailment, the skill of the pranic healer, the degree of cooperation from the patient and, in some cases, the use of other forms of healing or treatment to complement pranic healing. As stated earlier, the approach in healing should be integrated or wholistic.

The rate of relief for simple and severe ailments may range from a few minutes to a few days. Generally, the time it takes to permanently cure a simple ailment using pranic healing alone ranges from a few minutes to a few days. For chronic or more severe ailments, it may range from a few days to a few months. In some cases, the cure is even dramatic or "miraculous." However, not all ailments and not all patients can be cured.

For simple cases, relief usually means complete cure, while for severe ailments, it means that the patient is partially healed and relieved. This does not mean that the patient is completely healed but is in the process of being cured. Please take note of this.

IMMEDIATE RECURRENCE OF PAIN OR SYMPTOMS

Several factors may contribute to the immediate recurrence of the symptoms after pranic treatment.

   1. Localized sweeping was not applied and energizing was not done sufficiently. Since the part to be treated was not cleansed, fresh prana had difficulty penetrating fully

into the part being treated. It is like trying to put fresh water on a sponge filled with dirty water. This can be done by using a lot of prana and projecting them with a stronger force. However, there is the risk of a radical reaction which will cause more temporary discomfort to the patient. It would be a lot easier if the dirty water is removed first from the sponge before pouring fresh water on it.

2. General sweeping was not applied on the patient who has holes in the outer aura; therefore, prana continues to leak out, causing again pranic depletion on the treated part.

3. The projected prana was not stabilized, causing it to simply escape or leak out from the body.

4. A disposal unit was not used, and thus, the diseased energy is still connected to the patient's energy body. If the patient is not sufficiently energized, it may cause the diseased energy to be drawn back. And if the patient tries to recall or keeps recalling his ailment, the diseased energy will most likely be attracted again to his energy body.

5. The healer is too attached or too anxious with the result. Because of this, the projected prana was not released or only partially released and it returned to the healer.

6. The patient is suffering from a severe type of disease that consumes prana at a very fast rate or the prana projected was not sufficient. The patient should, therefore, be treated more frequently.

REASONS WHY SOME PATIENTS ARE NOT HEALED

1. All of the preceding factors that may contribute to the immediate recurrence of pain or symptoms after pranic treatment (See pages 205-206) may also be the contributing factors why patients do not get well.

2. The patient may not be receiving the right pranic treatment because of improper scanning. For instance, difficulty in moving the arm could be caused by pranic congestion on the heart and the solar plexus chakras or by pranic congestion on the meng mein chakra. So just treating the arm will give temporary relief but not a permanent result.

3. Energizing and frequency of pranic treatment are not sufficient. This is like giving a medication of insufficient dosage and at insufficient intervals.

4. Certain ailments require other forms of treatment. Examples are ailments caused by malnourishment and improper diet.

5. The patient is simply too old and too weak or too sickly. For certain unexplained factors, some aged patients just do not retain a large portion of the projected prana. This does not mean, however, that very old or very sickly patients should be ignored. On the contrary, they should be given proper care and treatment.

6. The disease is of karmic origin and the right time for complete healing has not yet arrived. The patient perhaps has not yet learned the lesson that he is supposed to learn.

PERSONAL HEALTH PROBLEMS THAT A HEALER MAY ENCOUNTER

1. Some healers may experience pain in their finger joints, hands or arms. This is due to the absorption of diseased energy or diseased etheric matter from the patients. This can be avoided by immediately washing the hands and the arms after general and localized sweeping and also after energizing. In the long run, not washing the hands and the arms immediately will result in regular partial absorption of diseased energy, resulting in turn in arthritis of the fingers. The healer may use salt and water to wash his hands and arms.

2. Some healers may experience the symptoms or the ailments of their patients. This is due to full absorption of the diseased energy into the system of the healer traceable to, first, not washing the hands and arms after healing and, second, not using the disposal unit when treating patients. Some of the diseased energy may have been absorbed by the legs from the surrounding area. It is advisable to take a shower after treating a lot of patients in one session to clean the entire body. The healer should wash his entire body with salt or with salty water. This process has cleansing effects on the entire body and the healer will feel his body becoming lighter.

3. Some healers may become sick with infectious diseases. This can be avoided by refraining from healing when feeling low, intense anger or irritation and after having an emotional outburst. These negative emotions cause temporary pranic depletion, drooping of the health rays and punctures on the outer aura. It is also advisable to wash the hands and the arms with germicidal soap right after treating a patient with infectious

disease to protect not only the healer but also the next patient.

4. The healer may become too tired or depleted after treating a patient or several patients due to several factors:

   a. The healer energizes intensely and at a very fast rate. The amount of prana projected is much more than the amount of prana drawn in or the rate of projecting prana is much faster than the rate of drawing in prana. This can be avoided by being patient and not in a hurry. Heal your patients slowly and gradually. There are some healers whose energy levels are very high. Their inner aura is about ten meters thick and very dense. They absorb or draw in a tremendous amount of prana at a very fast rate. Some healers are born with a very high energy level while others attain this through disciplined esoteric training. Following a certain lifestyle such as being a vegetarian most of the time, having a moderate sex life, living a well-regulated emotional life, possessing a clear, prudent but decisive mind, and doing plenty of regular physical exercises (especially tai chi and yogic exercises) will, in the long run, result in good health and a very high energy level. Through clairvoyant investigation, it has been observed that vegetarians usually have more refined energy bodies and brighter and denser inner auras. However, although it is advantageous, it is not necessary to become a full vegetarian. Pork has to be strictly avoided by pranic healers since the energy of pork is very dirty.

   b. The healer continues "energizing" his patients subconsciously. This can be avoided by visualizing the cord between him and his patient as being cut off after the treatment.

    c. The healer is closely surrounded by his patients and they tend to draw in prana from the healer subconsciously, thereby causing the healer to become depleted. This can be remedied by keeping a certain distance from the waiting patients.

It is advisable for the healer to take regular vacations to recharge his body.

AVOID USING TOO MUCH WILL IN HEALING

It has been observed by the author that as a healer practices pranic healing for quite sometime, a healer consequently develops a stronger "will power". Therefore, he will have the tendency to use too much "will" in healing which tends to overwhelm the cells, thereby slowing down the rate of healing.

On the other hand, when a healer regulates the "will" in healing and instead impregnates the projected pranic energy with loving-kindness, it has been observed that the rate of healing is faster and the projected pranic energy is easily assimilated by the body.

RATE OF VIBRATION OF THE ENERGY BODY

The rate of vibration of the energy body vary from person to person. If the energy body of the healer has a higher rate of vibration than that of the patient, the patient will feel light and may experience a pleasant feeling that is quite difficult to describe. If the energy body of the healer has a much lower rate of vibration than that of the patient, the patient may feel heaviness and discomfort and sometimes pain. The energy body of the healer is usually more refined than that of the patient.

Heavy smokers have coarser energy bodies. The energy body of a heavy smoker is filled with dirty brown spots. This brownish material partially clogs the nadis or meridians and, therefore, negatively affects the health of the smoker. The brown spots are located not only on the lungs but also on other parts of the energy body; they cause lung diseases and other ailments. When a healer with a more refined energy body is contaminated by a heavy smoker who has accidentally touched him, the healer will feel stickiness, heaviness and pain on the area being touched. It is very important that the healer should be a non-smoker or should give up smoking because, instead of becoming better, the patient might become worse, especially if the part being treated is quite delicate. To fully appreciate what the author has just stated, ask a heavy smoker to energize your arm and observe what happens.

Of course, the author does not make any moral judgment on smokers. He is just pointing out the negative effects of smoking on the body. And in this case of a pranic healer, smoking has possible harmful effects on the patient. However, the author knows of a few healers who smoke lightly, but have not reported any negative experience with their patients. Still, it is better to avoid unnecessary risks. Just imagine what will happen to the patient if some dirty, brownish matter are accidentally transferred to the eyes or the heart of the patient.

Sometimes the patient may feel slight pain and heaviness on the part being energized if the healer is tired and had an emotionally strenuous day. The healer should rest and resume healing the next day or until he feels better.

On rare occasions, the patient may have a very refined energy body or the rate of vibration of his energy body may be much higher than that of the healer. Such a patient, if treated by a healer whose energy body is coarser, would only experience more discomfort. He should be treated by a healer whose energy body is as refined or more refined than that of the patient.

As a healer continues to practice healing, his energy body is gradually being cleansed and refined. His inner aura becomes brighter and denser. He becomes a more powerful healer.

POPULARIZING PRANIC HEALING

Great benefits can be obtained by popularizing and adopting pranic healing to help and alleviate the suffering of sick people. This can be accomplished by translating this work on pranic healing to different major languages. To further disseminate and encourage the practice of pranic healing, a Pranic Healers' Association can be established in each country and in each major city. Workshops on pranic healing should also be conducted regularly to train people in this method.

It is further recommended that the Ministry or Department of Health or the corresponding government agency of every country should investigate the effectivity of pranic healing and, if found effective, adopt it as a complementary and economical form of treatment in government hospitals and clinics. Doctors and nurses will find it advantageous to learn and practise pranic healing since it can help them become more effective in their work. It is extremely beneficial if at least one person in every family knows pranic healing since it can be used as a "pranic first aid" to treat simple and difficult ailments when the need arises.

CHAPTER FIVE

Pranic Self-Healing and Pranic Invocative Healing

After long hours at my desk translating Chinese texts, I sometimes felt very tired and nearly exhausted. But five minutes of these yogic breathing exercises would renew my strength and enable me to get on with my work. It cured my rheumatism and gave me instant relief not only when I caught cold but also when I contracted the dreaded Asian flu many years ago.

– Luk K'uan Yu
The Secrets of Chinese Meditation

Self-scanning	214
Manual Technique	214
Pranic Breathing Technique	215
"Self-Distant Healing" Technique	216
Pore-Breathing Technique	217
Taoist Six Healing Sounds	217
Chakral Breathing Technique	218
General Cleansing and Energizing	220
Method 1 - Pranic Breathing	220
Method 2 - Visualization Technique	221
Method 3 - Meditation on the White Light	222
Pranic Physical Exercises	224
Physical and Mental Recharging	225
Water and Salt Bath	226
Avoiding Negative Emotions and Thoughts	228
Principle of Diversion or Releasing	229
Integrated Approach to Self-healing	230
Problems Encountered in Self-healing	233

Karma	234
Karma and the Golden Rule	236
Neutralizing Negative Karma	238
Suggested Ethical Guidelines	239
Terminology	240
Pranic Invocative Healing	241
Self-healing Affirmation	246
Assigning Healing Angels	247

In pranic self-healing, the same two basic principles of cleansing and energizing are used. There are several methods of healing oneself: the manual technique, pranic breathing technique, "distant healing" technique, the pore-breathing technique, taoist six healing sounds, chakral-breathing technique and others.

When doing pranic self-healing, you also have to stabilize the projected pranic energy, use a disposal unit for hygienic reasons, and wash your hands at the end of the treatment.

SELF-SCANNING

Although you can heal without scanning, feeling your own chakras and organs before and during pranic self-healing will help you treat yourself better and more effectively.

MANUAL TECHNIQUE

1. Scan the affected parts and chakras.

2. Pranic breathing is optional but definitely helpful.

3. With your hands, apply localized sweeping and energizing on the chakras and the parts to be treated. Throw the diseased energy into the disposal unit.

4. The whole process should be continued until healing is complete or the condition has greatly improved.

5. Stabilize the projected pranic energy.

6. For simple ailments or disorders, the relief is usually immediate. The following are a few examples:

In case of menstrual discomfort, just by manually applying localized sweeping 50 to 100 times on the sex chakra, a woman will usually experience partial or complete relief without even energizing.

For slight abdominal pain and mild loose bowel movement, manually applying thorough localized sweeping on the upper and lower abdominal areas will make the pain disappear partially or completely in a few minutes and the loose bowel movement will stop.

If a person has a headache, manually applying localized sweeping and energizing on the affected parts will usually bring partial or complete relief.

PRANIC BREATHING TECHNIQUE

1. Do pranic breathing.

2. Simultaneously visualize that you are cleansing and energizing the affected part and chakra. You may actually move your hand(s) to cleanse and energize the affected area.

'SELF-DISTANT HEALING' TECHNIQUE

In using the distant healing approach for self-healing, imagine in front of you a very short image of yourself. Do scanning, general sweeping, localized sweeping and energizing with your hands as though you were treating another person.

1. Imagine or visualize yourself in front of you about one foot tall during the entire treatment.

2. Scan yourself with one or two fingers.

3. Do pranic breathing during the entire pranic self-healing treatment.

4. Apply general sweeping on the front of your body by using your hands. Then turn yourself or the image around and apply general sweeping on your back.

5. Apply localized sweeping thoroughly and energizing on the chakras and parts to be treated with your hands.

6. Stabilize the projected pranic energy.

7. Use a disposal unit for the dirty diseased energy.

8. After healing yourself, wash your hands up to the elbow.

9. Repeat the treatment until healing is complete.

This technique is called "self-distant healing" technique because the method used is very similar to distant healing.

PORE-BREATHING TECHNIQUE

1. Do pranic breathing. Inhale and visualize prana or white light going into the pores of the affected part.

2. Hold your breath for a few seconds and visualize the grayish diseased energy as becoming lighter or the affected parts as becoming brighter.

3. Exhale and visualize the grayish diseased energy being expelled through the pores and through the health rays. Visualize the health rays being straightened. Through the straightened health rays the "used up" prana and diseased energy are expelled from the body. Your attention must be focused one or two meters away from the treated part to facilitate the healing process since energy, including diseased energy, follows where your attention is focused.

4. Hold your breath for a few seconds and visualize the treated part as becoming brighter.

In pore breathing, you just simply inhale fresh prana through the pore and exhale the grayish diseased energy. Pore breathing is practiced by some students of ki kung or esoteric martial arts and by some students of hermetic science.

TAOIST SIX HEALING SOUNDS

The Taoist six healing sounds is similar to the pore-breathing technique except that specific sounds are shouted out for specific organs to facilitate the expelling of diseased energy. Once you feel the affected part relatively cleansed, then you can breathe slowly and gently and utter the sound softly. Following are the six healing sounds (*The Secrets of Chinese Meditation* by Lu K'uan Yu):

Spleen	—	Hu
Heart	—	Ho
Lungs	—	Szu
Stomach	—	Hsi
Liver	—	Hsu
Kidneys	—	Ch'ui

The author, when healing himself, is not so particular about the specific sound used for a specific organ. Using the Taoist six healing sounds is similar to practicing martial arts. Every time the practitioner strikes and exhales, he shouts. What is important is the intention or the will to expel the diseased energy which is facilitated by shouting when exhaling.

Different teachers and authors have different variations on the six healing sounds. The technique is also varied. When the healing sound is shouted out, it has an explosive effect on the diseased energy. When done gently or almost inaudibly, there is a slow, gradual expelling of diseased or used-up energy. The shouting approach is more suitable for those who are sick, while the soft and gentle approach is for those who are healthy and only want to clean and energize their internal organs.

CHAKRAL BREATHING TECHNIQUE

1. Do pranic breathing. Inhale slowly and concentrate on the affected chakra. Visualize the chakra drawing in or inhaling fresh prana. Hold your breath for a few seconds and visualize the prana being assimilated. Exhale slowly and visualize the chakra throwing out or exhaling the grayish dirty matter. Hold your breath for a few seconds and visualize the chakra becoming brighter and healthier. Repeat the process several times.

2. Do pranic breathing. Inhale slowly and concentrate on the affected organ. Visualize the chakra and the organ inhaling or drawing in prana. Visualize the prana as passing through the chakra, then to the affected organ. Hold your breath for a few seconds and visualize the chakra and the affected organ becoming brighter. Exhale slowly and visualize the grayish dirty matter being thrown out by the affected organ through the chakra. Hold your breath for a few seconds and visualize the chakra and the affected organ becoming brighter. Repeat the process until there is substantial relief. This technique is called chakral breathing.

3. Instead of exhaling slowly, you can exhale forcefully and quickly. This may or may not be accompanied by shouting. The exhalation is done through the mouth. Simultaneously, visualize the grayish diseased energy being thrown out of the affected organ through the chakra.

4. If you feel heaviness or pranic congestion on the chakra and in its organ(s) after doing chakral breathing, just inhale without willing prana to go into the chakra and its corresponding organ(s). Exhale and visualize prana going out of the chakra and its corresponding organ(s). Visualize the chakra becoming dimmer. Continue doing this until the condition normalizes.

Chakral breathing technique is very potent and the relief is usually immediate for simple ailments. Overdoing this technique may result in pranic congestion on the chakra and its corresponding organs. Overdoing it for a prolonged period may result in physical and psychological ailments. The negative effect or effects are not usually felt immediately but only after a few hours or days. This is just like having a big overdose of a potent drug. Chakral breathing should be practiced with moderation.

Caution should be taken when doing chakral breathing on the head chakras, heart chakra and eye chakras since their corresponding organs are quite delicate and could easily be congested. Chakral breathing should preferably not be done on the meng mein, basic and spleen chakras unless supervised by a competent teacher. Doing chakral breathing on these three chakras may result in severe pranic congestion on the entire body which may manifest as weakening of the body, high blood pressure or allergy throughout the body.

Pregnant women should not practice chakral breathing on the navel, sex, spleen, meng mein and basic chakras because it may adversely affect the unborn child.

Patients suffering from venereal disease, cancer or leukemia should not do chakral breathing on the affected chakras since it may worsen their condition.

GENERAL CLEANSING AND ENERGIZING

If your body is quite weak or there is infection, apply general cleansing and energizing on yourself.

Method 1 - Pranic Breathing

Diffuse or scatter your consciousness to all parts of your body. Do pranic breathing for 10 cycles or more. Inhale slowly, hold, exhale slowly and hold. After pranic breathing, meditate on the navel for about five breathing cycles. Meditate on the secondary navel chakras which are about two inches below the navel and about two inches inside. Do this for about five breathing cycles. Imagine a light on the secondary navel chakras rotating seven times clockwise then three times counterclockwise. The clockwise and counterclockwise rotation is viewed from the outside.

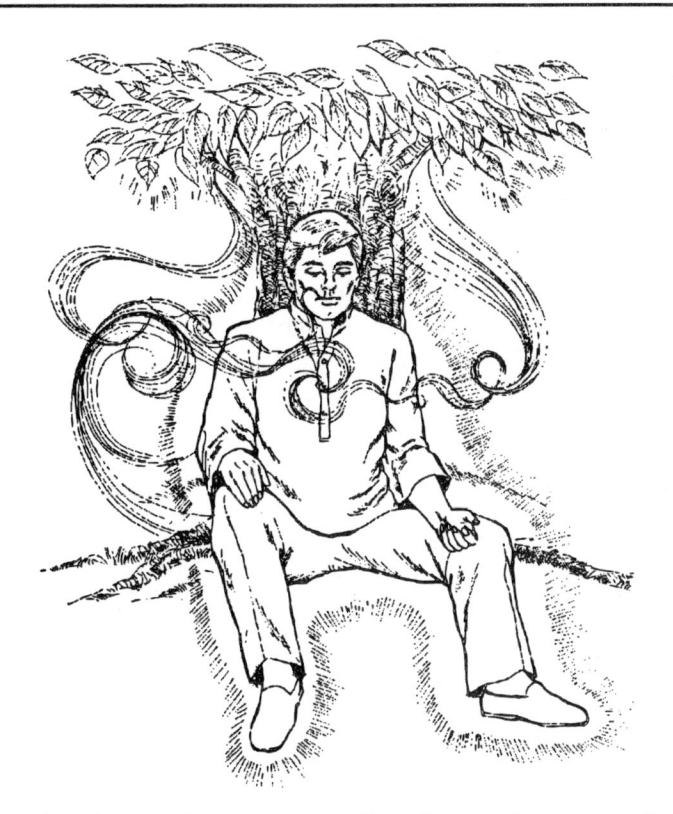

PRANIC SELF-HEALING AND PRANIC INVOCATIVE HEALING

Fig. 5-1 *Resting under a tree to absorb pranic energy from the tree and the ground*

Massage the kidneys and the meng mein chakra after the meditation. This is to avoid pranic congestion. When you become proficient, you will feel pranic energy going into all parts of your body.

Method 2 - Visualization Technique

This method is similar to "self-distant healing" technique. Do pranic breathing. Visualize yourself or another person applying general and localized sweeping and energizing with prana to your body. Visualize and will your body becoming brighter, the health rays disentangled, and the outer aura brighter. Be sure to use a disposal unit for the dirty diseased energy.

Method 3 – Meditation on the White Light

This method of general cleansing and energizing is usually called meditation on the white light or meditation on the 'middle pillar.' The middle pillar technique has been used by various Oriental and Occidental esoteric schools. This technique is divided into two parts, the first dealing with general cleansing and energizing, and the second with the circulation of prana.

Part 1: General Cleansing and Energizing

1. Do pranic breathing and simultaneously visualize a ball of intense bright light above the crown.

2. Visualize a stream of light coming down from the ball to the crown, then gradually down to the feet. Visualize the white light cleansing and energizing all the major chakras, all the important organs, the spine, and the bones of the body.

3. Visualize the white light coming out of the feet and flushing out all the grayish diseased energy.

4. Visualize a brilliant ball of light at the bottom of the feet. Draw in earth prana in the form of a stream of light from this brilliant ball of light. Inhale and draw in prana through the sole chakras up to the head. Exhale and let prana sprinkle out of the crown chakra. Repeat the whole process three times.

Part 2: Circulating Prana

1. Visualize prana circulating from the bottom of the feet, up to the back of the body, up to the head, down to the face, to the front of the body, then to the feet. Circulate prana from back to front thrice.

2. Reverse the circulation and circulate prana from front to back. Circulate thrice.

3. Circulate prana from left to right three times and from right to left three times. The purpose of circulating prana is to evenly distribute it throughout the body and to prevent pranic congestion in certain parts of the body.

This meditation can be used daily to improve and maintain one's health. It is also done by some esoteric students before engaging in activities that require a lot of prana. You may perform this meditation before healing a large number of people. Though it has many variations, this meditation presented here is simplified and easy to perform.

Once you become proficient in this meditation, some of you will literally feel your body tingle and feel a strong current moving within and outside your body. You may also use the excess prana generated to produce "biosynthetic ki" or navel ki by concentrating on the navel chakra for about several minutes. Store this biosynthetic ki in the three secondary navel chakras located about one and a half to two inches below the navel. This is done by simply concentrating on this area for about three minutes. Pranic breathing should be done simultaneously with the preceding instructions. Each secondary navel chakra has a big flexible meridian that is used for storing navel ki. In short, the three secondary navel chakras are warehouses for the biosynthetic ki. The three secondary navel chakras are called ki hai which means ocean of ki since these minor chakras are filled with biosynthetic ki. It must be repeated that biosynthetic ki or navel ki is different from prana. It is synthesized by the navel chakra and may apear as milky white, whitish red, golden yellow, and other colors. It varies in size and density. Ordinary persons have very little biosynthetic ki compared to spiritual aspirants and practitioners of ki kung or qigong (the Chinese art of generating internal power).

It would be advisable for you to learn meditation on the white light and practice it every day. It makes your energy body cleaner, brighter, and denser, thereby making you a better healer.

PRANIC PHYSICAL EXERCISES

Physical exercise plays a vital role in self-healing and maintaining one's health. Warm-up exercises, dancing, sports, hatha yoga, martial arts or tai chi promote circulation of prana in the body, and facilitate the drawing in of fresh prana and the expelling of used-up prana or diseased energy. This is seen clairvoyantly as white fresh prana being drawn in and grayish diseased energy being thrown out when one is exercising. It is better if pranic breathing is done when exercising. There are specific physical exercises in hatha or Taoist yoga to treat specific ailments. Which pose or exercise to use can easily be determined by observing and analyzing which part of the body is being moved, bent, compressed or stretched by a specific pose or exercise and what chakra(s) is located on the corresponding part(s) that is being exercised.

In fact, you can develop your own exercises or techniques to clean and energize a specific chakra by inventing certain motions which would move, bend, compress and stretch that part of the body where the specific affected chakra is located. Doing physical exercises also facilitate the assimilation of prana after pranic treatment. A good exercise should consist of a short series of motions that would clean and energize all the major and minor chakras on the arms and legs.

PHYSICAL AND MENTAL RECHARGING

Physical Recharging

When you feel physically tired, there are two chakras you must cleanse and energize: the solar plexus chakra and the navel chakra.

1. Apply localized sweeping on the solar plexus chakra for 30 times.

2. Energize the solar plexus chakra with your palms or the tips of your fingers by doing pranic breathing for about 10 cycles. When exhaling, be aware of the whole body. This is to facilitate the distribution of pranic energy to the different parts of the body.

3. Apply distributive sweeping on the solar plexus chakra to avoid congestion.

4. Stabilize the projected pranic energy.

When this is done properly, the body will be energized and recharged. However, if you are still exhausted, you can do more pranic breathing cycles.

To further strengthen and energize the body, the navel chakra may also be treated.

1. Apply localized sweeping on the navel chakra for 30 times.

2. Energize the navel chakra with your palms or the tips of your fingers by doing pranic breathing for five to 10 cycles.

3. Stabilize the projected pranic energy.

Mental Recharging

When you are mentally exhausted and you still have a lot of work, you can do the following:

1. Apply localized sweeping 30 times each on the ajna, forehead, crown, and the sides of the head.

2. Apply localized sweeping on your back head for 30 times.

3. Curl your fingers and place them at the back of your head. Then do deep pranic breathing for 5-10 times to energize the entire head. When exhaling, be aware of the ajna, forehead and crown chakras, the left and right brain, and the left and right eyes. This is to facilitate the distribution of pranic energy to the different parts of the head.

4. If you feel a bit dizzy or overenergized, apply some sweeping on the head to remove the excess energy.

WATER AND SALT BATH

Sea water or water with salt is very effective in removing diseased energy from the energy body, especially for patients suffering from cancer, leukemia, venereal disease, arthritis, paralysis and leprosy.

Cancer patients have very dirty energy bodies; the affected parts are congested with diseased energy. Patients with venereal diseases also have dirty energy bodies and very dirty and "sticky" sex chakras. Patients with leprosy have very dirty energy bodies and extremely dirty basic chakras. These patients will benefit greatly from bathing with sea water or water with salt every day.

PRANIC SELF-HEALING AND PRANIC INVOCATIVE HEALING

The water-with-salt treatment will substantially clean the energy body and gradually strengthen the body and its defense system. Although this treatment is simple, it is quite effective and therefore should be taken seriously.

This treatment has to be done once or twice a day because the energy body becomes dirty again after a while or a day. This is also why the treatment has to be done daily or thrice a week for at least several months or for a lifetime.

a. Take a swim in sea water for 20 minutes. This will substantially clean the energy body. If this is not possible, taking a bath with water and salt will do: After cleansing yourself with soap and water, rub your entire body gently with fine salt. Then wash it off after about one or two minutes.

If you have a severe ailment, you may prepare a mixture of salt and water. Put about one to two kilograms of sea salt or fine salt to a tub of warm water, at about 39 to 40 degrees centigrade. Soak yourself in it. This has to be done everyday.

b. To energize the body, just rest under a shaded area to absorb pranic energy from the surroundings through pranic breathing.

c. Do this every day for the first two weeks, then later thrice a week for several months or for as long as necessary.

For Arthritic or Paralytic Patients:

   a. Take a swim in sea water for about 20 minutes to clean the energy body.

   b. Cover your body up to the shoulders with sand to absorb ground prana. The sand should not be too hot for you to take.

   c. Repeat thrice a week for as long as necessary.

Meat and fish should be avoided in your diet to facilitate healing, since their pranic energy content is not so clean as vegetables and fruits.

Patients with cancer should avoid taking megadoses of vitamins E, A, C and royal jelly because they may aggravate the condition. Patients with venereal diseases should avoid taking megadoses of vitamins E, B12 and royal jelly.

AVOIDING NEGATIVE EMOTIONS AND THOUGHTS

The author has observed that many patients with severe ailments usually harbor negative emotions for a long period. An example is a patient who suffers from cirrhosis of the liver in spite of the fact that he does not drink alcohol. He has a bad temper and curses other people at the slightest provocation. Due to negative emotions, his solar plexus chakra malfunctioned and inevitably affected his liver.

It has also been observed by the author that many patients suffering from severe rheumatoid arthritis, damaged kidneys, and malfunctioning of the immune defense system have so much resentment and anger. Patients with cyst in the bust or armpit tend to have too much stress. Their solar plexus chakra is quite congested. Stress also affects the solar plexus chakra and liver and to a certain degree the cholesterol level of the body. It is therefore advisable for patients suffering from severe ailments to have more positive attitude and emotions and learn simple meditation.

PRINCIPLE OF DIVERSION OR RELEASING

One time, the author had a severe headache. Instead of healing himself or having a friend heal him, he decided to experiment by listening to soothing music with full concentration. He was curious as to what would happen to his energy body and the diseased energy.

The effect, based on a clairvoyant's observation, was amazing. The grayish diseased energy started to thin out gradually and slowly to the extent of almost disappearing. After 5 to 10 minutes, the author got up and felt a slight reduction in pain. He noted that when attention was withdrawn from the music and directed to the head area, his head suddenly became more grayish. The final condition, however, was much lighter than when the experiment started.

There are several possible explanations to what happened:

1. Relaxing the mind and the body facilitates self-healing.

2. Since the energy body is easily affected by the mind and emotion, anything that has positive effects on the mind must also have some positive effects on the energy body.

3. By diverting the attention to something that is pleasant or harmonious, the diseased energy was "released" or "the hold was loosened," thereby allowing the body to heal itself more effectively. This is why the grayish matter became thinner or lighter. It seems that when the attention is focused on the pain, this tends to hold

together the diseased energy, thus hindering the healing process.

4. By reconcentrating on the affected part, the diseased energy was drawn back so that the affected part became grayish again.

The author has observed that if he focuses his attention on the pain and tries to remove it, he finds it more difficult to heal himself. But if he just ignores the pain and concentrates fully on what he is visualizing, the rate of healing is very fast.

The principle of diversion or releasing is also applicable in healing others. When some patients become so engrossed with the strange movements of the healer, their concentration on the pain they are experiencing is temporarily distracted, thereby facilitating the healing process. At times when the attention of the patient is focused on the pain or the discomfort is so intense, then it would be very helpful to ask the patient to concentrate on soothing music or on a very nice picture.

> *People have little idea of how much they increase the potency of the disease by the constantly directed thought which they expend upon it (by thinking too much about the ailment), and the attention they pay to that area wherein the trouble is located.*
>
> *– Alice Bailey,* Esoteric Healing

INTEGRATED APPROACH TO SELF-HEALING

1. Do physical exercises for about 5 to 10 minutes.

2. Apply pranic self-healing.

3. Do physical exercises for the treated chakra and organ for a few minutes to facilitate the assimilation of prana

by the body. This is done by either moving, twisting, compressing, stretching or bending the part of the body where the specific chakra is located to further cleanse and energize it.

4. Drink energized water, or water that has been exposed to the sun.

5. Rest and recuperate under a big, healthy tree, preferably pine tree, to absorb excess prana from it and the ground. If possible, embrace the tree. This has very beneficial effects. It is advisable to change trees regularly because they may get sick or die in the long run because of absorption of too much diseased energy from the patient.

6. Expose your body to the morning sun for about five to 10 minutes and simultaneously do visualization and/or pranic breathing to draw in solar pranic energy. This should not be done more than once a week. If you do it everyday for about a year, it may have an adverse effect on the body and may result in cancer.

7. Take Chinese or Korean ginseng to increase the synthetic ki within the human body. Unlike other kinds of food, ginseng contains synthetic ki which is concretized pranic energy. The energy will last for about seven to eight hours if a person takes about one or two grams of ginseng. However, this depends upon the quality of the ginseng used and the health of the patient.

Healers will find it helpful to take ginseng before healing, especially when there are many patients and particularly in cases where the patient's ailment is severe and the absorption of pranic energy is very fast. Take another dose after healing to energize and strengthen the body and minimize depletion.

8. Engage in enjoyable and productive activities that are not strenuous rather than brood over your predicament or ailment. This will facilitate the release of the diseased energy.

9. All forms of negative emotions and thoughts should be avoided or minimized since this will only aggravate your condition.

10. Religiously inclined patients can pray regularly and request the Lord to make them whole and perfect again.

11. Take medication. Healing is faster by treating simultaneously both the energy and the visible physical body than by treating the visible physical body or the energy body alone. As stated previously, the treatment should preferably be wholistic or integrated.

12. For severe ailments, consult a reputable medical doctor and a certified pranic healer.

It is advisable for severely sick patients to be taught pranic self-healing even if they are treated by conventional methods or by pranic healing.

Eating the proper food, taking enough water, breathing properly, doing sufficient physical exercise, leading a moderate lifestyle, and having a calm disposition and a clear, decisive mind would greatly help maintain one's physical, emotional and mental well-being.

PROBLEMS ENCOUNTERED IN SELF-HEALING

Some healers may find it difficult to heal themselves. This could be due to several possible factors:

1. The body of the healer has become very weak and painful, making concentration and utilization of his will difficult.

2. The healer may be good in projecting prana but may have little practice in self-healing.

3. The healer is either too lazy, too tired, or too weak or just does not really care enough to heal himself. Or the healer simply prefers to rest and be healed by another healer.

4. The ailment requires treatment using other supplementary or more appropriate forms of healing combined with pranic healing.

5. On rare occasions, healing oneself of serious ailment is not possible due to karmic factors or negative karma.

Many healers sometimes find it difficult to heal themselves and the author is no exception; he does not hesitate to take medication whenever necessary, consult a medical doctor, get an acupressure massage, or seek the help of another healer if he does not feel too well. There are times when he prefers to rest and let another person do the healing.

KARMA

Some serious ailments are due to negative deeds, thoughts, and feelings in the present and past lives of the patient, or negative karma. This is why after healing, Jesus usually says, "Your sins are forgiven." But not all serious ailments are due to negative karma. No pranic healer should ever turn away a patient just because he thinks the ailment may be due to negative karma. Actually, there are very few clairvoyants who can see with great accuracy into the past karma of a patient. Even if it is due to negative karma, you are not in a position to know when the negative karma has been fully worked out; therefore, the patient is entitled to be healed. If the ailment is due to negative karma and it has not been worked out, then no amount of treatment can heal the patient. The healer can in no way interfere with the negative karma of the patient.

For instance, the author was approached by a woman with a seriously injured right leg, which was quite painful from the hip down to the foot. She could hardly move it, so pranic healing was applied for about 30 minutes. The pain was greatly reduced; she was able to partially bend her knee and move her hip without any pain. On the day she was scheduled to have her second treatment, she was involved in three freak accidents involving her right leg, causing the patient intense suffering. It was very difficult for her to visit the author. She has not returned for further treatment ever since. For these three "accidents" to occur in a matter of a few hours was probably a case of negative karma. (For more information on karma, please refer to reading materials of Edgar Cayce, Astara, Theosophy, Agni Yoga, Rosicrucian, and other esoteric groups.)

Karma, in its broadest sense, means what you sow is what you reap or what you give is what you receive (Galatians 6:7). It is the law of cause and effect as applied to an individual or a group of individuals such as a family, a corporation or a nation.

> God cannot be mocked. A man reaps what he sows.
>
> — Galatians 6:7

> For with the same measure that ye mete withal it shall be measured to you again.
>
> — Luke 6:38

> Thou shalt receive requital and reward in just return for whatsoever thou dost.
>
> — Koran

> Just as a farmer plants a certain kind of seed and gets a certain crop, so it is with good and bad deeds.
>
> — Mahabharata

> So long as an evil deed has not karmically matured, the fool thinks his deed to be sweet as honey. But, when his evil deed karmically matures, he falls into untold misery.
>
> — Dhammapada
> Wisdom of the Buddha

> Each man, by the action of unerring karma, receives in exact measure all that is due, all that he deserves, neither more nor less. Not one benevolent or evil action, trifling as it may be, as secretly as it may be done, escapes the precisely balanced scale of karma.
>
> — Helena Roerich
> Foundation of Buddhism

KARMA AND THE GOLDEN RULE

The law of karma, when applied positively, manifests as the *yang golden rule*: "Do unto others what you would have them do unto you." This rule can be applied to get what you want or desire. If you want to be prosperous, then you must give and practice charity. If you want cordiality and harmony, then be cordial and courteous to others.

The law of karma can be used to avoid undesirable things or events when applied as the *yin golden rule*: "Do not do unto others what you would not have them do unto you." If you do not want to be cheated or swindled, then treat others honestly and fairly. If you have worked out most of your negative karma and have not done anybody any harm, then you have nothing to fear. Nothing can harm you. The law of karma is unbreakable. This is the meaning behind the statement, "My righteousness is my shield." Literally, nothing can harm such a man. A thousand or a million people may fall beside him but not a single strand of his hair will be touched!

The golden rule, when applied positively and negatively (yang and yin), will produce harmony and prosperity in your life and protect you from the vicissitudes of life. When applied by most people and nations, it will bring about world peace. The law of karma is also the basis of the command given by Lord Christ to "love your enemy." To return hate with hate, anger with anger, spite with spite, malicious injury with malicious injury will only worsen things. But, to return hatred with kindness and love will inevitably result in harmony and peace. It is indeed a pity that after almost 2,000 years, the teachings of the Lord Christ are only given lip service and not put into action by the majority of His followers. The command to love one's enemy was taught not only by Christ but also by Lord Gautama Buddha and other world religious teachers.

The law of karma applies to individuals as well as to nations. Therefore, the law of karma and the golden rule can be used by the leaders of nations to solve some of the national and international problems in the long run.

The Golden Rule is also universally taught:

> *Do not do unto others what you do not want others do unto you.*
>
> – Confucius

> *As ye would that men should do to you, do ye also to them likewise.*
>
> – Luke 6:31

> *This is the sum of all true righteousness: Deal with others as thou wouldst thyself be dealt by. Do nothing to thy neighbor which thou wouldst not have him do to thee hereafter.*
>
> – Mahabharata

> *Whatever thou likest not for thine own self, for any person else, too, like it not.*
>
> – Dhammapada
> Wisdom of the Buddha

> *Noblest religion this – that thou shouldst like for others what thou likest for thyself; and what thou feelest painful for thyself, hold that as painful for all others too.*
>
> – Koran

NEUTRALIZING NEGATIVE KARMA

Negative karma can be neutralized through the Law of Mercy and the Law of Forgiveness:

1. Meditate and learn the lesson that is to be learned and make a firm resolution to do the right thing.

2. Use the Law of Mercy.

   Blessed are the merciful for they shall obtain mercy.
   — Matthew 5:7

   By showing mercy to others, mercy will be shown to you:

   a.) Give 10 percent of your income to charity for the rest of your life, especially in order to alleviate the sufferings of other people.

   b.) Avoid eating meat and fish: being a vegetarian would be very helpful. By showing mercy to the members of the animal kingdom, mercy will also be shown to you.

   c.) Avoid injuring, bullying, and being cruel to other people. Mercy cannot be shown to those who do not show mercy to others.

3. Use the Law of Forgiveness.

   As stated in the prayer of St. Francis of Assisi, "It is in pardoning that we are pardoned," and in the Lord's Prayer, "One must first forgive others before one can seek divine forgiveness" (Matthew 6:12). "...For if ye forgive men their trespasses, your Heavenly Father will also forgive you but, if ye forgive not men their trespasses, neither will your Father forgive your trespasses" (Matthew 6:14-15).

- a.) Make a list of all your enemies and those who have hurt you.

- b.) Mentally visualize forgiving each one of them.

- c.) Mentally bless each one of them with what is best for them. Example: "May you be blessed with what is best for you."

- d.) Mentally request for the Lord's mercy and forgiveness.

- e.) Repeat the entire process for as long as necessary until one feels an inner sense of forgiveness.

It is possible for patients with very severe or terminal illness to be healed through the law of mercy and the law of forgiveness.

SUGGESTED ETHICAL GUIDELINES

1. It is the duty of the healer to try his best most of the time to heal and alleviate the condition of his patients.

2. The healer is entitled to charge a reasonable rate for his services. He should avoid charging an excessive fee that would unduly burden the patient.

3. Under no circumstances should a healer turn away or neglect a patient because of his inability to pay.

4. The healer should withhold any information concerning the cases of his patients to others if the disclosure of

such information will or may cause their embarrassment.

5. Under no circumstances should a healer take sexual advantage of his patients. Whenever possible or permissible, healing should be done in the open or in front of others. Healing in a closed room with the healer and the patient alone should, as much as possible, be avoided or minimized.

Most patients are quite gullible or easily influenced. This is due to two factors: the ability of the healer to produce amazing results, and the absence of knowledge of some patients on what to expect or what will be required of them during pranic healing.

6. Under no circumstances should the healer misuse his power. Power or the ability to manipulate invisible subtle energies is neither good nor bad. Power is good when used constructively and bad when used for destruction. It becomes bad when there is evil intention and misapplication of power.

TERMINOLOGY

Pranic healing or ki healing has been called by so many names like magnetic healing, faith healing, psychic healing, and laying on of the hands. Unfortunately, these labels are inaccurate and misleading. They only make an accurate and deeper study difficult, if not impossible.

There is nothing magnetic about the hands. The left hand is not negative or receptive nor is the right hand positive or projective. Both hands or hand chakras are capable of absorbing and projecting prana. It is just a matter of intention or willing which hand chakra is to predominantly absorb and which one to predominantly project. The energy or prana projected is not magnetic but rather vitalizing and strengthening. This is why the term "magnetic healing" is inaccurate. This does not in any way minimize the effectivity of magnetic healing. The terms "psychic healing," "faith healing," "laying on of the hands," etc., are too broad and could mean and imply so many things to different people. Therefore, it is not advisable to use these terms loosely.

For example, laying on of the hands describes to a certain extent only the outward acts but does not explain or describe what is happening inwardly or invisibly. Therefore, it would give the misconception that the act of laying on of the hands causes the healing. It is actually the involuntary or deliberate projection of prana (life energy) from the hand to the affected part and the involuntary absorption of the diseased energy by the hand into the body of the healer that cause the healing.

Another term that can be used to describe pranic healing is "bioplasmic healing," since it is by healing the bioplasmic body that the visible physical body is correspondingly healed.

PRANIC INVOCATIVE HEALING

As a common practice, some pranic healers make an invocation or pray before starting to heal. The invocation may be directed to God, to divine beings or to their spiritual guides. There are some invocative healers who may not understand the principles and the mechanics behind the healing process. They simply feel tremendous power flowing into their body, causing it to vibrate and become warm. Some invocative healers may not be so sensitive as to feel the flow of energy into their body. This does not in any way alter the fact that the body is being used as a channel for healing energy. There are also cases where the inflow of "healing" power triggers temporarily the clairvoyant faculty of the healers. Those who practice invocative healing are usually called faith healers or "charismatic healers."

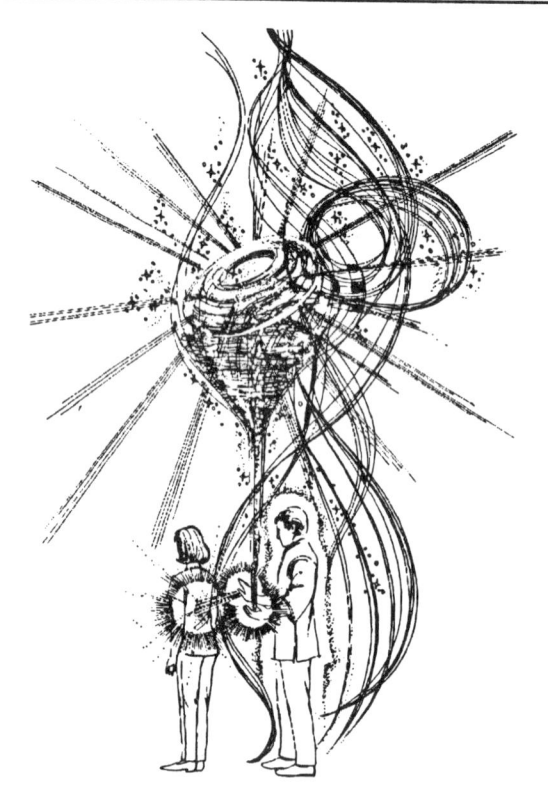

Fig. 5-2 *Pranic invocative healing: downpouring of spiritual healing energy*

In invocative healing, you invoke for the healing energy, and the healing ministers and healing angels who manipulate and control the healing energy and the energy body of the patients, and thereby ensure the safety of the patients. The invocative healer should maintain a receptive attitude in order to receive intuitive guidance or instructions. Healers who are quite willful should be careful when practicing invocative healing since there is the danger of overenergizing the patient.

If it is time for the patient to leave his body, the healing angels will not appear. The healer will usually be intuitively aware that there is no response.

PRANIC SELF-HEALING AND
PRANIC INVOCATIVE HEALING

Although some of these invocative or "faith" healers may not be knowledgeable about pranic healing, this does not in any way diminish the potency and effectivity of healing. Some of these healers can heal at a very fast rate and for so many hours without getting tired. Even advanced pranic healers would find it difficult to duplicate what some of these invocative healers are capable of doing.

If you intend to practice healing by prayer or pranic invocative healing, it is advisable that you meditate and pray regularly and request God to make you a divine healing instrument.

During pranic invocative healing, it is important to concentrate on the crown chakra and the center of your palms used for healing. In advanced pranic healing, this is called the crown-hand chakras technique. You can do sweeping and energizing with this technique. Be in tune for intuitive instructions. Before ending the treatment, the healer and the patient should give thanks to God and the higher beings.

The pranic invocative healing technique given is applicable to all persons of any religious denomination. It is quite potent and effective. One does not have to be "religious" for it to work. Just believe in God and trust that with God everything is possible!

Procedure:

1. Say for a few minutes any religious prayer you are used to. Then mentally recite this healing invocation:

   To the Supreme God,
   Thank you for making me
   Thy Divine healing instrument.
   Let my entire being be filled with
   compassion for others who are suffering.

> *To the Supreme God,*
> *Thank you for the healing and*
> *regenerating energy.*
> *With thanks and in full faith!*
>
> *To my spiritual Teachers,*
> *to the healing ministers, and holy angels,*
> *to the spiritual helpers, to all the great ones,*
> *Thank you for the divine guidance,*
> *divine love and mercy,*
> *Thank you for the healing.*
> *With thanks and in full faith.*

The invocation can be made once or twice with intense concentration, and with strong and full conviction. It should be done with humility, sincerity, and reverence.

2. Before starting the treatment, request the patient to use his own words to invoke for divine healing.

3. For those with background in pranic healing, apply pranic treatment on the patient. Concentrate on your crown chakra and your hand. Connect your tongue to your palate during the entire pranic treatment.

4. Another approach which is simpler is to place your hand either on the affected part, the ajna, forehead, crown or back heart chakra. Silently recite and invoke:

    > *To the Supreme God,*
    > *Thank you for healing this patient!*
    > *In full faith, so be it!*

5. You may do pranic breathing while healing. This is optional but helpful.

6. Say a short prayer of thanksgiving after the treatment. Silently say:

   To the Supreme God
   Thank you for your blessings
   and for healing this patient.

   To my spiritual Teachers,
   to the healing ministers, and holy angels,
   to the spiritual helpers, to all the great ones,
   Thank you for your blessings
   and for healing this patient.

7. At the end of the treatment, request the patient to say a prayer of thanksgiving on his own.

For simple ailments, the cure is usually instantaneous. For more severe ailments, the relief is fast but complete recovery may require several treatments or several months. Treatment has to be given several times a week, depending upon the needs of the patient. Invocative healing can be applied on a group of patients by a healer or it can be done by a group of pranic invocative healers on a patient. Care should be taken not to overenergize the patient.

Negative karma sometimes can be neutralized through divine intercession. For students who intend to go full time into healing and who want to practice pranic invocative healing, it is important that they undergo a period of refining or improving their character. The downpour of healing energy, together with the spiritual energy, magnifies many times the positive and negative characteristics of the healer; hence, the necessity for self-purification through the daily practice of inner reflection. Also, a person with refined or higher vibration tends to attract entities with similar or higher vibration while a person with gross or lower vibration or characteristics tends to attract undesirable entities with similar low vibration.

Spiritual chanting, singing and dancing are other forms of invocative healing. This type of invocative healing is universal and is used by some Christians, Sufis and persons of other religious faiths.

SELF-HEALING AFFIRMATION

> *God is Almighty,*
> *God is All-Merciful.*
> *God is healing me of all my ailments,*
> *With thanks and in full faith!*

1. Repeat this prayer for about five minutes with full concentration, humility, reverence and faith.

2. Be still, be receptive and wait for about 10 minutes.

3. When this is done properly, it will bring rapid or instantaneous relief for simple ailments.

4. For persons suffering from severe ailments, repeat this twice a day for as long as necessary, even if it takes several months or years.

5. Self-healing affirmation is complementary to Meditation on Twin Hearts. For those suffering from severe ailments, meditate on the twin hearts. After releasing the excess energy, do the self-healing affirmation. Combining both will make the rate of healing much faster.

6. End the session by saying a short prayer of thanksgiving:

> *To the Supreme God,*
> *Thank you for your blessings,*
> *your mercy and your healing.*
> *With thanks and in full faith!*

If symptoms persist or if the ailment is severe, please consult immediately a medical doctor and, also a certified pranic healer.

ASSIGNING HEALING ANGELS

After treatment, it is better to request God to assign a healing angel to remain with a patient suffering from a severe ailment in order to further accelerate the healing process. The patient should be instructed to be more receptive by invoking God's blessings several times a day. The receptivity of the patient will make the work of the healing angel a lot easier. The healer can request for a healing angel to be assigned to the patient by silently reciting this prayer:

> *To the Supreme God,*
> *thank you for assigning a healing angel*
> *to remain with the patient*
> *until he is completely cured.*
> *With thanks and in full faith.*
> *So be it!*
>
> *To the healing angel assigned,*
> *thank you for the healing.*
> *In full faith. So be it!*

It is important that the invocation should be done with humility, sincerity and reverence.

In the near future, healing angels and healers will be more actively cooperating to produce dramatic or miraculous healing on a wider scale.

– Choa Kok Sui

CHAPTER SIX

Pranic Distant Healing

The planetary-etheric body is whole, unbroken and continuous; of this etheric body, those of the healer and of the patient are integral, intrinsic parts.... The channels of relationship can be conductors of many different types of energy, transmitted by the healers to the patient.

– *Alice Bailey*
Esoteric Healing

Prana (life energy) colored by the thought of the sender may be projected to persons at a distance, who are willing to receive it, and the healing can be done this way.

– *Yogi Ramacharaka*
The Science of Psychic Healing

Energy follows thought.

– An esoteric maxim

Two Principles in Pranic Distant Healing 250
Distant Scanning 251
Pranic Distant Healing 252

TWO PRINCIPLES IN PRANIC DISTANT HEALING

Pranic Distant Healing is based on two principles:

1. The Principle of Interconnectedness

The mechanism of pranic distant healing is similar to that of the telephone. You are able to contact another person because your telephone line is linked to the other person's line. The healer and the patient are interconnected because their etheric or energy bodies are parts of the earth's etheric body. Therefore, the pranic healer can heal the patient at a distance because their energy bodies are interconnected.

2. The Principle of Directability

Pranic energy follows where your thought or intention is focused. When you think of a person, the pranic energy goes to him. Therefore, since "energy follows thought", when the healer focuses his attention to the patient, he can remove diseased energy and project pranic energy to him.

Pranic distant healing is similar to close-ranged pranic healing. The only difference is that in pranic distant healing, the psychic faculty of the healer has to be developed or sharpened further through regular practice for greater accuracy. Those of you who have been healing or experimenting on healing may have developed the skill to sense what part of the patient is affected with the use of distant scanning or even without scanning. Some may even have developed the psychic sense to feel or see vaguely the degree of healthiness of an organ that is being energized. The unfolding or gradual development of psychic faculty is a natural by-product of healing. It is advisable to at least gain proficiency in intermediate pranic healing before advancing to pranic distant healing.

DISTANT SCANNING

The ability to scan a patient at a distance is something that has to be gradually developed through regular practice.

Procedure:

1. When a patient comes to you for healing, do not scan him with your hands at close range and do not interview him immediately.

2. Let your patient sit in front of you at a distance of three or four meters. Close your eyes. Imagine the patient is near and in front of you. Distantly scan the energy body and the visible physical body of your "imagined" patient. You can do this with your physical hand or you can mentally scan the patient with your "imaginary or etheric hand." Scan the chakras, and the major organs from the crown down to the feet. Do you feel any congestion or depletion? Scan the spine from top to bottom. Do you feel any obstruction?

3. If you are partially clairvoyant, try to psychically see the chakras and the major organs from the crown down to the feet. Pay special attention to the major chakras. Are the chakras bright, grayish, muddy red or black? Are they thick or thin or just normal? Look over the important organs from top to bottom. Do they look good? Do they look too reddish or bluish?

    You do not have to feel strongly or see clearly to be accurate. Being able to scan or see vaguely is good enough. Relax, do it slowly but thoroughly. The patient will not mind waiting for a few minutes.

4. Open your eyes. Get up and scan thoroughly the patient.

5. Interview the patient. Evaluate the condition of the patient and compare it with the findings based on distant scanning and psychic diagnosis.

It is possible that you will achieve some degree of accuracy even on the first try. Continue practicing until you become not only relatively accurate but very accurate. This may require at least from several weeks to several months of regular practice. Proper and effective treatment depends upon accurate scanning.

Try actual distant diagnosis and scanning first on patients you have treated before. Then gradually try it on patients whom you have never met. Get a picture of the patient to help you establish "contact" with him.

PRANIC DISTANT HEALING

Method 1

1. Connect your tongue to your palate and do distant scanning on the patient. It is very important to rescan the patient during the treatment.

2. Do pranic breathing.

3. Visualize the patient in front of you about one foot to two feet tall. The visualization does not have to be clear. What is important is having a clear intention to heal the person.

   Do not visualize the patient as very far from you since

PRANIC DISTANT HEALING 253

this would tend to condition your mind that healing the patient is very difficult. This may discourage you in doing pranic distant healing. Or it may cause the healer to overreact by projecting the pranic energy with too much force or will when healing. Using too much will has damaging effects on the patient. Instead of getting better, he will become worse. This is similar to having overseas conversation. When you talk to the other party, you do not have to shout at him.

4. Mentally or verbally repeat the patient's name during the entire treatment.

5. Visualize or imagine that you are applying general sweeping on the front and the back of the patient's body. Apply localized sweeping on the affected part(s) and chakra(s). You may actually move your hands while cleansing the patient.

6. Dispose of the diseased energy by throwing it into the disposal unit. Continue cleansing until the affected part(s) and chakra(s) look brighter.

7. Energize the affected chakra(s) and part(s). Do five to ten cycles or more of pranic breathing and mentally repeat the name of the patient as you exhale. Continue energizing until the treated parts look quite bright and healthy or until you feel the treated parts have been sufficiently energized.

8. Stabilize the projected pranic energy.

9. Cut the etheric link between you and the patient.

10. Scan the patient to determine whether he has been

properly treated. If not, repeat the entire process until the treated parts improve substantially.

11. Wash your hands after healing to remove the diseased energy.

Method 2

1. Connect your tongue to your palate and do distant scanning on the patient. Be sure to rescan the patient during the treatment.

2. Close your eyes; visualize a brilliant ball of light on top of the patient, then visualize a stream of white light washing the head area and gradually going down and cleansing the entire body. Gather the diseased energy and throw them into the disposal unit.

3. Visualize the grayish matter in the affected part becoming less dense and lighter. Will it to come out or see it floating out.

4. The diseased energy can be disposed of by mentally throwing them into the disposal unit.

5. Energize the affected parts by visualizing a ball of light (pranic ball) being formed and gently projecting it to the affected part.

6. Stabilize the projected pranic energy.

7. Cut the etheric link between you and the patient.

8. Rescan the patient. Give further treatment if required.

9. Wash your hands after healing.

The difference between Method 1 and Method 2 is that in the former, prana is drawn to the body of the healer before projecting it to the patient; in the latter, prana is drawn from the surroundings and projected directly to the patient without passing through the body of the healer.

When you are already proficient, you can try healing old patients at a distance, then gradually try new ones.

"Like the bee gathering honey from the different flowers, the wise man accepts the essence of different scriptures and sees only the good in all religions."

– Srimad Bhaoavatam

Harmony through tolerance.

Diversity in forms, unity in essence!

– Choa Kok Sui

CHAPTER SEVEN

Testimonials

AMERICA (USA)
   1. Thrombocytosis 259
   2. Soft Stools/Bladder Incontinence 262
   3. Leg Injury Due to Accident. 264
ARGENTINA
   1. Scoliosis 265
AUSTRIA
   1. Stiff Neck 266
BRAZIL
   1. Impetigo 267
   2. Horse-kicking Accident 268
   3. Urinary Tract Infection; Allergic Reactions
      to Medicines 269
CANADA
   1. Left Knee/Shin Injury;
      Carpal Tunnel Syndrome; Hemorrhoids 270
   2. Herpes Zoster and Psoriasis 272
   3. Herpes Zoster and Right-Hip Pain Due to a Fall 273
FINLAND
   1. Neurologic Disorder 275
GERMANY
   1. Slipped Disk 276
   2. Ovarian Cysts/Infertility;
      Bladder and Urethral Infections 277
   3. Multiple Sclerosis 278
INDIA
   1. Kidney Stones 279
   2. Chronic Miscarriages 280
   3. Cataract 281
   4. Post-surgical Complications (Brain) 282
   5. Cervical Spondylitis 284
   6. Ulcerative Colitis/Night Blindness
      and Hearing Loss 285
   7. Chronic Vomiting 287

INDONESIA
- 1. Intermittent Blackouts 288
- 2. Pre- and Post-Liposuction Treatments;
  Post-Herpetic Neuralgia 289
- 3. Anal Fistula 291
- 4. Ulnar Bone Fracture with Dislocation 292
- 5. Acute Renal Failure 293

IRELAND
- 1. Lump on the Side of the Knee 294
- 2. Pneumonia/Acute Backpain 295

ITALY
- 1. Breast Cancer 296

MALAYSIA
- 1. Localized Arthritic Pain (Fingers) 297

MEXICO
- 1. Brain Tumor 298
- 2. Pneumonia; Backpain;
  Stress and Tension 299

NETHERLANDS
- 1. Arthritis/Migraine 300

PHILIPPINES
- 1. Emphysema 302
- 2. Abdominal Pain 303
- 3. Wound 304
- 4. Urinary Ailment 306
- 5. Kidney Ailment 308
- 6. Burn 310
- 7. Jaw Inflammation 312
- 8. Arthritis 313

SINGAPORE
- 1. Nose Bleeds, Allergic Reactions,
  Minor Cuts and Abrasions 315

SWITZERLAND
- 1. Skin Rashes 317
- 2. Throat Pain and Hoarseness 318

URUGUAY
- 1. Parkinson's Disease 319
- 2. Backpain 321

VENEZUELA
- 1. Migraine 322
- 2. Nasal Allergies 323
- 3. Chronic Sinusitis 324

TESTIMONIALS

NAME: Diane M. Smith
ADDRESS: 11009 W. Church St., Franklin, WI 53132, USA
AGE: 45
OCCUPATION: Part-time Administrative Assistant
CASE: Thrombocytosis*
HEALER: Stephen Co

In July 1996, I had been diagnosed with a rare blood disorder called thrombocytosis. This ailment has many side effects, the most harmful being an extremely high platelet count of over a million which could cause a heart attack or stroke. Some of the other side effects I experienced were extreme fatigue, heart palpitation, shortness of breath, bloating and swelling of my legs and ankles.

I was put on an experimental medication to bring down my platelet count. I spent three days in the hospital, undergoing tests to determine the cause of the ailment, including a bone marrow test for leukemia. There was no basis found for my illness.

After six months of dealing with oncologists, my platelet count was up and down, and I felt horrible. I read about Stephen Co's article in a woman's magazine. He talked about healing a young woman who was blinded with almost the same blood disorder that I had. I called his office in California and found out that he would be in St. Louis on February 8 and 9, 1997 for a Pranic Healing Workshop. I had a strong feeling that I needed to go even though I had never heard of Pranic Healing and had no idea what to expect.

---

*Thrombocytosis is a condition marked by an abnormal increase in the number of blood platelets.

Before I had this illness, my life was filled with pain and anger. On Sunday, February 9, my life changed forever. I remember so vividly and so powerfully as though it was yesterday. The actual healing took close to an hour. I felt a tremendous force, a pulling going on inside my body for quite some time. Stephen took my hands and kept telling me to let go. Finally, I experienced a tremendous white light throughout my entire body, an illumination so powerful I felt as though I could have floated to the ceiling. It was incredible. I felt an immediate sense of well being and peace, gratitude, blessedness, and complete joy.

I was late leaving for the airport and almost missed my flight going back to Milwaukee. I literally had to run through the St. Louis airport to catch my plane. When I finally sat down, the tears began to flow because I realized that the fatigue had left me and I felt incredibly well. This feeling continued each day to get stronger and all of the symptoms of my blood disorder disappeared. On my first visit to my oncologist, my platelet count remained about the same. The next visit, it went down quite a bit, and on my last visit my count was within the normal range. I had also decreased my medication to half the original dosage. My doctor was quite amazed. In addition, I just had my sixth-month visit to my dentist and he was also amazed because my diseased gum tissue was completely healed as well. Since then, I have read the Pranic Healing book, used all of the prayers in it, and I meditate with the Twin Hearts tape on a daily basis. I realize now that my blood disorder was a spiritual ailment brought on by my anger, resentment and negativity.

I have never felt better in my life, both physically and emotionally. I continue to grow in body, mind and spirit. I attended the Pranic Healing workshop for the second time and thanked Stephen Co for the gift that he has given me - a new life filled with love, joy, peace and well-being. I realized that since I have been given this blessed gift, I must now return it with love. He was able to free me of my pain and start my body on the healing process. I must also thank my Lord and Savior for, without Him, none of these blessings would have been possible.

(Signed) DIANE SMITH
May 3, 1997

NAME: Jimmy O'Donnell
ADDRESS: USA
AGE: 4
CASE: Soft Stools; Bladder Incontinence
HEALERS: Stephen Co and Natalie Shields

My son is four years and four months old. During his entire life, he has been in diapers and has had very soft stools. I hardly ever could dump his stool from the diaper into the toilet because it was so soft. When he turned four in February of this year, I felt I needed to work on this issue because no preschool would take him in diapers, plus the fact that perhaps, something was wrong with his digestive tract. I had him muscle-tested by a naturopath and pranic healing came up very strongly as the modality to address this problem. (Muscle-testing involves asking nonverbally the client's body what it needs for its benefit.)

After I had taken the introductory Pranic Healing course, about early April during the first session, Natalie worked on him for an hour and his first bowel movement after that was wonderfully firm. After four years of creamy stools, this felt like a miracle! She did distant healing later that week as well. His stools never totally regressed — unless his diet was not healthy that day — though they often were a mixture of soft on the outside with some firmness to them. In early June, Natalie worked on him once in person and once distantly, still focusing on the quality of the stool. In mid-June, I told her that the stool was consistently firm enough that he should be able to tell us he has to go to the toilet.

I felt he needed pranic psychotherapy as well. There were two issues that needed addressing: One, he refused to wear big boy underpants and, two, he *never* initiated going to the toilet for either pee (to urinate) or poop (to move the bowels). When asked if he was a big boy or a baby, he usually answered "baby." There was a big part of him that did not want to grow up.

TESTIMONIALS

Natalie did pranic healing on him twice that week. Two days after his last session, he asked to be in big boy pants and has never worn diapers since. However, if we ask him to go pee in the toilet, he reluctantly will but refuses to go poop in there. Also, if we forget to have him pee and he starts to pee on the floor, he cannot stop himself and empties his bladder where he stands.

Ten days after Jimmy's last session with Natalie, Stephen Co did pranic healing on him. Later that day, Jimmy started to pee twice in his big boy pants but stopped himself and asked to be put on the toilet to finish. The next day, he had not wet his bed as usual. At lunch, he ran to my daughter and said, "Poo-poo." Thinking he had pooped in his pants as usual, she said, "Oh no!" Jimmy shook his head and she realized that he wanted to use the toilet to go poop. He had his first bowel movement in the toilet and it was initiated by him. A double win!

I am so grateful to Stephen Co and Natalie for this gift.

(Signed) KATHY O'DONNELL
(Mother)
June 29, 1997

NAME:	Cynthia Guerrero de Leon
ADDRESS:	306 Dunkerhook Road, Paramus, NJ 07652 USA
AGE:	46
OCCUPATION:	Pianist/Director of Finance
CASE:	Leg Injury due to Accident
HEALER:	GM, Physician

On January 14, 1997, while I was standing at a bus stop, I was hit by a car that had lost control after it had hit another car. My injuries included multiple lacerations, subcutaneous swelling on the right leg and foot, and a broken fibula.*

Going through the crutch, cane and limping stages in the course of five months, I gradually regained the ability to do basic physical leg movements, except full knee bends and squats.

On June 15, GM did a special pranic healing session on my right leg and foot. Immediately after that, I was able to bend my knee to a full squat. My physical activities involving the affected leg are now back to normal.

(Signed) CYNTHIA GUERRERO DE LEON
August 1, 1997

---

*The fibula is one of two bones on each leg.

NAME:	Dara Sonia Filipof
ADDRESS:	Avenida Rivadavia 6387 5 A1
	Capital Federal, Buenos Aires
	ARGENTINA
OCCUPATION:	Acupuncturist and Pranic Healer
CASE:	Scoliosis*

Karina Gonzalez, a 22-year old student, had scoliosis. For 12 years, she had been suffering so much pain that she found it difficult to sleep. Her family took her to different alternative therapies, but the only course of action given was a surgery in which a bar of metal would be implanted in her vertebral column to straighten her spine.

When she came to consult me, nobody could touch her back because it was so sensitive and painful. I applied pranic healing and the pain diminished by 80 %. After 12 sessions, she could sleep and go to the gym. The improvement is dramatic and she's undergoing regular pranic treatment.

(Signed) DARA SONIA FILIPOF
July 18, 1997

---

*In scoliosis, the spine, instead of being straight, is S-shaped. Thus, the spinal bones compress on the spinal nerves, causing pain and limitation of motion.

NAME:	Franz Danninger
ADDRESS:	Lebensquelle Universelle
	Energie Gesundheitszentrum
	A-5164 Seeham 6 2
	AUSTRIA
OCCUPATION:	Pranic Healer
CASE:	Stiff Neck

Petra Wolftaler, a 12-year old schoolgirl, could not move her head for half a year because the nerve in the neck area was pinched. After just one 30-minute pranic treatment, the problem was completely gone and the patient could already move her head as if she never had the ailment.

(Signed) FRANZ DANNINGER
June 3, 1997

NAME: Camilla de Gouvea Bezerra dos Santos
ADDRESS: Av. Oswaldo Cruz, Apt. 1.401
Flamengo, Rio de Janeiro RJ, BRAZIL
AGE: 3
CASE: Impetigo*
HEALER: Araci Ag. Monteiro

In January 1996, my daughter Camilla, who at that time was two and a half years old, had a skin disease diagnosed as impetigo. Her body was full of eruptions which, according to the pediatrician, were as painful as second-degree burns. Camilla became a very restless and aggressive kid.

For almost a month, I tried homeopathic and allopathic treatments but none of them solve the problem. I decided to try pranic healing. After two sessions of cleansing and energizing by Araci, the skin eruptions regressed, declining progressively and making Camilla's behavior normal again.

(Signed) PATRICIA DE GOUVEA
BEZERRA DOS SANTOS
(Mother)

(Signed) ARACI AG. MONTEIRO
May 22, 1997

---

*Impetigo is an acute contagious skin disease characterized by small blisters with pus which rupture and develop distinct yellowish crusts.

NAME:	Pedro Baldratti
ADDRESS:	Rua Dr. Eduardo de Souza Aranha,
	140 No. 64 Vila Olimpia
	CEP 04543-120 Sao Paulo, BRAZIL
AGE:	56
OCCUPATION:	Real Estate
CASE:	Horse-kicking accident
HEALER:	Lela Jordao

In 1988, a horse kicked me on the face, injuring my chin and jaw in the process. My teeth were torn away together with my gums.

I went to the Hospital da Face where my chin was recomposed. Steel threads were used to join the bones. After some years, these steel threads became oxidized and rusted, resulting in a strong inflammation. Doctors advised the removal of the threads.

On April 19, Mrs. Lela Jordao, a pranic healer, begun to treat me. After 45 days,* the inflammation disappeared completely.

(Signed) PEDRO BALDRATTI
July 23, 1997

---

* This testimonial is supported by a certification from Dr. Weivel Joao Sozzo, Pedro Baldratti's dentist. According to Dr. Sozzo, "After 45 days, a new control x-ray surprisingly showed a local bone development instead of a normal recuperation which should be about eight to 10 months! I was informed that he had taken pranic treatments which in my technical opinion was fantastic."

NAME:	Carlos Eduardo de Maio
ADDRESS:	R. Batataes, 262 - Jardim Paulista CEP 01423-010 Sao Paulo, BRAZIL
OCCUPATION:	Pranic Healing Therapist
CASES:	Urinary Tract Infection; Allergic Reaction to Medicines

Cristiani Magalhães Costa, a 32-year old psychologist, was diagnosed with urinary tract infection in October 1996. Her medical doctor prescribed allopathic medicines, but the infection did not subside. The patient had a strong headache and felt dizzy, and also had kidney and abdominal pains. She told the doctor about her reactions to the medication and how she felt her condition was getting worse. The doctor told her to stop one of the medicines but the other treatment she had to continue.

The patient got worse for the next two days and started vomiting excessively, making her very weak. She had to go twice to the hospital for administration of glucose. Back home, she could neither eat nor get out of bed. The strong pain persisted.

Her mother called me up. When I went to the patient's house on a Friday evening, I applied advanced pranic healing for about 45 minutes. At the end of the session, she felt better and got out of bed with no sign of pain.

The following Sunday, I did another healing on her upon her request. The result of the second session was excellent. The pain and the infection disappeared and she felt good. She was completely cured.

(Signed) CARLOS EDUARDO DE MAIO
July 21, 1997

NAME: Elliot Gose
ADDRESS: 303 Ross-Durrance Rd., Victoria
V9E 2A3, CANADA
AGE: 71
OCCUPATION: Retired University Professor
CASES: Left knee/shin-tendon pulled;
Carpal Tunnel Syndrome;*
Hemorrhoids
HEALER: Dorothea Vickery

When I retired in 1991, I looked forward to an active life on what had been our summer property. I enjoyed clearing the land of dead trees, sawing and chopping them up for firewood. I also looked forward to hiking in the surrounding hills. Unfortunately in October 1995, by the time I was 69, I had pulled a tendon behind my left knee and had to stop hiking. The anti-inflammatory drug prescribed by my doctor gave me no relief. But a month of pranic healing treatments by Dorothea Vickery brought a remission of symptoms. I have hiked pain-free for the past 18 months.

When I developed carpal tunnel syndrome on my right hand, I feared I would no longer be able to chop firewood, especially when my doctor told me that there was no cure for it. After a couple of months of pranic healing by Dorothea, the symptoms were gone. When they return in a mild form, following strenuous exercise, the symptoms disappear within two days of rest without re-treatment. I am now clearing trees on our extensive property and sawing wood.

---

*Carpal Tunnel Syndrome is due to the compression of the median nerve characterized by pain upon bending of the wrist, excessive accumulation of fluid in the tissues of the fingers, tense and shiny skin and atrophy of the muscles of the palm.

TESTIMONIALS

Dorothea's treatment of a bout of hemorrhoids this past spring was nothing short of magical. After the first treatment, I was 100 percent cured! I had two follow-up treatments and had no reappearance of symptoms since then. This had never been my experience with hemorrhoids in the past.

(Signed) ELLIOTT GOSE
May 18, 1997

NAME:	Maria Cristina "Nona" Castro
ADDRESS:	Pranic Healing Services Canada
	207-1455 Robson Street, Vancouver
	BC V6G 1C1 CANADA
OCCUPATION:	Pranic Healer
CASE:	Herpes Zoster* and Psoriasis**

The patient, Ernesto Gatchalian of Ontario, Canada, was suffering from shingles, a viral disease medically known as herpes zoster. The diseased affected the left side of his body. His prostate was also inflamed and this made it impossible for him to urinate for three days. After pranic treatment, the body pains disappeared and urination was normalized.

The healer also found out that the patient had been suffering from psoriasis for 30 years. The patient had tried prescribed creams and pills which had several side effects on the blood, but none of the medications were successful.

Psoriasis was heavy on the arms and legs. As an experiment, pranic healing was done for three days on the arms but not on the legs. A daily salt-apple cider vinegar bath was also recommended.

The skin on the arms had become smooth with no trace of psoriasis. The legs, however, were still affected with the skin disease. Pranic healing will also be applied. Meanwhile, the patient has taken the course.

(Signed) MARIA CRISTINA "NONA" CASTRO
August 2, 1997

---

*Herpes Zoster is a painful inflammation of the nerve endings that is due to a virus infection. It is marked by small blisters on the skin that follow the path of the affected nerve.

**Psoriasis is a chronic skin disease characterized by red, scaly patches.

TESTIMONIALS

NAME:	Helen Zamfir
ADDRESS:	Copetown, Ontario, CANADA
AGE:	57
OCCUPATION:	Retired (Teacher/Counsellor for 35 years)
CASES:	1. Herpes Zoster
	2. Right-Hip Pain Due to a Fall

1. *Herpes Zoster*

When I arrived to do pranic healing on Marie Hulme, a 50-year old medical secretary, I was very concerned because the area around her eyes was a reddish-purple color and there were sores under the eyelids. I knew that shingles (Herpes Zoster) around the eyes were extremely dangerous, possibly causing blindness. The left side of her body from the armpit to the waist and around the navel was raw flesh and very painful. While working on the affected areas, the patient indicated that the pain had subsided. Upon completion of the first treatment, I went back to scan it and happened to glance up at her eyes. I was astounded! The reddish-purple color from under the eyes had disappeared and so had the sores. The patient quickly went to the mirror. When she came back, she was in awe, saying, "This is amazing. The sores have disappeared as well as the discoloration."

The next day, the patient indicated that the sores on her body had turned from the red rawness to a healed over-pinky color. After the third treatment, the patient's energy level had returned. She is very grateful for the success of pranic healing.

2. *Right-Hip Pain Due to a Fall*

A year ago, Jean Finch, an 83-year old caregiver to a 105-year old mother until last fall, had fallen down a set of cement stairs and had badly hurt her head as well as the right side of her body, especially the back and hip area. Hip replacement was recommended and surgery was set for August 8, 1997.

Apparently, the patient was not thrilled about the operation so she inquired about other possibilities. Her reflexologist, who had been working on her feet once a week but was unable to get the pain to subside suggested that I might be able to help her.

She was in severe pain when I arrived. She was limping as she tried to use a walker to assist her. After the first treatment, she was astounded that the leg and hip area was free of pain. "I can't believe this pain has gone!" she exclaimed.

After eight treatments, the patient was walking freely with little pain. She cancelled her operation because she felt so much better. Now, she works in the garden, does her own washing and ironing and hopes to be able to scrub the floors. It's wonderful to see the sparkle in her eyes. Thanks to pranic healing.

(Signed) HELEN ZAMFIR
August 7, 1997

NAME:	Kristina Andersson
ADDRESS:	Sjöllén, 00200 Helsinki, FINLAND
AGE:	44
OCCUPATION:	Teacher
CASE:	Neurologic Disorder
HEALER:	Tor-Fredric Karlsson

Having suffered a neurologic disorder that affected my face, mouth and throat, with cramps around the eyes, I sought pranic treatment. There was no big change during the first two treatments. After a break of four weeks, two more pranic treatments followed. I felt a notable change around the mouth. It felt relaxed and, although I had a very stressful period at work, my energy increased remarkably. Now I feel almost completely recovered with only a slight tension in the throat every now and then. I have also regained my joy for life.

(Signed) KRISTINA ANDERSSON
July 1997

NAME: Elisabeth Veihöver
ADDRESS: Uhlandstr. 20
52349 Düren, GERMANY
OCCUPATION: Retired
CASE: Slipped Disk
HEALER: Bernhard Späth

I had a slipped disk in the lower spine that required an operation in 1996. After this, I had severe pain for several months, especially in the upper legs. Without a cane or a wheelchair, it was not possible to move. My legs were weak and my ankles were numb. I also had burning pain on the soles of the feet. A doctor administered injections twice a week to relieve the pain. No result.

In May 1997, I underwent pranic treatment. After four sessions, my pains were relieved. This enabled me to walk without a cane. The numb feelings and burning sensations are almost gone.

(Signed) ELISABETH VEIHÖVER
July 1997

NAME: Raphaele Berglar
ADDRESS: Gleuelerstr. 373, 50935 Köln
GERMANY
CASES: 1. Ovarian Cysts and Infertility
2. Bladder and Urethral Infections

Case 1: Ovarian Cysts and Infertility

Karin Voigt who is 26 years old had cysts in her ovaries. Before pranic healing was applied to her, she had prolonged menstrual cycles and did not ovulate. The diagnosis was infertility.

After pranic treatment, she is now on the third month of her pregnancy!

Case 2: Bladder and Urethral Infections

An 11-year old schoolchild, Anncharlott Berglar, had severe pain on her abdomen while urinating. The doctor said that she had an infection of the bladder and the urethra.

On April 7 and 8, 1996, pranic healing was done, using the advanced technique. After two days, the symptoms disappeared. Her urine became clear as attested by the results of a urinalysis.

(Signed) RAPHAELE BERGLAR
July 1997

NAME: Sabine MaBfeller
ADDRESS: Antwerpener Str. 5, D-13353 Berlin, GERMANY
AGE: 31
CASE: Multiple Sclerosis
HEALER: Hannelore Kugel

I had been diagnosed with multiple sclerosis. Before I underwent pranic treatment, I suffered from disturbances in equilibrium, walking and coordination problems, partial numbness of the legs and feet, strong low back pain, stiff cervical spine, urine incontinence, periodical eye infections (iritis), easy fatigability, lack of energy, depression and aggressiveness. These symptoms brought on a sense of powerlessness.

After I went in for pranic healing, my energy level has become more stable. I have more power and drive and can think more positively. My low back pains have disappeared and my metabolism is now normal. Although my walking and equilibrium problems are still existent, and relapses still occur, walking is much easier and the equilibrium is more stable after each pranic treatment. I feel better than ever.

(Signed) SABINE MaBFELLER
May 22, 1997

TESTIMONIALS

NAME:	Nandita Srinath George
ADDRESS:	12 Amritavanam, 23 Temple Avenue
	Srinagar Colony, Saidapet
	Chennai - 600 0015 INDIA
AGE:	29
OCCUPATION:	HRD Executive
CASE:	Kidney Stones
HEALER:	Cliff Saldanha

I retired to bed as any other day, albeit exhausted, but was awakened by the need to empty my bladder in the middle of the night and there was also a good deal of pain accompanying the discomfort. This went on almost nonstop for over an hour. As soon as it was possible, my husband took me to a hospital.

The doctors diagnosed my condition as kidney stones and this was later confirmed by a sonogram report that showed eight stones, four to five millimeters in size. I was put on allopathic medication, but knowing of pranic healing, I underwent this therapy too, in addition to disintegration of the stones.

From the very first session, pranic healing relieved me totally of pain and discomfort. However, since the doctor was considering surgical intervention, two weeks later I went in for an MRI scan. To everyone's surprise and much to my relief and joy, the report showed only one stone, reduced in size and in an insignificant position. Result: *No surgery!*

No pain or discomfort have I experienced ever since. My probem has been solved in just about a forthnight. Many thanks to the timely intervention of pranic healing.

(Signed) NANDITA SRINATH GEORGE
July 1997

NAME: Geetha Sukumar
ADDRESS: No. 9, 1st Street, Shakti Nagar
Choolaimedu, Chennai - 600 094
INDIA
AGE: 30
OCCUPATION: Housewife
CASE: Chronic Miscarriages
HEALER: Sushama Saldanha

I had been married for seven years and like any married couple, my husband and I were looking forward to having our baby, but as luck would have it, even though I would conceive, I would have a miscarriage in a month and a half or so.

This happened on four to five occasions and the longest I was able to hold the foetus was three months, despite good medical care and assistance. Medical opinion varied from doctor to doctor and though we gave all of it a fair try, no benefit seemed to accrue. This brought about despondency in my life and a lot of disharmony in my relationship with my husband.

We heard of pranic healing from a friend of ours. After talking to Ms. Sushama Saldanha of the possibilities that pranic healing could offer, for the first time, we saw a ray of hope. We began therapy right away and in a couple of sessions, I was already beginning to feel a different person and deep within, something was happening to me which I cannot put into words.

Three months of pranic healing and I was pregnant again. I took treatments regularly for another couple of months or so. My pregnancy continued normally and all medical tests proved fine. I was blessed with a beautiful baby girl in nine months. Our life now has a different dimension, thanks to Sushama Saldanha and to pranic healing.

(Signed) GEETHA SUKUMAR
July 18, 1997

TESTIMONIALS

NAME:	Prema Srinivasan
ADDRESS:	H-8/6, IInd Avenue, Indira Nagar Chennai - 600 020 INDIA
AGE:	37
OCCUPATION:	Housewife/Seamstress
CASE:	Cataract
HEALER:	Radhika Reddy

It was the end of October 1995 when my eyes began to give me trouble. On medical examination, it was diagnosed as early cataract to the extent of about 35 %. The doctor advised me to wait till the cataract was fully matured and then to undergo surgery.

Having heard of pranic healing, I decided to try it out in the meantime and went to the Pranic Healing Center at Adyar. I began therapy on November 2, 1995 and took 15 sessions till December 8, 1995, after which upon the advice of the healer, I went to my ophthalmologist for a test.

I was very happy to hear his findings that my eyes were totally normal and that I had nothing to worry about. I continued pranic healing sessions for some more time and then took the basic course.

I went on to do the Advanced and Psychotherapy courses too and am now a regular healer at the same center.

What a tremendous contribution to well being this art and science is!

(Signed) PREMA SRINIVASAN
July 18, 1997

NAME: Goverdan Das
ADDRESS: M/s Bala Tourist Service
132 A Kodambakkam High Road
Chennai - 600 034 INDIA
AGE: 46
OCCUPATION: Business Clerk
CASE: Post-Surgical Complications (Brain)
HEALER: Severine Menezes

I had undergone brain surgery for removal of a blood clot as a result of intradural bleeding. I also had hemiplegia (paralysis of one side of the body). Though technically the surgery was declared successful, I was worst off after it, suffering loss of memory, numbness of the limbs, giddiness, chronic constipation and ulceration in the mouth and throat.

This made me totally dependent on others and I was unable to eat solid food, making me very weak and miserable. I was sure my end was near and I was preparing myself and the members of my family for what seemed the inevitable. To my good luck, I was introduced to Pranic Healing and though I did not know what to expect from it, I was willing to undergo this treatment for whatever it was worth.

This was God-sent; after the very first treatment, I experienced a tremendous relaxation in my body and was already feeling pretty good. A few sessions later, it was a miracle that the ulceration in my mouth and throat had almost disappeared and I was able to eat solid food. After a few more sessions, my bowel movements began to improve and in a couple of days, there was no trace of constipation too.

I had definitely improved. Pranic healing brought me back from the mouth of death and despair and now after a few weeks of regular treatment, I am absolutely normal and am travelling all around on my own. I am back to living life fully. Many thanks to pranic healing and more so to Ms. Severine.

(Signed) GOVERDAN DAS
July 19, 1997

NAME: N. Manoharan
ADDRESS: 12C, Pocket A13, Kalkaji Extension
New Delhi - 110 019, INDIA
AGE: 62
OCCUPATION: Engineer
CASE: Cervical Spondylitis*
HEALER: P. G. Krishnamachari

I used to suffer from cervical spondylitis for many years. I tried allopathy, homeopathy and Tibetan medicines. One day, while strolling in the neighbouring park, an acquaintance, Krishnamachari, noticed my discomfiture. He offered and gave me a healing right there at the park. I felt an immediate sense of relief, unlike pain killers which used to take almost an hour to relieve any pain.

I decided to have a few more sessions of pranic healing. Within about eight healings, I was fully relieved of the pain, almost unbelievable to me.

In the meantime, I had found that Pranic Healing is simple for me to learn. I decided to take it up with the hope that I will also be able to help others in the way I had been helped. Looking back to my decision, I find that it had virtually changed my life to something happier.

(Signed) N. MANOHARAN
July 17, 1997

---

*Cervical Spondylitis is the inflammation of the neck vertebrae.

TESTIMONIALS

NAME:	N. Manoharan
ADDRESS:	12C, Pocket A13, Kalkaji Extension
	New Delhi - 110 019, INDIA
AGE:	62
OCCUPATION:	Engineer
CASE:	1. Ulcerative Colitis*
	2. Night Blindness and Hearing Loss

CASE 1: Ulcerative Colitis

Anita Keshari, who is in her early 20s from Type IV, NRC-48, PUSA Campus, New Delhi, has been suffering from blood-stained diarrhea. She had tried all forms of therapies but they all proved to be in vain. Finally, she was advised to undergo surgery to remove most parts of her large intestine and was told to return within one week.

It was at this time that she heard about pranic healing. Her worried mother took Anita to the Pranic Healing clinic. Within a few healings, there was indication of relief. The attending physician advised postponement of surgery. After some more healings, her condition improved and the doctor agreed that clinically she was fit and could avoid surgery.

Many months after, Anita is now healthy and feels that she has overcome her problem fully. Interestingly, many visits to the Pranic Healing Center induced confidence in her to take Pranic Healing courses. Today, she is a good healer.

---

*Ulcerative Colitis is the chronic inflammation of the linings of the colon manifested by recurring bloody diarrhea, abdominal cramps and anemia. Associated symptoms may be bone, skin and blood abnormalities.

Case 2: Night Blindness and Hearing Loss

Paresh Awasthi, a 29-year old businessman, of E-17, Greater Kailash-II, New Delhi, had been living with the problem of night blindness and hearing impairment. He had difficulty moving around by himself in lowly-lit areas. To overcome his hearing impairment, he used a hearing aid. He consulted medical doctors but received no positive assurance of a solution to his problems.

Having heard about pranic healing, he visited the Sri Aurobindo Pranic Healing Center. When he came to me for treatment, he was receptive to the suggestion of continued healing for a few days. In three weeks, he started to feel some improvement in his sight. After nearly three months, he could see better at night also. His hearing improved and slowly he got rid of the hearing aid as well.

He is grateful for the help of pranic healing and thanks Master Choa Kok Sui and this healer. He is already taking steps to learn this great art and science so he can help others to benefit from it too.

(Signed) N. MANOHARAN
July 17, 1997

NAME:	Preethi Mythili
ADDRESS:	HZ Ring Road Apartments
	Periyar Pathai Vadapalani
	Madras - 94 INDIA
CASE:	Chronic Vomiting
HEALERS:	T.K. Mythili and Padmini Sharma

My daughter Preethi had been vomiting for the past five months. She became very weak and was not able to eat anything. At that time, I started doing pranic healing with the help of Ms. Padmini Sharma. I did it regularly with full confidence. Slowly, I saw her condition improving. Now she is totally free from vomiting. I am happy about it. I thank God for introducing pranic healing to me because through it I was able to cure my child.

(Signed) T.K. MYTHILI
(Mother)
July 17, 1997

NAME: Handoyo Gazali
ADDRESS: Pinang Suasa 3/UA 31 Pondok Indah
Jakarta 12310
INDONESIA
AGE: 47
OCCUPATION: Project Manager
CASE: Intermittent Blackouts

Dwi A. Srijanti, who is 33 years old, sought medical help for her on and off blackout spells. The neurologist's diagnosis indicated that there were leakages found in the bridges of fine blood vessels leading to the cerebellum, causing dysfunction of the optic nerves. Surgery was recommended but with a very risky health benefit to the patient. She objected to this and preferred to solve her problem through alternative medicine, pranic healing in particular.

The patient underwent pranic treatment three times a week for the first three months, followed by two times a week for one year. This approach resulted in the total recovery of the patient.

We have all the medical data of the patient which were taken before, during and after the pranic treatments to support the effectiveness of this alternative medicine approach.

(Signed) HANDOYO GAZALI
July 23, 1997

NAME:	Dr. Indah Yulianto
ADDRESS:	Jl. Adisuciato 46. Solo, INDONESIA
AGE:	45
OCCUPATION:	Dermato-venereologist
CASES:	1. Pre- and Post-Liposuction Treatments
	2. Post-herpetic Neuralgia

1. Pre- and Post-liposuction Treatments

After doing liposuction (Surgical removal of local fat deposits) for lipostructure in more than 150 patients, I have experienced that they would be restless and would complain of pain for three days. The liposuction takes about two hours and has to be performed by three doctors.

After I learned pranic healing in March 1997, I applied it to my 10 latest patients. Before doing liposuction, I would clean the affected part with light green prana and then energized it with light blue prana. Suctioning the fat deposit became easier and painless. The operative process is also faster and I can do it alone in 45 minutes. Even after the operation, my patients told me that they did not suffer from any pain.

2. Post-herpetic Neuralgia

The patient had been suffering from herpes zoster facialis-dextra for the last three months. He had undergone a two-week treatment as an in-patient in the department of ophthalmology in the hospital. Later, he became an out-patient of a neurologist for three months due to unbearable pain in the affected area. He would always experience nightmares and could not have a good sleep. Though other doctors had given him tranquilizers and painkillers, the suffering persisted. As a result, his weight was down by five kilograms.

I applied general sweeping and localized sweeping on all his major chakras using electric violet and energized the affected part and all the upper chakras with light green and light blue.

After two days, the patient, who had been assisted by his son during the previous session, came to me half-running for his second treatment. Overjoyed, he tapped happily on my table. The chronic diabeticum neuritis and arthritis in his two crippled fingers was now normal. His high blood pressure and uric acid level, also previously high, were also normal.

I applied the same treatment as the first session, but I added whitish green and whitish violet on both hands, liver, pancreas, heart, back head, spine and the thymus, thyroid, pituitary and pineal glands.

After three treatments, given every two days in one week, the blood pressure became 140/95 and the blood sugar was 135 mg./100 ml. All complaints of pain has disappeared and his condition has normalized. He is now back working as a farmer.

Pranic Healing is very complimentary to my dermatologic practice. I find it very useful.

(Signed) DR. INDAH YULIANTO
July 1997

NAME:	Ir Hardoyo
ADDRESS:	Jl Usip Sumoharjo 91 Solo
	INDONESIA
AGE:	46
OCCUPATION:	Architect
CASE:	Anal Fistula

A 49-year old medical doctor who had been suffering from a fistula in his anus came to me for pranic healing treatment. Due to the "hole" in his perineum, he had to wear a a sanitary napkin everyday to prevent the smell of the secretions from coming out. This has caused him so much distress.

Earlier, he had consulted a surgeon in Singapore who suggested surgery for his condition. The doctor said, however, that there was no guarantee that he would be cured and there might be the possibility of a relapse. Scared, he tried to look for an alternative treatment and found pranic healing.

During the first treatment, I followed the procedure in Master Choa's *Advanced Pranic Healing* book. Using green prana, I cleansed the affected part and then I mentally visualized that I was sewing the hole with a surgical thread until it was perfectly closed. Later, I projected yellow prana, followed by violet prana as an "antibiotic".

The patient felt that he was already cured after two treatments but he continued to undergo pranic healing for about ten sessions more. Wanting to be certain about his recovery, he went back to his surgeon in Singapore for a final assurance. The surgeon signed a certificate which confirmed that he was now completely healed.

(Signed) IR HARDOYO
July 1997

NAME: Dr. Nani Wigati
ADDRESS: Jl. Usip Sumoharjo 91, Solo
INDONESIA
AGE: 43
OCCUPATION: Medical Doctor and Pranic Healer
CASE: Ulnar Bone Fracture with Dislocation

Mrs. Hendrati who is 57-years old came to me with a severe swelling in the right elbow joint, caused by a fall. X-ray results showed a fracture of the ulnar bone with dislocation, a part of it pointing sideward. According to the orthopedist, the swollen part had to be treated first, after which the fracture would have to be operated.

The patient came to the Solo Pranic Healing Center for treatment. I cleansed the affected area carefully and thoroughly with whitish green and whitish orange. I also visualized the fractured bone returning to the right position and normalizing. Then I energized it with whitish green and whitish blue. To cement the broken bone, I used yellow and whitish orange, and a combination of whitish orange and whitish red.

After three times of pranic treatment, the patient was cured totally as attested by the results of x-ray tests.

(Signed) DR. NANI WIGATI
July 1997

NAME:	Dr. Petrus Lukmanto
ADDRESS:	Jalan Kayumanis VIII/51, Jakarta Timur
	Jakarta 13130, INDONESIA
AGE:	44
OCCUPATION:	Medical Practitioner and Pranic Healer
CASE:	Acute Renal Failure

My patient, Ir Haryanto who is 55 years old, has been diagnosed with Acute Renal Failure. He had symptoms of severe nausea and vomiting, fever and weakness. Laboratory values showed an elevated urea level of 280 (normal value is up to 50) and creatinine was 11.2 (normal value is up to 1-2).

I treated him thrice a day for 14 days. The symptoms gradually disappeared and after 12 days, the urea and creatinine levels returned to their normal levels. At present, the urea and creatinine are still normal.

In the beginning, I myself almost did not believe in my ability to heal patients with pranic energy because the response is quite fast. I have treated some patients who suffered from stroke or cerebrovascular accident and they became normal after one or two sessions only.

I find pranic healing very useful in accelerating the natural healing process of the body. It is a powerful healing tool and the result is often miraculous.

(Signed) DR. PETRUS LUKMANTO
July 1997

NAME:	Bernadette Hickey
ADDRESS:	33 Pineview Drive, Aylesbury D-24, IRELAND
AGE:	40
OCCUPATION:	Curtain maker
CASE:	Lump on the side of the knee
HEALER:	Bernadette Sheridan

I went to my doctor in April 1996 with a large lump on the side of my knee. This lump was giving me so much discomfort. At night, it felt like sand moving about inside. My doctor was very concerned and sent me immediately for x-rays.

On my return to his clinic, he could not believe that the results of the tests were negative and the lump had disappeared. He told me that he had been afraid that the lump was cancerous. I told him that since I had last seen him and before my x-rays, I had gone to Bernadette Sheridan, a pranic healer. He told me to stay with her since whatever she was doing was right. He could not believe the results she had achieved. To this day, I have had no problems and my knee is perfect!

(Signed) BERNADETTE HICKEY
May 21, 1997

NAME:	Christine Walsh
ADDRESS:	Breaffy, Castlebar, Co. Mayo
	IRELAND
AGE:	48
OCCUPATION:	Primary School Teacher
CASES:	Pneumonia; Acute Backpain
HEALERS:	Jack and Lulu Hynes

In July 1996, I suffered from severe pain under my left shoulder blade and had difficulty breathing. I went to my doctor who diagnosed me with pneumonia in the left lung. She put me on a course of antibiotics. This, however, failed to alleviate my condition so the doctor suggested that I should be confined in the hospital. I refused and she put me on a different course of antibiotics.

This was when I began pranic treatment. After just two sessions of pranic crystal healing, the pain under my left shoulder disappeared and has never recurred. The pneumonia cleared and my doctor was very surprised at how quickly I have recovered from my illness.

In May 1997, I had acute back pain which totally immobilized me. After just one session of pranic healing, the pain eased substantially and I was able to move freely again. It was like a miracle.

I am so grateful that I was priveleged to be introduced to Pranic Healing.

(Signed) CHRISTINE WALSH
August 18, 1997

NAME:	Milena Panzavolta
ADDRESS:	Via Carradori 19, Carpinello (FO), ITALY
AGE:	41
OCCUPATION:	Employee
CASE:	Breast Cancer
HEALER:	Loretta Zanucolli

A cancer in my right breast had been diagnosed on October 7, 1996. Since my son was already being assisted and given therapies for his allergies at the center (*Gruppo Romagna Pranic Healing*), I asked Loretta to treat me too.

Six months later, when I went for another medical check up, the doctors were astonished and couldn't believe that the cancer had disappeared.

I believe that this healing method is very valid and wonderful. I think that everybody should undergo this new technique.

(Signed) MILENA PANZAVOLTA
May 21, 1997

NAME:	David Cheah
ADDRESS:	3 Jin Abang Haji Openg Satu,
	Taman Tun Dr. Ismail
	60000 Kuala Lumpur, MALAYSIA
AGE:	34
OCCUPATION:	Architect/Painter
CASE:	Arthritic pain on the fingers

I was finishing some paintings for my first exhibit when I experienced arthritic pain on the joints of the fingers of my left and right hands. I felt that the problem could be psychological or anxiety- and stress-related, occurring at a time when I was branching out into a new career direction. Initially, it would come and go, especially when I was painting, washing brushes, etc., making it difficult to use my hands and fingers. Later, the pain was almost constantly there — not excruciating but irritating pain — even when I wasn't using my hands and fingers.

After one healing session, all of the pain on the right hand has vanished and my left hand only experiences occasional discomfort when I wash brushes, etc. for a long time. Apart from that, it's back to painting as normal!

(Signed) DAVID CHEAH
May 22, 1997

NAME:	Maria de la Luz Bautista Rivera
ADDRESS:	Calle Nogal 205, Colonia Corralejo, Zuazua, N.L., MEXICO
AGE:	55
OCCUPATION:	Housewife
CASE:	Brain Tumor
HEALER:	Dr. Domingo Garcia Hernandez

Two years ago, I had bouts of a terribly strong headache. My hands and arms trembled. I could neither keep them still nor could I take hold of anything with my hands. I could not also sleep well.

I consulted a neurosurgeon at a public health hospital. His diagnosis, according to a computerized scan, was a brain tumor. He scheduled me for surgery on May 26, 1997, but I did not accept the idea of undergoing the procedure. Instead, I decided to look for an alternative treatment.

I started pranic healing sessions with Dr. Domingo Garcia Hernandez on May 6, 1997. He detected a severe congestion on the left side of the head. The treatments were done in 10 sessions in a span of one month — three times per week during the first and second weeks, and two times per week during the third and fourth weeks. The symptoms disappeared completely just after a week of healing.

After pranic treatment a month later, another computerized scan was taken. The result of the test showed that the tumor was almost gone. Now the surgery has been postponed for six months while I continue with the pranic treatments until the tumor disappears completely.

Thanks to Pranic Healing as an alternative healing. I have recovered my normal way of life and avoided a high-risk surgery.

(Signed) MARIA DE LA LUZ BAUTISTA RIVERA
August 1, 1997

TESTIMONIALS

NAME:	Monica Lozano Garza
ADDRESS:	Andadores 38 Edificio Vallecito Dep. 1 Col. Cumbres, Monterrey, N.L., MEXICO
AGE:	43
OCCUPATION:	Actress
CASE:	Pneumonia; Backpain; Stress and Tension
HEALER:	Victor Longoria

I had been experiencing severe back pain since I was young. I was also under a lot of stress and I felt tense most of the time. I contracted pneumonia and went to see some doctors.

At the same time, I underwent pranic treatment — three sessions every five days. In the first session, Mr. Victor Longoria treated my back pain, the stress and tension and the pneumonia. Since then, the back pain disappeared completely; my breathing problem subsided as well as the stress and tension. During the next sessions, Mr. Longoria treated just the pneumonia. After the three sessions, I have recovered and feel very happy.

Thanks to Pranic Healing. It is the fastest technique I have ever tried to regain my health.

(Signed) MONICA LOZANO GARZA
August 2, 1997

NAME:	Edith Meex
ADDRESS:	Spijkerweg 5
	6584 AB Molenhoek
	THE NETHERLANDS
OCCUPATION:	Pranic Healer, Rebalancer, Teacher, Reader-healer
CASE:	1. Arthritis
	2. Migraine

As I am already working professionally with body-mind-spirit awareness, it is interesting to see what pranic healing has added to the whole.

Since I took the pranic healing workshop, sessions with clients take less time and are more effective and sufficient. In the past, I was guided more by intuition and often did not know what or why healings worked the way they did. Now I know how it works and what I can use in special cases. I also had often felt limited to handle situations with clients in pain but now I believe pranic healing, if used in the proper way, has unlimited possibilities. Also, before the course, I was quite worn out and longed for days off. Pranic healing provided me with practical and simple tools on how to take care of myself as a healer and therapist.

Before Pranic Healing came into my life, I often felt I worked alone. Now, I have "teamed up" with the Divine. It feels like a nice way to express it. I actually experience the connection with the Divine and I can use my own intelligence as well — for example, knowing what colors to use. Pranic healing gives a sort of "finishing touch" to the sessions. I have never come across a stronger healing art.

TESTIMONIALS

Case 1: Arthritis

Mrs. M has some arthritis in her left knee and could not walk properly. I practiced distance healing on her. She did not know about this. A few days later, she called me and *en passant* said, "You'll never guess what I did. I went for a long walk as the pain on my knee is gone." I was very amazed at first and it took a few minutes to realize what was happening here. It filled me with gratitude, but there was also some fear. This is so powerful.... Two weeks later she called; she ruptured her left-knee ligaments. Then I remembered the part in the book that tells about the phenomenon. Again, I was amazed.

Case 2: Migraine

Mrs. H has severe migraine attacks every month for about four or five days. During the first session, I followed the procedure as recommended in the book. I asked her to give me a ring if the migraine occurs. A few days later, when she had the migraine, the aura of the head area was really hot and I gently swept it with green and blue till it cooled down. She felt relieved. While energizing, I implanted the thought that the relief would increase during the next few hours and the veins would relax and go back to their healthy state. That was exactly what happened. The next day, the migraine was history. She was very happy to have had it for one day only.

Until then, migraine was one of the ailments I did not know how to handle with clients. I am very please with the result. We will do some more sessions to see whether she can let go of it totally.

(Signed) EDITH MEEX
June 17, 1997

NAME: Edgardo Anacan
ADDRESS: 10 Tiamson St., Midtown Subdivision
Paranaque, Metro Manila
PHILIPPINES
OCCUPATION: Retired Businessman
CASE: Emphysema

Sometime in 1988, I had difficulty breathing and was coughing severely, causing my shoulders to hunch. I shed off five kilos and lost my voice. I was very, very weak. I could hardly walk and talk because of breathing difficulty. I had to rest every time I climbed each step of the stairs to catch my breath.

Due to my very poor health condition, I went to the Philippine Lung Center for a medical checkup. My doctor told me I had emphysema. This disease is not alien to me. Two of my best friends and an uncle of my wife died of it. I knew that there was no cure for this illness, so I resigned myself to my fate and told myself that if I die, so be it. I then gave instructions to my wife and sons about my burial and gave my business to one of my sons.

One day I came upon a book on pranic healing. After reading it, I went to the pranic healing center every day for treatment. After several sessions, my voice returned and I was full of energy. I noticed a big improvement. So I continued with the pranic treatments three times a week, then twice a week, for about six months.

After six months, I went back to the Philippine Lung Center for my medical checkup and my doctor pronounced that I was 90 percent healed!

I still continued to submit myself to pranic treatment for several more months until I already felt normal. Today, after a year, I can say that I am completely healed.

(Signed) EDGARDO B. ANACAN
September 2, 1989

NAME:	Jose Pangngay, Sr.
ADDRESS:	Mt. Data, Bauko
	Mountain Province, PHILIPPINES
OCCUPATION:	Security Officer
CASE:	Abdominal Pain
HEALERS:	Hermie Corcuera and Faith Sawey

On December 3, 1995, my abdomen suddenly became painful. A few hours later, the pain became very severe. I could hardly stand up and walk because of the piercing sensation that was localized on the right lower portion of my abdomen. I was also having high-grade fever and chills, and I vomited several times.

I felt blessed, however, that at the time there were two teachers, Hermie Corcuera and Faith Sawey, who were conducting a Pranic Healing seminar in Mt. Data. I requested them to heal me and was partially relieved. Approximately 60 % of the pain was still there, especially on the right lower portion. I decided to seek medical help and was confined at the Lutheran Hospital in Abatan, Bugias, Benguet at 12:00 midnight of the same day. The doctor's impression was to rule out acute appendicitis. He advised further observation and appendectomy (surgical removal of the appendix) should the signs and symptoms worsen. I requested to be transferred to Baguio Medical Center where there was more advanced equipment. Shortly after my release from the Lutheran Hospital, I asked my companion to take me back to Mt. Data to continue the pranic healing treatment.

After the treatment, I was taken to Benguet Laboratories in Baguio City. Several laboratory examinations were made to validate the previous findings at Lutheran Hospital and to consider the possibility of an appendectomy. When the results came out, the medical director was surprised to find out that everything was normal!

(Signed) JOSE PANGNGAY, SR.
March 1997

NAME: Allan C. Cañete
ADDRESS: 3-I Stanford Street, Cubao
Quezon City, PHILIPPINES
AGE: 24
OCCUPATION: Student
CASE: One-Day-Old Wound

The width of the wound on the sole of my left foot was about 1/4 of an inch. There was a little bleeding but it was very painful because of a small seashell particle left inside the wound (I had stepped on a sharp seashell in one of the beaches at Agoo, La Union). I tried hard to remove it but to no avail. No medicine was administered before, during, and after the application of pranic healing.

The wound was one day old, but I could no longer use my left foot. Although it was not infected, symptoms showed that infection might set in.

I was given two successive pranic treatments, first, by some pranic healing students. Actually, the procedure was just an experiment on rapid healing suggested by the author.

The second treatment was administered by the author and it took him only one and a half hours to rapidly and completely heal my wound right before my eyes! During both the first and the second treatments, I could feel a tickling, tingling sensation even if there was no skin contact because the distance between the healer's hand and my wound was about one centimeter apart. After the second treatment, I could feel very little pain and could use again my left foot for walking even if the seashell particle was still inside the healed wound. After two days I removed the seashell with my fingernails. The healing mentioned took place in a running vehicle.

I find this healing technique very strange but the result is amazing and very effective. In the ordinary method of treating a wound, it would take several days to have it healed, besides the possibility of having it infected during the process. With pranic healing, it took only about three and a half hours to heal the wound right before my eyes without much ado and without infection during and after the treatment.

                                     (Signed) ALLAN C. CAÑETE
                                          December 26, 1986

NAME: Alvin de los Santos
ADDRESS: 207 Interior Reparo St., Baesa
Quezon City, PHILIPPINES
AGE: 7
CASE: Urinary Ailment

When my son was five years old, he had a kidney ailment and his attack was severe. He had high blood pressure, high fever, generalized edema, difficulty in breathing and discharging urine from the body, and pain in the area around his urinary bladder and ureters. His urine was reddish. He got tired very easily and his studies in preparatory school were disrupted because of his ailment.

After an interval of about six months from the first attack, his ailment recurred. The second attack was not so severe as the first. He had pain in the area around the urinary bladder and ureters, and had difficulty urinating and the color of his urine was deep yellow.

I took him to a kidney specialist for treatment. The medication given for the first and second attacks was the same and it greatly relieved him of most discomforts, except for the pain around the urinary bladder and ureters. He was advised to avoid too much physical exertion, which meant no playing — a torment for any child like my son.

When his ailment recurred for the third time, he experienced a piercing pain in the area around the urinary bladder and ureters. He still had difficulty discharging urine, which was yellow-orange in color. I did not let him take any pills or medications. I took him instead to a pranic healer for treatment. The pranic healer advised me not to include salty foods in Alvin's diet. He gave pranic treatments thrice within a two-week period.

After the treatments, my son experienced a dramatic change and improvement in his health condition; his ailment has not recurred up to this time. Before, he got tired very easily. But now, he plays like any other children. The difficulty in passing urine and the piercing pain he had felt completely disappeared. So far, there has been no disruption in his studies.

(Signed) MERLITA DE LOS SANTOS
(mother)
January 15, 1987

NAME: Marilou Gatchalian
ADDRESS: 4 Bedana St., San Nicholas
Pasig City, PHILIPPINES
AGE: 35
OCCUPATION: Housewife
CASE: Kidney Ailment

I first experienced pain during urination on May 30, 1989. The next day, my urine was already tainted with fresh blood. I then took a sample of my urine to a laboratory for urinalysis. Then I took the results to a lady physician for proper advice and medication. I was given a pain killer and told that the urinalysis indicated no infection and that bleeding might have been due to kidney stones. I was then advised to see a urologist.

On the third day, the pain became more intense and the bleeding continued. It was also on this day that the urologist prescribed first aid medicines to ease the pain. I was also advised to undergo laboratory testing to determine whether bleeding was due to kidney stones or hemorrhagic cystitis. The laboratory testing was supposed to be done in the afternoon. Unfortunately, some of the medicines needed for the procedure were not available in the laboratory and had to be bought outside. Sadly too, some of the medicines needed were not available in Quezon City. The laboratory testing was rescheduled. That same day, I went straight to the pranic healing center for treatment.

Pranic treatment was continuously administered for nine days except one Sunday when the center was closed. On the fifth day of pranic treatment, I experienced considerable relief and was able to urinate with greater ease.

Every morning, after the previous afternoon's pranic treatment, my urine showed traces of minute, grainy substances similar to a pulverized brownish powder with some blood clots. This was the case for four to five days. I did not anymore subject myself to further laboratory testing. On Thursday, June 8, 1989, the bleeding stopped completely. Although I could still feel a little discomfort, the pain was gone and so were the grainy substances. I received more pranic treatments on June 9 and 10. Now, I am back to my normal self again. But this time, I am very careful with my diet. I also avoid doing strenuous physical activities.

While I was undergoing pranic treatment, I had always kept my lady physician-friend posted of my daily improvement (she has attended the Pranic Healing workshop given by the Institute for Inner Studies), and was equally ecstatic about how I got well and avoided a possible operation to remove the kidney stones which, according to her, would have cost from 25,000 to 35,000 pesos.

I am truly thankful and very grateful that pranic healing has provided relief not only to me but also to many others equally afflicted. Each treatment is an experience where one feels closer to God – indeed an experience of Thanksgiving.

(Signed) MARILOU GATCHALIAN
July 20, 1989

NAME:	Lolita S. Ramos
ADDRESS:	5 K-JJ Kamias Road
	Quezon City, PHILIPPINES
OCCUPATION:	School Teacher
	Quirino Elementary School
	Quezon City
CASE:	Burn
HEALER:	Hector Ramos

My left hand was burned by boiling cooking oil which I had poured from the frying pan. I cried because of the severe pain. Three of my fingers - the middle, ring and little fingers - and almost one third of my palm were swollen red. My little finger became as big as my middle finger.

Hector, my son, offered to heal me, but I kept on crying. My son had already cured me on a number of occasions in the past but they were all minor ailments like toothaches and colds. So, I really had my doubts because I felt that, in this case, the injury was a severe one.

This was the longest time he spent curing me. After almost forty-five minutes, I could bend my three fingers with the help of my right hand. The pain had been greatly reduced.

The next morning, my palm had only three tiny red spots. Hector healed it again and after a while, my swollen eyes (due to crying) were the only evidence of my experience. There was not even a dark spot on my hand which usually happens when tiny drops of cooking oil would splash on it while frying food.

That same day, I assisted in giving the Civil Service Examination held in the school. My co-teachers asked why my eyes were swollen. I told them of my very unusual experience but there was no trace of it on my hand. Some of my co-teachers started to ask help from my son so that they might be cured too. He spent time with them last summer of 1989.

(Signed) LOLITA S. RAMOS
September 7, 1989

NAME: James Ansell Castañarez
ADDRESS: 274-C Esquivel Apt., P. Mariano St.
Ususan, Taguig, Metro Manila
PHILIPPINES
AGE: 3
CASE: Jaw Inflammation

Though I had read of Choa Kok Sui from a Philippine Daily Inquirer article by Nick Joaquin and got hold of his book on pranic healing, it was months later when I got to meet him personally.

I met him auspiciously in one of the meditation meetings conducted by his group. That night, he healed my three-year-old son of a jaw inflammation which was set for operation at Makati Medical Center. The jaw inflammation caused by anaerobic infection was gone in three days without recourse to operation. Since then I became an avid believer of his healing ability after this episode.

(Signed) GREG CASTAÑAREZ
(father)
September 2, 1989

NAME:	Mary G. Lee
ADDRESS:	123 Scout Lozano St.,
	Quezon City, PHILIPPINES
AGE:	69
OCCUPATION:	Housewife
CASE:	Arthritis

Sometime in 1984, I experienced pain on both legs, from the knees down to the feet. My knees, especially, were quite painful and swollen. Between 1985 and this year (1989), the arthritic pain went up my right hip. My right elbow too became painful but not swollen. During severe arthritic attacks, I had difficulty getting up. There were times when I would be bedridden for two weeks.

Unfortunately, I did not consult any doctor because I was afraid to know their findings. For four years, I just took pain killers and herbal medicines.

In May 1989, my arthritis became very severe. The pain became so intense and my knees became more swollen. Finally, I decided to consult a medical doctor at the University of Santo Tomas Hospital. After two weeks of taking the prescribed medicines, I noticed that I developed a slur in my speech. My mouth and face became slightly twisted. My attending physician was alarmed and directed me to see a neurologist who immediately instructed me to stop taking all my medicines. At that very moment, he confined me in the hospital because he said I was about to have a stroke — caused by the medicines I had taken.

The neurologist gave me another set of medications to lower my blood pressure which was then 160/100. It went down to 130/80. After being confined for two and a half days, I was sent home.

About the last week of May, a friend who had been going to the pranic healing center for her kidney problem visited me. She said that she felt relieved after every treatment. Since I did not know anything about pranic healing, I decided to wait and see how it could help my friend before going to the healing center myself. So, for quite sometime I would call my friend regularly to ask if there was any improvement in her condition. I learned later that her ailment had not recurred.

On June 22, I finally decided to go to the healing center for treatment. I was very weak and was limping. The first time I was treated, I felt something warm going inside my body. The pain on my knees diminished and the pain on my right elbow disappeared. From that time on, I went to the healing center three times a week.

On the first week of August, after more than a month of treatment, the pain on my knees became mild and the swelling disappeared. As instructed by the healer, I took a bath with water and salt to cleanse my body. On August 15, all the pain disappeared and I felt a cool, soothing sensation or some energy circulating inside my legs.

Now some of my friends comment that I look healthier, stronger and younger. To this date, I have not experienced any pain or relapse. I walk a lot now. I can walk to the market alone which used to be impossible. Before, just walking two blocks from our house made me very tired. But now, I can walk a few kilometers a day without any problem at all. I walk from our place to Kamuning market and back for three rounds.

I still visit the pranic healing center regularly for recharging.

(Signed) MARY G. LEE
August 24, 1989

NAME:	Vicki Seng Pek Armes
ADDRESS:	18 Jalan Lembah Thomson, S.577489 SINGAPORE
AGE:	38
OCCUPATION:	Forensic Scientist - Scenes of Crime Officer, Police (U.K.) Manager - Pranic Workshop Pte. Ltd. (Singapore)
CASE:	Nose Bleeds, Allergic Reactions, Minor Cuts and Abrasion

My seven-and-a-half-year old son had been suffering for years since the age of three from frequent nose bleeds. On the average, it would take about 15-20 minutes of ice packs, nose pinching and pressure to stop the bleeding.

Such a nose bleed occurred the day after I took the Master Choa Kok Sui Pranic Healing Course. I reacted quickly by applying localized sweeping to the ajna. To everyone's amazement, the nose bleed stopped after three sweeps. I continued to apply a dozen or more local sweeps to the ajna, then energized with a little white prana. Since that day I've treated his now-quite-rare nose bleeds with the same technique, but now I use color prana. This has, of course, lessened the healing time.

Some other experiences of almost instant healings have occurred in the schools that I have taught in. Here cuts, abrasions, allergic reactions, aches and sprains occur numerously. One seven-year old girl had reacted to facial make-up at a school concert. Although she had removed the make-up half an hour before seeing me, her face, eyes, cheeks and neck were still swollen, itchy and painful. Upon scanning, the affected areas were hot and prickly. I applied localized sweeping immediately with light whitish green and light whitish blue on all the affected areas. Within one minute, the swelling and the puffiness subsided. I continued sweeping until the areas were thoroughly cleansed. Her face and neck returned to their normal color. She walked away as if nothing had happened.

I also found that in cases of minor cuts and abrasions, using advanced pranic healing worked wonders in stopping the bleeding and in alleviating pain.

Of all the patients that I have healed, I have always found children — no matter what age — to be the most receptive.

(Signed) VICKI SENG PEK ARMES
August 3, 1997

NAME:	Patricia Rüesch
ADDRESS:	Matthofring 26, 6005 Luzern (CH)
	SWITZERLAND
AGE:	33
OCCUPATION:	Homeopathist, Energy Work
CASE:	Skin rashes
HEALER:	Cheryl Weiss

Three weeks ago I had a skin rash that began on my shoulders, spread over my back and then finally over the upper part of my arms and also around the hip area. The rashes were reddish but didn't itch. I thought about going to the doctor for diagnosis. But then I thought that now I could give Pranic Healing a chance.

I called Cheryl Weiss and she told me to take a salt water bath the night before the treatment and to make sure to massage my body properly with a cloth and salt in the bath and then lie in the saltwater bath for at least one hour. The following day, Cheryl worked on me a good two hours.

Three days after the treatment, the rash was gone! And ever since then, it has never come back. Also, another skin rash – or what I believe was a skin fungi – that had itched for a long time on the abdominal area also disappeared. That was a very good and helpful treatment. Thank you.

(Signed) PATRICIA RÜESCH
May 25, 1997

NAME:	Max Krausler
ADDRESS:	Kirchmattstr. 34, 6312 Steinhausen
	SWITZERLAND
AGE:	62
OCCUPATION:	Mechanic/Controller
CASE:	Throat Pain and Hoarseness
HEALER:	Stefan Weiss

I smoked up to two packs of cigarettes as well as a pipe several times everyday until 1984. After I quit smoking, symptoms of throat pain and hoarseness occurred with continual recurrence thereafter. To alleviate the pain at night, I had to tie a bandana around my neck.

In January 1997, I met Stefan Weiss who did a short pranic treatment on me. I was totally freed from the throat pain, hoarseness and a choking feeling in the throat area. Another positive effect reached thereafter, I dropped another four kilos of bodyweight.

(Signed) MAX KRAUSLER
July 1997

NAME: Isaac Gomez Cabrera
ADDRESS: Obligado 1296, Montevideo
URUGUAY
AGE: 65
CASE: Parkinson's Disease

In May 1996, I underwent surgery for removal of a "water cyst" from my left kidney. The surgeon told me that I could have some pain in this area for a long time. Some time later, I started feeling cold and painful along the left leg which started to lose strength and weight. I began to limp. The left arm lost vitality and I felt very tired. Allopathic medicine could not provide the cause for my condition. A homeopath diagnosed it as Parkinson's Disease. Besides homeopathic remedies, I was treated with acupuncture, macrobiotic diet, Reiki, Yoga and Ayurveda with no result. New symptoms appeared such as weakened arms and legs, trembling and contraction, hunching of the back, rigidity, difficulty in breathing due to contraction of the diaphragm, weight loss, insomnia, constipation, loss of sexual desire, accelerated aging, overall body weakness and mental confusion.

In July 1977, I attended an introductory conference by Mr. Del Pe, announcing Pranic Healing courses. I immediately sensed that the curriculum was relevant to my problem. I attended the basic and advanced seminars. On the first day, I experienced weakness and fatigue initially. However, as the day ended, I noticed that after doing Meditation on Twin Hearts, I recovered my strength. During the following days, my condition improved considerably. As a result, the dosage of Levo-Dopa, the drug I was taking for Parkinson's, was reduced. On the last day of the Advanced Pranic Healing workshop, I was able to dance the salsa. My voice became stronger and my intellectual capacities began to normalize. By learning and experiencing with Mr. Del Pe the meditation and self-healing techniques, I could feel as if a flow of fresh and pure air has impregnated my whole body, releasing my tense muscles and making them obey my mind's orders.

I have continued practicing everything that I have learned in the workshops — the physical exercises, pranic breathing, meditation and self-healing. I feel I am being born again. My physical appearance is now of a man my age, perhaps even younger.

(Signed) ISAAC GOMEZ CABRERA
July 23, 1997

NAME: Maria Elena Garcia
ADDRESS: Garcia Lago 12, Paso Carrasco
Montevideo, URUGUAY
AGE: 37
CASE: Back Pain
HEALER: Del Pe

Senior Pranic Healer Mr. Del Pe healed my chronic lumbar back pain in five minutes. He taught me a technique to cleanse my chakras to maintain the healthy state of my back. I have been using it successfully ever since. This technique was also applied to remove menstrual cramps. What a relief! Thank you for sharing and teaching us such invaluable information.

(Signed) MARIA ELENA GARCIA
May 15, 1997

NAME: Marisol de Armas
ADDRESS: Calle Los Caciques, Qta "Peluza" Urb El Llanito, Caraca, Miranda, VENEZUELA
AGE: 53
CASE: Migraine
HEALER: Alejandra Graterol

Before July 1996, I suffered from severe migraine which sent me to bed everytime it hit me. The pain was so strong that I cried and thought my head was going to explode. I went to some doctors and they ran tests on me, including tomographies to rule out the possibility of a tumor. There was nothing but the strong pain.

In July 1996, Alejandra Graterol was in my house when I had another migraine attack. She did a healing on me and in just one session, the pain not only disappeared but I haven't had migraine anymore since then for almost a year now. After that, I became a pranic healer also.

(Signed) MARISOL DE ARMAS
May 23, 1997

NAME:	Judy Parra
ADDRESS:	Ave. Ppal Urb. Lomas de Prados del Este, Res. Cybele, Apto 8-D Caracas, Miranda, VENEZUELA
AGE:	40
CASE:	Nasal Allergies
HEALER:	Alejandra Graterol

I have been suffering from nasal allergies for the past 18 years. The frequent attacks has become a major problem for me. The mucus was green and bloody and would turn denser everyday. It got to a point where I had difficulty breathing and I could hear strange sounds in my chest. I was feeling very bad when I met Alejandra Graterol who healed me completely in the first session. With her knowledge, she applied a great healing and I don't know how to repay her. Thanks to all the Masters who prepared her for our good. So be it.

(Signed) JUDY PARRA
May 12, 1997

NAME: Berta Arrico
ADDRESS: Urb. Los Samanes, Calle 13,
Edf. Navacerrada Apto B2
Caracas, Miranda, VENEZUELA
AGE: 53
CASE: Chronic Sinusitis
HEALER: Bonnie Guevara

Since I was 36 years old, I have been suffering from a nasal obstruction that reduced my breathing capacity by 100 percent. This has required me to breathe through my mouth. Since then, I have lost my sense of smell, in addition to a recurring state of unconsciousness.

I have visited several doctors and all of them concluded that I have a congenital allergic condition.

By chance, Mrs. Bonnie Guevarra offered a pranic healing treatment which yielded excellent results. After four sessions, I was able to breathe 100 percent normally. I regained my sense of smell and am more alert to my surroundings.

(Signed) BERTA ARRICO
May 11, 1997

CHAPTER EIGHT

Meditation on Twin Hearts

Without leaving the house, one may know all there is in heaven and earth. Without peeping from the window, one may see the ways of heaven. Those who go out learn less and less the more they travel. Wherefore does the sage know all without going anywhere, see all without looking, do nothing and yet achieve (the Goal)!

– *Lao Tzu,* Tao Te Ching

Meditation should be directed toward the realization of oneness with God. Your entire attention should be given to the realization of God, always bearing in mind that the kingdom of God is within you, neither lo here nor lo there, but within you.

– *Joel Goldsmith*

Illumination Technique or Meditation on Twin Hearts	326
How to Activate the Heart Chakra and the Crown Chakra	332
Increasing One's Healing Power	339
Arhatic Yoga	341
Testimonials	342
Character-Building: The Five Virtues	351
Suggested Schedule	355

ILLUMINATION TECHNIQUE OR MEDITATION ON TWIN HEARTS

Illumination technique or Meditation on Twin Hearts is a technique aimed at achieving cosmic consciousness or illumination. It is also a form of service to the world because the world is harmonized to a certain degree through the blessing of the entire earth with loving-kindness.

Meditation on Twin Hearts is based on the principle that some of the major chakras are entry points or gateways to certain levels or horizons of consciousness. To achieve illumination or cosmic consciousness, it is necessary to sufficiently activate the crown chakra. The Twin Hearts refer to the heart chakra which is the center of the emotional heart, and the crown chakra which is the center of the divine heart.

When the crown chakra is sufficiently activated, its 12 inner petals open and turn upward like a golden cup, golden crown, golden flower or lotus to receive spiritual energy which is distributed to other parts of the body. It is also symbolized as the Holy Grail. The crown worn by kings and queens is but a poor replica or symbol of the indescribable resplendent crown chakra of a spiritually developed person.

The golden crown which is rotating very fast appears as a brilliant flame of light on top of one's head. This is symbolized by the miter worn by the pope, cardinals, and bishops.

When the crown chakra is highly activated, a halo is produced around the head. This is why saints of different religions have a halo around their head. Since there are different degrees of spiritual development, the size and brightness of the halo also vary.

When a person does Meditation on Twin Hearts, divine energy flows down to the practitioner filling him with divine light,

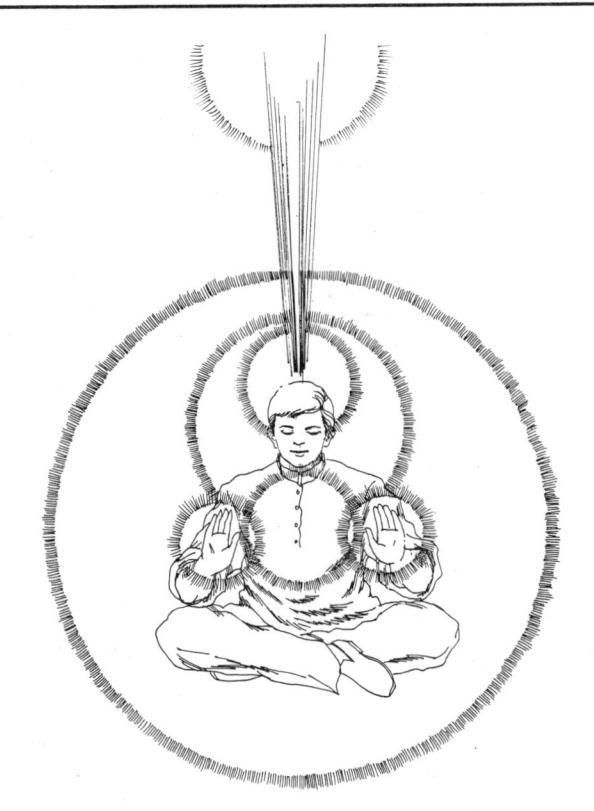

Fig. 8-1 *The Descent of Divine Energy during Meditation on Twin Hearts: In Christian tradition, this is called the descent of the Holy Spirit; in Taoist Yoga, the descent of the Heaven Ki or energy; in Kabbalistic tradition, the pillar of light; in Indian Yoga, the spiritual bridge of light or antakharana.*

love and power. The practitioner becomes a channel of this divine energy. In Taoist Yoga, this divine energy is called "heaven ki." In Kaballah, this is called the "pillar of light," referring to what clairvoyants literally see as a pillar of light. The Indian yogis call this pillar of light as the spiritual bridge of light or "antakharana." The Christians call this the "descent of the Holy Spirit" which is symbolized by a pillar of light with a descending dove. In Christian arts, this is shown in pictures of Jesus or the saints having a pillar of white light on top of their head with a descending white dove. This is to symbolize the coming down of divine energy. Spiritual aspirants who have practiced this meditation for quite sometime may experience being enveloped by dazzling, sometimes blinding, light or his head filled with dazzling light. This has been a common experience among advanced yogis and saints of all religions. If you study the holy scriptures of different religions, you will notice the similarity in their experiences.

The crown chakra can only be sufficiently activated when the heart chakra is first sufficiently activated. The heart chakra is a replica of the crown chakra. When you look at the heart chakra, it looks like the inner chakra of the crown chakra which has 12 golden petals.

The heart chakra is the lower correspondence of the crown chakra. The crown chakra is the center of illumination and divine love or oneness with all. The heart chakra is the center of higher emotions. It is the center for compassion, joy, affection, consideration, mercy and other refined emotions. It is only by developing the higher refined emotions that one can possibly experience divine love. To explain what is divine love and illumination to an ordinary person is just like trying to explain what color is to a blind man.

There are many ways of activating the heart and crown chakras. You can use physical movements or hatha yoga, yogic breathing techniques, mantras or words of power, and visualization techniques. All of these techniques are effective but are not fast enough. One of the most effective and fastest ways to activate these chakras is to do Meditation on Loving-Kindness, or bless the whole earth with loving-kindness. By using the heart and crown chakras in blessing the earth with loving-kindness, they become channels for spiritual energies, thereby becoming activated in the process. By blessing the earth with loving-kindness, you are doing a form of

MEDITATION ON TWIN HEARTS

world service. And by blessing the earth with loving-kindness, you are in turn blessed many times. It is in blessing that you are blessed. It is in giving that you receive. This is the law!

A person with a sufficiently activated crown chakra does not necessarily achieve illumination for he has yet to learn how to use the activated crown chakra. This is just like having a sophisticated computer but not knowing how to operate it. Once the crown chakra has been sufficiently activated, then you have to do meditation on the light, on the mantra om or amen, and on the intervals between the oms or amens. Intense concentration should be focused not only on the mantra om or amen but especially on the interval between the two oms or amens. It is by concentrating on the light and the interval (moment of stillness or silence) between the two oms or amens that illumination or samadhi is achieved!

In yoga, there is a common saying that if the water is turbulent, it is difficult to see what is under it. If the water is calm, one can easily see what is under the water. Likewise, when the mind and the emotions are chaotic, self-realization is not possible. When the mind and the emotions are still, however, it is possible to achieve what Indian yogis call "self-realization," or what is known in Buddhism as "becoming aware of one's true nature" or "illumination" in the Christian religion.

With most people, the other chakras are quite activated. The basic chakra, sex chakra, and solar plexus chakra are activated in practically all persons. Their instincts for self-survival, sex drive and their tendency to react with their lower emotions are very active. With the pervasiveness of modern education and work that require also the use of the mental faculty, the ajna chakra and the throat chakra are developed in a lot of people. The heart chakra and the crown chakra, however, are not developed in most people. Modern education, unfortunately, tends to overemphasize the development of the throat chakra and the ajna chakra, or the development of the concrete mind and the abstract mind. The development of the heart has been neglected. Because of this, you may encounter a person who is quite intelligent but very abrasive. This type of person has not yet matured emotionally or has a heart chakra that is quite underdeveloped. Although he is intelligent and may be "successful," his human relationships may be very poor, hardly having any friend and may have no family. By practicing Meditation on Twin Hearts, a person becomes harmoniously balanced. This means that the major chakras are more or less balancedly developed.

Whether the abstract and concrete mind will be used constructively or destructively depends upon the development of the heart chakra. When the solar plexus chakra is overdeveloped and the heart chakra is underdeveloped or when the lower emotions are active and the higher emotions are underdeveloped, then the mind would likely be used destructively. Without the development of the heart in most people, world peace will not be possible. This is why the development of the heart should be emphasized in the educational system.

Persons below 18 years old should not practice the Meditation on Twin Hearts since their bodies cannot yet withstand too much subtle energies. Doing so may even manifest as physical paralysis in the long run. However, there are exceptions to this rule. There are many highly evolved souls who have incarnated and whose bodies are now in the adolescent stage. These advanced adolescents have big chakras and can start doing Meditation on Twin Hearts at the age of 14 or 15, but their condition should be monitored to avoid unnecessary problems. Persons with heart ailment, hypertension or glaucoma should not also practice Meditation on Twin Hearts since it may worsen their condition. It is important that those who intend to practice Meditation on Twin Hearts regularly should practice self-purification or character-building through daily inner reflection. Meditation on Twin Hearts not only activates the heart chakra and the crown chakra but also the other chakras. Because of this, both the positive and

MEDITATION ON TWIN HEARTS

negative characteristis of the practitioner will be magnified or activated. This can easily be verified by the practitioner himself and through clairvoyant observation.

For those who intend to practice Meditation on Twin Hearts regularly, the following will have to be avoided:

1. Eating pork, eel and/or catfish
2. Smoking
3. Excessive consumption of alcoholic drinks
4. Addictive and hallucinogenic drugs

Eating pork, eel and/or catfish while doing this meditation regularly may result in kundalini syndrome. Pork oil or lard should definitely be avoided. Kundalini syndrome may manifest as:

1. Chronic fatigue (or chronic extreme general weakness)
2. Overheating of the body
3. Chronic insomnia
4. Depression
5. Skin rashes
6. Hypertension and others

Heavy smokers may experience chest pain while doing Meditation on Twin Hearts since their front and back heart chakras are dirty. There is also the possibility of developing hypertension if one smokes regularly. Therefore, smoking has to be avoided if a person intends to do this meditation on a regular basis.

Excessive consumption of alcoholic drinks, and the use of addictive and hallucinogenic drugs have to be avoided also because they make the energy body dirty. Meditating with a dirty energy body will cause pranic congestion.

HOW TO ACTIVATE THE HEART CHAKRA AND THE CROWN CHAKRA

1. *Cleansing the Etheric Body through Physical Exercise.* Do physical exercises for about five minutes to cleanse and energize your etheric body. By exercising, light grayish matter or used-up prana is expelled from the etheric body. It also minimizes possible pranic congestion since Meditation on Twin Hearts generates a lot of subtle energies in the etheric body.

Sometimes when a spiritual aspirant meditates, he may experience unusual physical movements for a limited period of time. This is quite normal since the energy channels are being cleansed.

2. *Invocation for Divine Blessing.* You can make your own invocation. Here is one example the author usually uses:

> *To the Supreme God,*
> *Thank you for Your Divine Blessings!*
> *For guidance, help, protection and illumination!*
> *With thanks and in full faith!*
>
> *To my spiritual teachers,*
> *To the holy angels, spiritual helpers,*
> *and all the great ones,*
> *Thank you for your divine blessings!*
> *For guidance, help, protection and illumination!*
> *With thanks and in full faith!*

Invoking the blessing of Divine Providence and one's spiritual guides is very important. Every serious spiritual aspirant usually has spiritual guide(s), whether he is consciously aware of them or not. The invocation is required for one's guidance, help and protection. Without the invocation, the practice of any advanced meditational technique can be dangerous.

MEDITATION ON TWIN HEARTS

3. Activating the Heart Chakra by Blessing the Entire Earth with Loving-Kindness. Press your front heart chakra with your finger for a few seconds. This is to make concentration on the front heart chakra easier. Concentrate on the front heart chakra and bless the earth with loving-kindness. When blessing, you may visualize the earth as very small in front of you. Blessing the earth should not be done mechanically but with feelings. You may use the prayer of St. Francis of Assisi in blessing the earth:

To the Supreme God,
Make me an instrument of your peace.
(Feel the inner peace and bless the earth with peace.)

Where there is hatred, let me sow love.
(Feel the divine love. Allow yourself to be a channel of divine love and bless the earth with love.)

Where there is injury, pardon.
(Feel the spirit of reconciliation and bless the earth with the spirit of reconciliation, understanding, harmony and peace.)

Where there is despair, hope; doubt, faith.
(Feel the divine hope and faith, and bless the earth with hope and faith. Bless people who are having a difficult time with hope and faith.)

Where there is darkness, light; sadness, joy.
(Allow yourself to be a channel of divine light and joy. Bless the earth with divine light and joy. Bless people who are sad and in pain with divine light and joy.)

When blessing, feel and appreciate the implications of each phrase. You may also use visualization. When blessing the earth with loving-kindness, visualize the aura of the earth becoming dazzling golden pink. This blessing can be directed to a nation or a group of nations. Do not direct this blessing to specific infants, children or persons during the main meditation because they might be overwhelmed by the intense energy generated by the meditation. Infants, children or other persons can be blessed after releasing the excess energy. This is safe.

Do no overdo this blessing at the start. Some may even feel a slight pranic congestion around the heart area. This is because your etheric body is not sufficiently clean. Apply localized sweeping to remove the congestion.

4. *Activating the Crown Chakra by Blessing the Earth with Loving-Kindness.* Press the crown with your finger for several seconds to facilitate concentration on the crown chakra and bless the entire earth with loving-kindness. When the crown chakra is sufficiently opened, some of you will feel something blooming on top of the head and some will also feel a certain pressure on the crown. The following blessing may be used:

> *From the center of the heart of God,*
> *Let the entire earth be blessed*
> *with loving-kindness.*

(Feel loving-kindness. Allow yourself to be a channel of divine love and kindness and share these with the whole earth.)

> *Let the entire earth be blessed with*
> *great joy and happiness.*

(Feel the joy and happiness and share these with the entire earth. Visualize people with heavy, difficult problems smiling, their hearts filled with joy and happiness. Visualize their problems becoming lighter and their faces lightening up.)

*From the center of the heart of God,
Let the entire earth be blessed with
understanding, harmony, and divine peace.*
(Allow yourself to be a channel of understanding, harmony and peace. Visualize people or nations that are on the verge of fighting or are fighting reconciling and living in harmony with each other. Visualize people putting down their arms, shaking hands and embracing each other.)

*Let the entire earth be blessed with
goodwill and the will to do good.*
(Imagine people not only filled with good intentions, not only talking about doing something good but actually carrying out these good intentions. This is the meaning of the "will to do good.")

5. *Meditating and Blessing the Earth with Loving-kindness through the Heart and Crown Chakras Simultaneously.* After the crown chakra has been activated, concentrate simultaneously on the crown and heart chakras, and bless the earth with loving-kindness for a few minutes. This will align both chakras, thereby making the blessing much more potent. Imagine the small earth in front of you. You may use this blessing:

*From the center of the heart of God,
Let the entire earth, every person, and
every being be blessed with divine love
and kindness.*
(Feel the divine love and kindness and share these with the whole earth, every person and every being.)

*Let the entire earth, every person,
and every being be blessed with
warmth, caring and tenderness.*
(Feel the sweet, loving feeling and share it with the whole earth.)

> From the center of the heart of God,
> let the entire earth, every person, and
> every being be blessed with healing,
> inner beauty, divine bliss and
> divine oneness.

(Feel the divine bliss and divine oneness, and share these with every person and every being.)

6. *Achieving Illumination: Meditating on the Light, on the Mantra Om or Amen, and the Interval between the Two Oms or Amens.* Gently imagine a brilliant white light or golden light on the crown. Feel the quality of the energy emitted by the light. Feel the inner peace, stillness and bliss emanating from the light. Be aware of the light, the inner stillness and the bliss for a few minutes. Gently and silently chant the mantra "Om" or "Amen." Meditate simultaneously on the light and the mantra. When meditating on the interval between the two oms or amens, simultaneously be aware of the light, the stillness and the bliss. Continue with the meditation for about 10 minutes.

Do not be frightened if you experience an inner explosion of light on the head area. When you are able to be aware simultaneously of the point of light and the interval between the two oms, you will experience this. Your entire being will be filled with light! You will have your first glimpse of illumination and first experience of divine ecstasy. To experience Buddhic consciousness or illumination is to experience and understand what Jesus meant when He said the following: "If thine eye be single, thy whole body shall be full of light" (Luke 11:34); "For behold, the kingdom of heaven is within you" (Luke 17:21).

If you feel like you are being pulled out of the body or you are moving inside a tunnel, just allow the experience to unfold on its own until you experience oneness with the light. Should you experience pervasive darkness or The Great Void, this is good. This is simply a transition between ordinary consciousness and expansion of consciousness. Just relax and be calm. Invoke for the blessing of the Supreme God and your spiritual teachers to bring you to a higher level of consciousness.

For some people, it may take years before they can experience an initial glimpse of illumination or Buddhic consciousness. For others, it may take only months, while for some, only weeks. In a few cases, they achieve initial expansion of consciousness on the first few tries. This is usually done with the help of the Guru.

When doing this meditation, the aspirant should be neutral. He should not be obsessed with results or filled with too much expectations. Otherwise, he will be actually meditating on the expectations or the expected results rather than on the point of light, the om and the interval between the two oms.

7. *Releasing Excess Energy.* After the meditation, release the excess energy by blessing the earth with light, loving-kindness, peace and prosperity for several minutes until you feel your body is normalized. You may bless specific persons or your family and friends after releasing the excess energy. Otherwise, the etheric body will become congested and the meditator will experience headaches and chest pains. The visible body will deteriorate in the long run because of too much energy. Other esoteric schools release excess energy by visualizing the chakras projecting out the excess energy and the chakras becoming smaller and dimmer. However, this approach does not utilize the excess energy productively.

8. *Giving Thanks.* After meditation, always give thanks to the Divine Providence and to your spiritual guides for divine blessings.

9. *Further Release of Excess Energy and Strengthening the Body through Massage and More Physical Exercises.* Shake the body for 30 times, massage the different body parts, then do physical exercises

for a few minutes. This is to further release the excess energy, expel more used-up prana from the body and thus, cleanse and strengthen the visible body. This will also facilitate the assimilation of the pranic and spiritual energies, thereby enhancing the beauty and health of the practitioner. Massaging and exercising after meditation also reduce the possibility of pranic congestion in certain parts of the body. This may lead to illness. You can also gradually cure yourself of some ailments by doing exercises after doing the Meditation on Twin Hearts. It is very important to exercise after meditation; otherwise, the visible physical body will inevitably weaken. Although the etheric body will become very bright and strong, the visible physical body will become weak because it will not be able to withstand the leftover energy generated by the meditation in the long run. You have to experience this yourself to fully appreciate it.

Some have the tendency not to do physical exercises after meditation but continue savouring the blissful state. This tendency should be overcome; otherwise, one's physical health will deteriorate in the long run.

After the physical exercises, stand with your legs shoulder width apart and your knees bent. Be aware of the soles of the feet. Project your consciousness down deep into the earth and bless the earth by silently saying:

> *Let Mother Earth be blessed with*
> *divine light, love and power.*
> *Let Mother Earth be regenerated.*
> *I am rooted and connected to Mother Earth.*

This will bring your consciousness down to the physical body. It will enable the meditator to deal with the affairs of daily life and earn a decent living. Many spiritual practitioners have problems maintaining their practicality because they are not rooted or grounded.

MEDITATION ON TWIN HEARTS

The instructions may seem quite long but the meditation is short, simple and very effective! It requires only about 30 minutes, excluding the required time for the physical exercises.

There are many degrees of illumination. The art of "intuiting" or "direct synthetic knowing" requires constant meditation for a long duration of time.

Blessing the earth with loving-kindness can be done by a group as a form of world service. When it is done for this purpose, bless the earth with loving-kindness through the heart chakra first, then the crown chakra and finally through both chakras. Release the excess energy after the end of the meditation. The blessing can be directed not only to the entire earth but also to a specific nation or a group of nations. The potency of the blessing is increased many times when it is done as a group rather than individually. Another way of blessing the earth with loving-kindness as a group is through daily radio broadcast at an appropriate time with some or most of the listeners participating.

Just as pranic healing can "miraculously" cure simple and severe ailments, the Meditation on Twin Hearts, when practiced by a large number of people, can also miraculously heal the entire earth, thereby making the earth more harmonious and peaceful. This message is directed to readers with sufficient maturity and the will to do good.

INCREASING ONE'S HEALING POWER

When a person practices Meditation on Twin Hearts daily or regularly, his major chakras and auras will increase in size, making his energy body stronger and more dynamic.

It has been observed by the author that pranic healers can heal patients very fast after doing Meditation on Twin Hearts. The healing results are just simply amazing.

You may perform this simple experiment to verify the validity of what has been stated:

1. Ask somebody who is proficient in this meditation or has been practicing this meditation for at least about two or three weeks to perform this experiment with you.

2. Scan his major chakras, inner and outer auras before doing the meditation.

3. While the person is meditating, wait for about three minutes before scanning his major chakras, inner and outer auras. Note the difference in their sizes before and during the meditation.

   When scanning the auras, gradually move five meters or more away from the subject and try to feel his energy body. You may feel a tingling or mild sensation on your hands and fingers. Others may feel some sort of a mild electrical current or sensation.

Several hours after meditation, the chakras and the inner aura will gradually reduce in size; however, they are still bigger than their former sizes. If this meditation is practiced daily for about a year or longer, the size of each chakra and the inner aura will increase substantially because of the cumulative effects of regular meditation.

A healer with big chakras and inner aura is powerful and can heal most minor ailments very quickly and almost instantaneously. A proficient intermediate pranic healer should have an inner aura of at least one meter in radius, and an advanced pranic healer, about five meters or more. A powerful master pranic healer can have an inner aura of at least several hundred meters in radius. A person with big chakras and inner aura is just like a big pump while a person with small chakras and inner aura is just like a mini pump. So, it is very advantageous to practice this meditation daily or regularly.

Having a powerful and dynamic energy body not only enhances one's healing powers but also increases one's effectivity and productivity in his work. Having taught many students and met all kinds of people, the author has observed that successful people and top executives usually have bigger chakras - about five or six inches or more - and an inner aura of about one or more meters. A person who has a magnetic personality or great charisma usually has bigger chakras and inner aura than ordinary people and tends to have a strong influence over most people.

Furthermore, a person who meditates regularly becomes more intuitive and intelligent. When he is faced with a problem, he will have the increased ability to see directly through the problem and find the right or proper solutions.

ARHATIC YOGA

There are other meditation techniques more advanced than Meditation on Twin Hearts. One of these is Arhatic Yoga which is only for a chosen few. Arhatic Yoga is called the "yoga of synthesis." It deals with the activation of the chakras, and awakening of the kundalini through a safe and systematic method. One of the common and serious mistakes among esoteric practitioners is to try to awaken the kundalini in order to activate the chakras. A truly advanced yogi or chi kung practitioner is aware of the necessity of purifying oneself and substantially activating the chakras first before awakening the kundalini. Otherwise, serious pranic congestion will occur if too much kundalini energy goes to the relatively underactivated chakras which are still small in size, resulting in serious physical ailments or discomforts. Hence, the practice of arhatic yoga should preferably be under the guidance of an advanced guru or master.

TESTIMONIALS

NAME: Imelda P. Viloria, M.D., FPCCP*
ADDRESS: 19 Emerald St., Nelsonville, Batasan Hills
Quezon City, Philippines

Q : *Please relate your experiences when you did Meditation on Twin Hearts.*

A: My very first experience with Meditation on Twin Hearts was during a pranic healing orientation held at the Veterans Memorial Medical Center. I remember my tears flowing profusely during the meditation. Perhaps, healing occurred. I felt light after the meditation, as if I had unburdened something heavy that I had been carrying.

The second time was in the Master Choa Kok Sui Pranic Healing Course I took at the Institute for Inner Studies. After the meditation, I felt very tired. Two hours following that, I felt so happy for no particular reason at all. It was easy to laugh and share the joy I was feeling then. The same thing happened on the second day of the workshop.

Q : *How long have you been practicing this meditation?*

A : I have been doing Meditation on Twin Hearts regularly for about a year now.

---

*Fellow of Philippine College of Chest Physicians

Q : *How has this meditation affected your life?*

A : I have become more understanding of myself and others, more tolerant and less easily angered. I feel more peaceful within, more forgiving of myself and others. I start my day with the Twin Hearts Meditation. It makes me feel secure of God's love. Even if things do not work out the way I expect them to, I still feel in control and expectant of the good that will come to me. It is easier to smile, to work and to give. Life is good!

(Signed) IMELDA VILORIA
March 16, 1997

NAME: Steven Martin
ADDRESS: Suite 275, Unit 5, State Condominium II
117 Aguirre Street, Legaspi Village
Makati City, Philippines

Q : What was your first experience with Meditation on Twin Hearts?

A : I was introduced to Meditation on Twin Hearts sometime in 1994 when I took the Master Choa Kok Sui Pranic Healing Course offered by the Institute for Inner Studies. The first time I did this meditation, many of my fellow participants in the course had incredible experiences of seeing brilliant white light and lots of colors. I had NONE! You can just imagine how left out I felt then. I trusted in my instructor's advice to keep doing the meditation.

Q : How has this meditation affected your life and your consciousness?

A : After I made it a habit to meditate on my own regularly, I began to notice certain changes in myself - changes which I was completely oblivious to before when I was meditating with a group and was very self-conscious. The first, and probably the most important change I noticed was a transformation in the way I interacted with people. Whereas before I view others with suspicion and deal with them in varying degrees of aggression, I found myself becoming more open to them and more tolerant of their behavior. Eventually, it dawned upon me that I had missed the point of the meditation completely. The meditation is not meant to dazzle the practitioner with incredible psychic pyrotechnics but to develop his capacity to love. As I slowly internalized this truth and trained myself not to have unreasonable expectations of the meditation, I began to experience certain phenomena. One time, I felt I was becoming slightly detached from my physical body during the latter part of the meditation. Another was a slight tickling sensation on the top of my head, which would correspond to the opening of the crown chakra. Occasionally, my body would also sway slightly in a circular motion. And finally, I would feel an intense whirling sensation on the center of both palms all throughout the meditation.

Happy as I am to be blessed with these incredible experiences, and hopeful to be able to experience more as I continue to practice this meditation, I value above all else the incredible feelings of love, harmony and goodwill I get from the practice of this wonderful meditation.

(Signed) STEVEN MARTIN
March 20, 1997

NAME: Marilette Liongson
ADDRESS: No. 28 Tampingco Street, San Lorenzo Village
Makati City, Philippines

Q: *How did you come across Meditation on Twin Hearts? What were your inner experiences?*

A: When I started Meditation on Twin Hearts during the Master Choa Kok Sui Pranic Healing class, I did not know what to expect. For the first time in my life, however, I became aware of an uncommon stillness in my mind. With regular practice, this became a usual occurrence. There is also a general feeling of well-being. Once while doing this meditation, I thought I heard a truck engine running in a steady hum, rising gradually to a higher pitch. I stopped my meditation (or so I thought) and looked out of our eighth floor window to see what the truck was doing. No truck. I ran around our whole condominium unit, looking out each window down the street, and looking for the source of the sound that went on and on. Of course, there was no truck.

There were times when my joy would bubble up from the heart to my head and all over my body. When I opened my eyes to see if any one was looking at my expression, I saw only points of light surrounding me like an ocean. As I focused on it at one point, the flame of light engulfed me. Everything else happened at an instant. Everything was just perfectly okay. I felt there was a burst of knowledge and acknowledgement of my being!

Q: *How has Meditation on Twin Hearts affected your life?*

A: After doing Meditation on Twin Hearts regularly for a short period of time, I noticed a feeling of centeredness and focus on my goals -- the bigger picture of things. At times, I even wondered how come I no longer reacted as adversarially towards unpleasant situations/people when ordinarily I would have been instantly "rabid." I found myself more patient and understanding towards myself and others since my connection with myself and others seems to have gone deeper than the apparent. Also, my initial reactions have become more mental rather than immediately emotional. I also noticed a heightened sensitivity towards the finer energies; I have, therefore, become also more sensitive towards other's thoughts and feelings as well as my own and the environment, thus enabling me to relate better with them.

(Signed) MARILETTE LIONGSON
May 3, 1997

Meditation on Twin Hearts
A Personal Experience, A Revelation

by Dr. Rolando A. Carbonell, Ph.D., D.D., Litt.D.

Meditation is an individual experience and, therefore, unique and different to everyone. Every meditative experience partakes of a deeply personal and individual spiritual adventure, an odyssey into the realms of one's inner and mysterious beingness. It is a moment-to-moment realization with the God-presence – which is in everyone.

What I have to share is, therefore, my own kind of experience based on few experiments on the meditation on "twin hearts." And as such, further practices on it may evolve into another kind of experience – as unexpected or as surprising as the previous one. It may be more expansive, or may even partake of an inner revelation. But always, as far as I am concerned, it leaves behind its "pathless path" a silent thrill, a fragrance, an incandescence, a "high feeling."

But that is going ahead of my story ...

First, I must state here that since 1962, when I was first initiated into yoga by my first guru, I have undergone various experiments in meditation. Also, the evolutionary process was not an easy one for me. It was an uphill struggle trying to tame the "bull" that is the mind – and the battle to conquer the ego was as great. The quest for transcendence was never an easy path for me.

Then, as if planned out by divine destiny or will, I was introduced to this unique Meditation on Twin Hearts. Perhaps

MEDITATION ON TWIN HEARTS

conditioned by my previous preparations, I eagerly and easily allowed myself to let go and be in the total flow by following the instructions given in this book.

As soon as I entered into my "inner space" – simultaneously visualizing a brilliant white light in my heart and crown chakras, and at the same time regulating my breathing to a rhythmic, deep, and almost musical cadence — outpouring blessings and loving-kindness to the entire universe — I seemed to have been whirled out of space feeling almost bodiless ... I felt the crown center opening up like a lotus-cup unfolding bigger and bigger, irradiating and containing more light ... spilling out all over my entire being. At the same time, the lotus petals in my heart center were pulsing with an even greater light.

For some inexplicable reason, beyond logic - almost beyond words - I felt an outreaching love for all mankind as if I wanted very much to permeate them with this light of love and kindness, of understanding and wisdom. It was as if light had become boundless. Or perhaps it was more an expansion of consciousness – for in that instant there seemed to have been a feeling of temporary omniscience. This was very humbling, indeed, yet, overpowering.

If this were an experience of illumination, indeed, then I must say here that "I have seen the Light." But even more "shocking" was experiencing myself as a "being of light" — I felt every cell of my entire being filled with light or has become light itself. I emerged from this brief initial experience of the Meditation on Twin Hearts feeling cleansed, purified, and energized by the stream of light, nay, I would even daresay by a flood of light!

That single meditative experience was memorable. Succeeding experiments on this meditation technique, though not necessarily so dramatic as the first one, gave me several valuable insights too vast for words. It was like falling in love; however you attempt to describe the feeling, one falls short of expression. No wonder the mystics remain silent about it. It is a wordless experience of the mysterious ... of the miraculous. And yet, how truly simple, easy, and comforting. One needs only to let go the ego, to have a sincere attitude of humility, of inward purity, of authentic love for God - or whatever name you may call Him. There is that intimate feeling of oneness with everyone, with the entire universe (which is permeated with light).

Meditation, which is an inward journey into the realms of one's own being, is truly the language of ecstasy, of bliss consciousness, of Divine presence.

My prayer is for everyone to have his own unique and individual experience of this powerful and effective meditation technique on twin hearts. And for each one to bear witness to that incandescence, that luminescence of inner light, that overwhelming realization that we are "the light of the world" - and that this light is the only hope in our despairing world. This light gives wisdom, love, understanding, and inner peace.

I may have said something or nothing. As I mentioned earlier, meditation is beyond words. It is better experienced than explained.

(Signed) ROLANDO A. CARBONELL

CHARACTER-BUILDING: THE FIVE VIRTUES

Pranic healers are supposed to be models for patients and their communities. As such, the development of the virtues is very important:

1. *Loving-kindness and Non-injury:* Loving-kindness and non-injury simply means absence of cruelty. Loving-kindness may be expressed physically, verbally and mentally. Being polite, courteous and helpful are acts of loving-kindness. Verbally, you can say words that are nurturing and encouraging. People are just like plants that need to be nurtured to bloom and grow. For instance, you can show appreciation or give recognition for the achievements of a person. In this way, he is inspired to become better. Mentally, loving-kindness means blessing other people.

In pranic healing, loving-kindness means healing a patient, even if the patient cannot afford to pay. It is healing others out of kindness and compassion.

Non-injury is refraining from hurting other people physically, verbally and psychically. On a physical level, non-injury means "Thou shalt not kill" or hurt other people out of anger or malice. The practice of harmlessness towards other creatures is also very important. Sometimes, however, a person may have to take the life of an animal to provide food for his family. The act of killing should not involve any cruelty, malice or enjoyment in seeing the animal suffer. Termination of rats, cockroaches, mosquitoes and insects is permissible for hygienic reasons.

Verbal injury is avoiding the use of harsh or injurious words which often take a longer time to heal than physical injury. A physical wound takes only one or two weeks to heal but the wounds caused by a tactless or malicious remark can take years to heal, if ever they do get healed at all. Therefore, watch your words that they do not hurt others. If you have to criticize another person, do it with love and softness. In other words, criticize with a heart. You will notice that this is more effective because the person will be more receptive.

On a more subtle level, non-injury means minimizing or abstaining from excessive mental criticism. Avoid enviousness also. In other words, one should strive to practice mental harmlessness. A person may not be physically and verbally injurious but in his mind he is always criticizing the faults and defects of other people. This does not mean that you should not be aware of the flaws or weaknesses of another person but there is no reason why you should dwell on his negative qualities 10 or 20 times a day for 365 days a year. When you do this, you create a negative image of the other person, thus making his progress more difficult. By being constantly critical, you prevent him from changing, even if he wants to change. Repeated mental criticism can, therefore, obstruct development. It will not help but will just delay the progress of another person. Before criticizing, one should realize that almost nobody is perfect and that it takes time to change and progress. Spiritual development implies a process and process implies time.

In pranic healing, non-injury means not misusing one's psychic powers.

Loving-kindness and non-injury are necessary for proper and harmonious interhuman relationships. If everybody practices them, the world would be a better place to stay.

2. *Generosity and Non-stealing:* Generosity means sharing or giving. On the physical level, it means sharing or giving money wisely. The key to prosperity is in giving. Donating a part of your income to spiritual and charitable institutions is a physical act of generosity. It has been observed that patients who give generously to the healer usually recover very fast from their ailments. This is because by giving, they are entitled to receive the healing energy. Therefore, when a patient gives generously, his capacity to receive

and assimilate the healing energy is greatly increased, thereby accelerating the healing process. The author has observed that in many instances, just paying a powerful pranic healer in advance will cause partial or complete healing even before the pranic treatment is consciously done. Blessing the earth is also a form of generosity. On an emotional level, you can be generous by being warm, nurturing and supportive. Mentally, you can share knowledge and skills to people who are ready and willing to learn. You will notice that your understanding of a certain subject becomes deeper when you do this. This is because you do not master a subject until you start teaching it.

Non-stealing means that a person should not take anything that does not belong to him. On the level of relationships, one should not steal affection or covet the spouse of another. It also means, on a more subtle level, that one should not steal the merit or credit that is due to other people. In pranic healing, non-stealing means that the healer must heal the patient very thoroughly if the healer has been properly paid in advance or will be paid later. It also means that the patient should properly compensate the pranic healer for the great healing benefit that has been received. In some instances, underpaying or not paying the healer, even if one has the financial capacity to do so, will result in a very slow healing rate or no healing at all.

3. *Honesty and Non-lying:* Honesty should be practiced in such a way that it will not harm or injure others. One should not use honesty or frankness as a tool or weapon to cause emotional pain or injury. Honesty should not be used out of malice. This is misusing the virtue of honesty. If there is a conflict between the virtue of honesty and the virtues of kindness and non-injury, the virtues of kindness and non-injury should prevail over honesty.

Non-lying means that one should not make untrue or false statements out of malice or with the intent to take advantage of other people.

4. *Industriousness and Non-laziness:* In pranic healing, industriousness means studying pranic healing books thoroughly. It also means practicing different pranic healing techniques regularly so that one becomes very skillful. It also means healing the patient thoroughly. Industriousness also implies a strong sense of responsibility. If one is given a certain task to do, one has to perform it properly and completely. It also means non-procrastination. Another term for industriousness is "constancy of aim and effort."

Constancy of aim and effort and non-laziness is the key to success and spiritual development.

5. *Moderation and Non-excessiveness:* It is important that one should avoid extreme or excessive behavior and practice moderation. In pranic healing, healing and helping a lot of people is very good – but not to the point of exhausting one's self. To do this five or six days a week is definitely excessive and bad for the health. There are healers who have become very sick or have died at a young age due to this type of excessiveness. A healer can be more useful to society for a longer period of time by practicing moderation in healing.

Having sex is good but one should practice moderation and non-excessiveness. Too much sex for a prolonged period of time will cause a dramatic decrease in one's healing power.

Financially, it means that one should avoid excessive and wasteful spending. If possible, one should save and invest 20 % to 30 % of one's net earnings after tax and tithing. This is one of the keys to prosperity.

SUGGESTED SCHEDULE

Inner reflection and firm resolution: One should try to master one virtue at a time. Preferably, one should try to practice and concentrate on one virtue for about two months. Meditate on what you have done the whole day in relation to the virtue. Be aware of the good things you have done. This will develop your self-esteem. At the same time, be aware of your mistakes. This is called inner reflection. Mentally erase the negative event and imagine you are doing the right thing at least five times. This is called firm resolution. The mechanism behind this is that repeated wholesome thought manifests as wholesome action. Repeated wholesome action will in the long run manifest as virtue. One should intensively practice inner reflection and firm resolution for at least two years.

Chapter Eight

That is why the major problem is not the pupil, but the educator, our own hearts and minds must be cleansed if we are to be capable of educating others.

Without a change of heart, without goodwill, without the inward transformation which is born of self-awareness, there can be no peace, no happiness for men.

– J. Krishnamurti,
Education and the Significance of Life

... Love always draws forth what is best in child and man.

Enlightenment is the major goal of education.

– Alice Bailey,
Education in the New Age

THE LORD BUDDHA HAS SAID:

Let us inspect our thoughts that we do no unwholesome deed; for as we sow, so shall we reap.

Hatreds never cease by hatreds in this world. By love alone they cease. This is an ancient law.

Goodwill towards all beings is the true religion: cherish in your hearts boundless goodwill to all that lives.

Go and do your duty: show kindness to thy brothers and free them from suffering.

THE LORD CHRIST HAS SAID:

So every good tree bears good fruit; but a bad tree bears bad fruit. A good tree cannot bear bad fruit, neither can a bad tree bear good fruit . . . Thus, by their fruit you will know them.

— Matthew 7: 17-20

Love your enemies, do good to those who hate you, bless those who curse you, pray for those who mistreat you.

— Luke 6: 27-28

Love the Lord your God with all your heart and with all your soul and with all your mind. This is the first and greatest commandment. And the second is like it: Love your neighbor as yourself.

— Matthew 22: 37-39

Go and heal the sick.

— Matthew 10: 8

APPENDIX ONE

Courses on the Inner Sciences
by Master Choa Kok Sui

1. Pranic Healing
2. Advanced Pranic Healing
3. Pranic Psychotherapy
4. Pranic Crystal Healing
5. Psychic Self-Defense
6. Kriyashakti for Prosperity and Success
7. Arhatic Yoga: Preparatory, 1, 2, 3, 4, 5 and higher levels
8. Clairvoyance
9. Others

For more information, contact:

INSTITUTE FOR INNER STUDIES, INC.
P.O. Box 4903
Makati Central Post Office
Makati City 1289
Philippines

Tel. Nos: (63-2) 819-1874; 812-2326; 813-2562
Fax No: (63-2) 731-3828

APPENDIX TWO

Pranic Healing Centers and Organizations

Below are the addresses, telephone and fax numbers of pranic healing centers and organizations worldwide with corresponding contact persons:

GLOBAL COORDINATING CENTERS:

1. **INSTITUTE FOR INNER STUDIES, INC.**
   P.O. Box 4903
   Makati Central Post Office
   Makati City 1289
   Philippines
   Tel. Nos: (63-2) 819-1874; 812-2326; 813-2562
   Fax No: (63-2) 731-3828

2. **WORLD PRANIC HEALING FOUNDATION, INC.**
   P.O. Box 9101
   Makati Cinema Square Mailing Center
   Makati City 1289
   Philippines
   Tel. Nos: (63-2) 812-4283; 812-5001
   Fax No: (63-2) 893-6144

3. **WORLD PRANIC HEALERS ASSOCIATION, INC.**
   P.O. Box 9101
   Makati Cinema Square Mailing Center
   Makati City 1289
   Philippines
   Tel. No: (63-2) 814-0977

ARGENTINA

1. *DARA SONIA FILIPOF*
   Avenida Rivadavia 6387 5° A1
   Capital Federal
   Buenos Aires, Argentina
   Tel-Fax No: (54-1) 631-8851

2. Anna Maria Adorati de Sosa
   La Pampa 1468
   Bo. Residencial Olivas 5000
   Cordoba, Argentina
   Tel. No: (54-51) 609-642

AUSTRALIA

1. *LEENA McGREGOR*
   "Avalon", Stoney Shute Road
   Nimbin, NSW 2480
   Australia
   Tel. No: (61-66) 337-196
   Fax No: (61-66) 897-445

2. Dr. Stan Ross and Wendy MacDonell
   84A North West Arm Road
   Gymea NSW 2227
   Australia
   Tel. No: (61-02) 954-501-70
   Fax No: (61-02) 954-507-71

AUSTRIA

1. ***ALFON SCHERR and BURGI SEDLAK***
   Mullner Hauptstr.36
   5020 Salzburg
   Austria
   Tel-Fax No: (43-662) 422-265

2. ***GABRIELA BAUMGARTNER***
   Grill Parzerstrasse 6
   A-8010 Graz, Austria
   Tel No: (43-316) 322-161
   Fax No: (43-3127) 423-33

BELGIUM AND LUXEMBOURG

1. ***PETRA CONTRADA***
   PRANIC HEALING CENTER GERMANY
   Gschrifterstr. 7
   87629 Füssen, Germany
   Tel. No: (49-8362) 921-645
   Fax No: (49-8362) 921-647

2. (For Belgium Only)
   INEZ VERHEYEN
   Nachtegalenlaan 19
   8630 Veurne, Belgium
   Tel-Fax No: (32-58) 316-497

PRANIC HEALING CENTERS AND ORGANIZATIONS

BRAZIL

1. ***SANDRA GARABEDIAN***
   Rua Iubatinga
   84 Apt. 41
   Cep 05716-110
   SP - Brazil
   Tel-Fax No: (55-11) 846-6476

2. Sao Paulo:
   Ruth Nobuko
   Jorge Secco, 118
   Taubate, 12062-250
   SP - Brazil
   Tel. No: (55-122) 320- 579

   Rachel Franco de Souza
   Gov. Pedro de Toledo, 12 Ap 41
   Santos 11045-550
   SP - Brazil
   Tel. No: (55-132) 357-163

3. Rio de Janeiro:
   Cristina Sotto Mayor Ribeiro Moller
   Senador Furtado, 29 Ap 301
   Rio de Janeiro 20270-021
   RJ - Brazil
   Tel. No: (55-21) 228-7652

   Alice Alves Domingues
   Oscar Valdetaro, 94 Ap 1606
   RJ - Brazil
   Tel. No: (55-21) 438-1994

Celia Maria Guedes de Araujo
Silveira Martins, 68 Bloco 1, Ap 201
RJ 22221-000 Brazil
Tel. No: (55-21) 205-5104

Sergio A. Teixeira Braga
Av. Das Americas, 2678 Casa 68
RJ 22694-102 Brazil
Tel. No: (55-21) 325-1345

Gabriel Habib Filho
Av. Alexandre Ferreira, 110 Ap 302
RJ 22270-000
RJ - Brazil
Tel. No: (55-21) 286-1473

Vera Lucia Pedrosa Matos
Jose Vicente, 27 Ap 104
RJ 20540-330
RJ - Brazil
Tel. No: (55-21) 571-6713

Amalita Monteiro
Estrada Alarilo de Souza, 549
24315-050
Niteroi - RJ - Brazil
Tel. Nos: (55-21) 714-7385; 711-5031

Jose Antonio Correa Patricio
Adelia Cintra, 146
Sao Gonsalo, RJ
Brazil
Tel. No: (55-21) 712-9251

4. ***YARA FLEURY VAN DER MOLEN***
   CENTRO VISVARAM
   R. Coari, 52 - V. Pompeia
   Sao Paulo, Brazil
   Tel. No: (55-11) 871-1344
   Fax No: (55-11) 813-8511

5. Sao Paulo:
   Ailton Honorato da Silva
   Anita Ruth Vaskevicius
   Cleonice M. Monteiro
   Essencia - A Integracao Do Ser
   Av. Onze de Junho, 1395 - V. Mariana
   Sao Paulo, Brazil
   Tel. No: (55-11) 573-03719

   Carlos Eduardo de Maio
   Espaco Terapeutico Equilibrio Maio
   Batatais, 262 - J. Paulista
   Sao Paulo, Brazil
   Tel. No: (55-11) 885-4898

   Rogerio Luciano Pacioni
   Nosso Espaco Bio
   Cumanachos, 88 - Penha
   Sao Paulo, Brazil
   Tel. No: (55-11) 684-0477

6. Santa Catarina:
   Maria Aparecida da Rocha
   Alvarenga Peixoto, 251
   Joinville, Brazil
   Tel. No: (55-47) 435-2846

7. Minas Gerais:
   Irene A. Goncalves Tamietti
   Madureira, 117- B. Aparecida
   Belo Horizonte, Brazil
   Tel. No: (55-31) 442-5961

   Maria Jose G. Gomes Candido
   Olimpio de Assis, 302 - C. Jardim
   Belo Horizonte, Brazil
   Tel. No: (55-31) 291-0029

   Jose Emerson Faria
   Luis Ferreira Campos, 245 - C. Eliseos
   Varginha, Brazil
   Tel. No: (55-35) 221-2714

8. Associacão de Terapeutas Pranicos
   Rua Coari, 52
   05022-030 Sao Paulo
   SP - Brazil

CANADA

1. **NONA CASTRO**
   PRANIC HEALING SERVICES, CANADA
   207-1455 Robson Street
   Vancouver, BC V6G 1C1
   Canada
   Tel. No: (1-604) 681-9088
   Fax No: (1-604) 681-5165

PRANIC HEALING CENTERS AND ORGANIZATIONS

2. *Duncan and Marilee Goheen*
   Global Institute
   1269 Begley Road
   Kelowna, BC
   V1P 1K8, Canada
   Tel. No: (1-250) 491-1228
   Fax No: (1-250) 491-1219

3. *Dorothea Vickery*
   Belmont Avenue
   Victoria, B.C.
   V8R 4A5, Canada
   Tel. No: (1-250) 595-1203

4. *Aleks and Gordona Radojcic*
   Harmony and Health
   5 Carscadden Drive
   North York, Ontario
   M2R 2A6, Canada
   Tel. No: (1-416) 512-2992; 636-8444
   Fax No: (1-416) 636-8676

5. *Marcus Abram*
   Box 160, 253 College Street
   Toronto, Ontario
   M5T 1R5, Canada
   Tel. No: (1-416) 410-9451

6. *Antjie Halim*
   Center for Peace and Pranic Healing
   P.O. Box 23, Salem, Ontario
   N0B 1S0, Canada
   Tel-Fax No: (1-519) 846-0804

7. *Sanjoy and Sujata Choudhuri*
   15 Garden Ave.
   Richmond Hill, Ontario
   L4C 6L5, Canada
   Tel. No: (1-905) 709-8635

8. *Janet Mierau*
   6981 Hycroft Road
   West Vancouver, B.C.
   V7W 2K6, Canada
   Tel. No: (1-604) 921-6981
   Fax No: (1-604) 921-6901

9. Canadian Pranic Healers' Association
   P.O. Box 5871
   Victoria, BC
   V8R 6S8, Canada
   Tel. No: (1-250) 380-2228
   Web Site: http://www.pranichealing.bc.ca
   E-mail: Pranic CA@aol.com

COLOMBIA

SANTIAGO AVILES LEE, M.D.
SANACION PRANICA COLOMBIA
Transversal 38 No. 101A - 48 Oficina 502
Santafe de Bogota, D.C., Colombia
Tel. Nos: (57-1) 635-2191; 635-7470
Fax No: (57-1) 635-7595

CZECH REPUBLIC

LENKA VOLMUTOVA
Detska '19, Prague 10
100 00 Czech Republic
Tel. No: (42-2) 773-565

EASTERN AND CENTRAL EUROPE

CHARLOTTE ANDERSON
14431 Ventura Blvd.
Suite 401
Sherman Oaks, Ca 91423
U.S.A.
Tel. No: (1-818) 380-3424
Fax No: (1-818) 783-9469
E-mail: omlove@aol.com

FINLAND

1. *TOR-FREDRIC KARLSSON*
   FINSK PRANIC HEALING
   Smedjeviksvagen 4 A9
   00200 Helsinki
   Finland
   Tel-Fax No: (358-9) 682-2876

2. *Magnus and Hannele Johansson*
   Kivimäentie 15B2
   01620 Vantaa, Finland
   Tel. No: (358-9) 878-3815

3. *Pekka Kääriäinen*
   Donnerinkatu 10C18
   05800 Hyvinkää
   Finland
   Tel. No: (358-19) 432-125

FRANCE

JACQUELINE LEGRAND
PRANIC HEALING FRANCE
10 Avenue de Wailly
78290 Croissy-sur-Seine
France
Tel. No: (33-1) 3976-2022
Fax No: (33-1) 3976-0355
E-mail: Jacqueline@ntt.it

GERMANY

1. *SAI CHOLLETI and RUTH EBBINGHAUS*
   SRI SAI SPIRITUAL SATSANG
   Sollner Str. 71
   81479 Munchen, Germany
   Tel-Fax No: (49-89) 795-290

2. *PETRA CONTRADA*
   PRANIC HEALING CENTER GERMANY
   Gschrifterstr. 7
   87629 Füssen, Germany
   Tel. No: (49-8362) 921-645
   Fax No: (49-8362) 921-647

PRANIC HEALING CENTERS AND ORGANIZATIONS

3. Augsburg and Heilbronn:
   Elisabeth Gilgen-Ammar
   Friedberger Str. 117
   86163 Augsburg, Germany
   Tel. No: (49-821) 668-314
   Fax No: (49-821) 668-585

4. Baden-Württemberg
   Edeltraud Mosthaf
   Hohenstaufenstr. 9
   73033 Göppingen, Germany
   Tel. No: (49-7161) 969-126
   Fax No: (49-7161) 969-127

5. Bremen:
   Manfred Wordemann
   Dorfstr.9
   28816 Stuhr, Germany
   Tel. No: (49-421) 803-786

6. Hamburg:
   Eiko Krebs
   Bilser Str. 28
   22297 Hamburg, Germany
   Tel. No: (49-40) 517-269

   Michaela Friedrich
   Bilser Str. 32
   22297 Hamburg, Germany
   Tel. No: (49-40) 511-4082

   Windfried J.J. Pfliegel
   Hartwig Hesse
   Str. 27 20257
   Hamburg, Germany
   Tel. No: (49-40) 493-303

7. Hannover:
   Frank Seipke
   Friedrichstr. 14
   27472 Cuxhaven, Germany
   Tel-Fax No: (49-4721) 381-80

   Igor Rosegger
   c/o Christa Preis
   Hauptstr. 11
   21376 Salzhausen, Germany
   Tel. No: (49-4172) 8771
   Fax No: (49-4172) 8336

8. München and Süd-Bayern:
   Beate Stoyanoff
   Prinzregentenstr. 64
   81675 München, Germany
   Tel. No: (49-89) 470-5880
   Fax No: (49-89) 470-5888

9. Niedersachsen:
   Elke Pocza
   Möwensteert 12
   26723 Emden, Germany
   Tel. No: (49-4921) 658-47

10. Rheinland-Pfalz:
    Adelheid Weber
    Am Haseberg 4
    56414 Herschbach/Oww, Germany
    Tel. No: (49-6435) 2428
    Fax No: (49-6435) 3671

PRANIC HEALING CENTERS AND ORGANIZATIONS

11. Schleswig-Holstein:
    Barbara Lohfert
    Simrockstr. 135
    22589 Hamburg, Germany
    Tel-Fax No: (49-40) 872-722

INDIA

1. **MR. C. SUNDARAM**, President
   DR. RAMESH SINGH CHOUHAN,
   Executive Secretary
   ALL INDIA PRANIC HEALING
   FOUNDATIONS TRUST
   2nd Floor, Sona Towers
   71 Millers Road, Bangalore
   Bangalore - 560 052, India
   Tel. Nos: (91-80) 220-4783; 220-4784
   Fax No: (91-80) 228-1480

2. *C. Sundaram*
   Pranic Healing Foundation of Karnataka
   2nd Floor, Sona Towers
   71 Millers Road
   Bangalore 560 054
   Karnataka, India
   Fax No: (91-80) 220-4783

3. *Sushil and Ramani Joseph*, Trustees
   Pranic Healing Foundation of Tamil Nadu
   Colt Computer Center, Round Table House
   69, Nungambakkam High Road
   Chennai 600 034,
   Tamil Nadu, India
   Tel No: (91-44) 825-7113
   Fax No: (91-44) 483-4794

Cliff and Shushma Saldanha, Trustees
Pranic Healing Foundation of Tamil Nadu
c/o (Anugrah) No. 1 First Link St.
Karpagam Gardens, Adyar, Madras
600 020, India
Tel. No: (91-44) 491- 8460; 491-2004
Fax No: (91-44) 491-0958

4. *Swamy Paramananda*
   Sri Sahaja Foundation for Pranic Healing
   Puranikattu Patti, Valavanthi Nadu
   Namakkal
   Kolli Hills 637 411
   Tamil Nadu, India
   Tel. No: (91-48) 264-7459

5. *Jayanti Patel*, Managing Trustee
   Pranic Healing Foundation of Maharashtra
   3 Gandhi Bunglaw, First Flr., LBS Marg.
   Karnani Line Junction, Ghatkopar West
   Mumbai - 400 077
   Maharashtra, India
   Tel. No: (91-22) 511-6914
   Fax No: (91-22) 511-4872

6. *Krishnan Veerappan*, Managing Trustee
   Pranic Healing Foundation of Delhi
   B-26, Gitanjali Enclave
   Delhi - 110 017
   Delhi, India
   Tel. Nos. (91-11) 461-5400
   Fax No: (91-11) 462-6597

PRANIC HEALING CENTERS AND ORGANIZATIONS

7. *Dr. Saradamba*, President
   Pranic Healing Foundation of Andhra Pradesh
   8-2-676/1/B/5, Deccan Gardens
   Sriram Nagar, Road 12, Banjara Hills
   Hyderabad - 500 034
   Andhra Pradesh, India
   Tel. No: (91-40) 339-8261
   Fax No: (91-40) 247-671

8. *Sr. Eliza Kuppozhackel*
   Pranic Healing Foundation of Kerala
   Bakker Hill, Kottayam, 686 001
   Kerala, India
   Tel. No. (91-481) 564-119

9. *Sri Pat Sharma*
   Pranic Healing Foundation of Uttar Pradesh
   32/48, Lowther Road
   George Town
   Allahabad
   Uttar Pradesh, India
   Tel Nos: (91-) 660-717; 600-261

INDONESIA

YAYASAN PRANA INDONESIA
P.O. Box 615 Jak.or
Sekretariat: Getsung Perintis Lt. IV,
JL. Kebahagiaan 4-14
Jakarta 11140 Indonesia
Tel. No: (62-21) 260-1234
Fax No: (62-21) 634-8475

IRELAND

LULU HYNES
Geashill, Curragh
Castlebar Co. Mayo, Ireland
Tel. No: (353-94) 232-55
Fax No: (353-94) 248-44
c/o Geraldine Joyce

ITALY

1. **ROBERTO ZAMPERINI**
   CENTRO ITALIANO DIFFUSIONE PRANIC HEALING
   Piazza C.A. Scotti 20
   0051 Roma, Italy
   Tel. No: (39-6) 582-314-18
   Fax No: (39-6) 582-314-19

2. **LORETTA ZANUCCOLI**
   GRUPPO ROMAGNA PRANIC HEALING
   Viale Malva Nord, 30
   Cervia (RA), Italy
   Tel. No: (39-544) 971-553
   Fax No: (39-544) 970-494

3. Bologna:
   Elena de Pace
   Gruppo Emiliano Pranic Healing
   Via Massarenti 155
   40138 Bologna, Italy
   Tel. No: (39-51) 535-441
   Fax No: (39-51) 532-680

PRANIC HEALING CENTERS AND ORGANIZATIONS

4. Gorizia and Trieste:
   Giovanni Perin
   Gruppo Pranic Healing Trieste
   Via Aris 44 - 34074
   Monfalcone (GO), Italy
   Tel-Fax No: (39-481) 778-512

5. Latina:
   Maurizio Parmeggiani
   Gruppo Apriliano Pranic Healing
   Via Giambattista Grassi 14
   Aprillia (LT), Italy
   Tel. No: (39-6) 927-278-99

6. Milano:
   Loretta Zanuccoli
   Pranic Healing Milano
   Viale Malva Nord, 30
   Cervia (RA), Italy
   Tel. No: (39-544) 971-553
   Fax No: (39-544) 970-494

7. Padova:
   Paulo Iusi
   Gruppo Pranic Healing Padova
   via L. Faggin 26 -35100
   Padova, Italy
   Tel. No: (39-49) 606-250

8. Torino:
   Giuseppina Serra
   Lungopo Antonelli 41 - 10153
   Torino, Italy
   Tel. No: (39-11) 835-907

9. Venezia:
   Filippo Daniele
   Gruppo Veneto Pranic Healing
   c/o Essex-via Grandi 16A - Caselle S.M. di Sala
   30035 Venezia, Italy
   Tel. No: (39-41) 573-1865
   Fax No: (39-41) 573-0150

10. (For English-speaking Students)
    Tor-Fredric Karlsson
    Via D. Silveri 11 - 00165 Rome, Italy
    Tel-Fax No: (39-6) 393-660-93

MALAYSIA

SAW QUEE KIM
PRANIC WORKSHOP SDN. BHD.
B2 Annex, Pusat Bandar Damansara
Damansara Heights
50490 Kuala Lumpur, Malaysia
Tel. No: (60-3) 253-1000
Fax No: (60-3) 253-2000
E-mail: aleph@pc.jaring.my

MEXICO

FERNANDO ALCOCER
Elena Arizmendi No. 25-201
Col. del Valle
Mexico, D.F. 03100
Tel. No: (52-5) 543-0201
Fax No: (52-5) 687-8144

NETHERLANDS

KIRSTINE POSTMA
Schaepstal 2, 1251 MZ Laren,
The Netherlands
Tel. No: (31-35) 531-8166
Fax No: (31-35) 531-5102

NIGERIA

REVEREND FR. IGNACIO SAWEY
Christ The King Catholic Parish
P.O. Box 211, Ilesa Osun State
Nigeria
Tel. No: (234-36) 460-757

SCANDINAVIA
(DENMARK, ICELAND, NORWAY, SWEDEN)

1. **TOR-FREDRIC KARLSSON**
   FINSK PRANIC HEALING
   Smedjeviksvagen 4 A9
   00200 Helsinki
   Finland
   Tel-Fax No: (358-9) 682-2876

2. (For Sweden Only)
   Pia Arman
   Slaggatan 41A
   79170 Falun, Sweden
   Tel-Fax No: (46-23) 130-33

SINGAPORE

SAW QUEE KIM
PRANIC WORKSHOP PTE LTD
P.O. Box 371
Thomson Road Post Office
Singapore 915713
Tel-Fax No: (0-65) 455-4593
E-mail: aleph@mbox3.singnet.com.sg

SWITZERLAND

STEFAN WEISS
PRANIC HEALING SCHWEIZ
Weinberglistrasse 7
CH-6005 Luzern, Switzerland
Tel-Fax No: (41-41) 360-7753

THAILAND

DR. WANNEE LIKHITTAM
PRANA FOR HEALTH CENTER
4132 Dindaeng Road, Dindaeng District
Bangkok 10320
Thailand
Tel. No: (66-2) 642-9148 to 9

PRANIC HEALING CENTERS AND ORGANIZATIONS

UNITED STATES OF AMERICA

1. **STEPHEN CO**
   AMERICAN INSTITUTE OF ASIAN STUDIES
   23555 E. Golden Springs Road Ste. Kl-2
   Diamond Bar, Ca 91765 U.S.A.
   Tel. No: (1-909) 860-5656
   Fax No: (1-909) 860-7595
   Internet: www.pranichealing.com

2. **DEL PE**
   THE CENTER FOR PRANIC HEALING, INC.
   Suite 142, 600 Meadowlands Parkway
   Secaucus, New Jersey 07094 U.S.A.
   Tel. Nos: (1-212) 713-5564; (1-201) 863-7816
   Fax No: (1-201) 863-7916

3. Connecticut:
   Suzanne Jarvis
   34 Sunset Road,
   Easton, Connecticut 06612 U.S.A.
   Tel. No: (1-203) 459-0296

4. Florida:
   Margarita Maristany
   6401, N.W. 57 Lane
   Parkland, Florida U.S.A.
   Tel. No: (1-954) 345-0723
   Fax No: (1-954) 345-8484

   Alejandra and Jaime Graterol
   14880 South West 104th Street
   Miami, Florida 33196 U.S.A.
   Tel. No: (1-305) 380-0910

Elsie Blanco
1250 SW 22 Terrace
Miami, Florida 33145 U.S.A.
Tel. No: (1-305) 856-5513
Fax No: (1-305) 858-6612

Juliet Ortiz
19500 South West 127th Ct.
Miami, Florida 33177 U.S.A.
Tel. No: (1-305) 238-4704

5. Massachusets:
   Del Pe
   THE CENTER FOR PRANIC HEALING, INC.
   Suite 142, 600 Meadowlands Parkway
   Secaucus, New Jersey 07094 U.S.A.
   Tel. Nos: (1-212) 713-5564; (1-201) 863-7816
   Fax No: (1-201) 863-7916

6. New Jersey:
   Dr. Glenn Mendoza and Marilag Mendoza
   THE CENTER FOR PRANIC HEALING, INC.
   Suite 142, 600 Meadowlands Parkway
   Secaucus, New Jersey 07094 U.S.A.
   Tel. No: (1-201) 652-4620
   Fax No: (1-201) 652-7917

7. New York:
   Carolyn Wilder
   c/o The Center for Pranic Healing, Inc.
   Suite 142, 600 Meadowlands Parkway
   Secaucus, New Jersey 07094 U.S.A.
   Tel. Nos: (1-212) 713-5564; (1-201) 863-7816
   Fax No: (1-201) 863-7916

URUGUAY

MARIA ELENA GARCIA
Garcia Lagos 12
Paso Carrosco
Montevideo, Uruguay
Tel. No: (598-2) 611-423

VENEZUELA

ALEJANDRA GRATEROL
FUNDACION CURACION
PRANICA DE VENEZUELA
Final Calle Milan, Edificio Canaca, Piso 4
Los Ruices Sur, Caracas 1071, Venezuela
Tel. Nos: (58-14) 315-943; (58-2) 214-976;
(58-2) 222-490/91

APPENDIX THREE

Recommended Readings

There are thousands of titles of esoteric books. Beginners would normally be overwhelmed by the vast amount of reading materials. Different books may contain different information which may contradict each other. This is rather confusing for the reader. Some books are substantial; some are not. The author has, therefore, recommended a list of reading materials.

1. *Autobiography of a Yogi* by Paramahansa Yogananda. Self-realization Fellowship, 3880 San Rafael Avenue, Los Angeles, California 90065 U.S.A.

2. *First Principles of Theosophy* by C. Jinarâjadâsa. The Theosophical Publishing House. 1921. Adyar, Madras, India.

3. *The Etheric Double* by Arthur E. Powell. Quest Book. The Theosophical Publishing House, Wheaton Illinois 60187 U.S.A.

4. *The Astral Body* by Arthur E. Powell. Quest Book. The Theosophical Publishing House, Wheaton Illinois 60187 U.S.A.

5. *The Mental Body* by Arthur E. Powell. The Theosophical Publishing House, London Ltd., 68 Great Russel Street, London, W.C. 1, England.

6. *The Causal Body and the Ego* by Arthur E. Powell. The Theosophical Publishing House, England.

RECOMMENDED READINGS

7. *The Solar System* by Arthur E. Powell. The Theosophical Publishing House, England.

8. *The Secret Science at Work* by Max Freedom Long. 1953. DeVorss and Co., P.O. Box 550, Marina del Rey, CA 90294 U.S.A.

9. *Esoteric Healing* by Alice Bailey. Lucis Publishing Company, 113 University Place, 11th Floor, New York, N.Y. 10003 U.S.A.

10. *The Secret Path* by Paul Brunton. DeVorss & Co., Publishers.

11. *The Secrets of Chinese Meditation* by Lu K'uan Yu. 1964. Samuel Weiser, Inc., 740 Broadway, New York, N.Y. 10003 U.S.A.

12. *Kosher Yoga* by Albert L. Schutz & Hilda W. de Schaps. Quantal Publishing. P.O. Box 1598 Goleta, CA 93117-1598-0.

13. *Initiation into Hermetics* by Franz Bardon, trans. by A. Radspieler. 1956. Dieter Ruggeberg, Wuppertal, Western Germany.

14. *The Practice of Magical Evocation* by Franz Bardon. Dieter Ruggeberg, Wuppertal, Western Germany.

15. *The Key to the True Quabbalah* by Franz Bardon. Dieter Ruggeberg, Wuppertal, Western Germany.

16. *The Yoga of Light* (*The Classic Esoteric Handbook of Kundalini Yoga – Hatha Yoga Pradipika*) by Hans Ulrich Rieker. The Dawn Horse Press, Star Route 2 Middletown, California 95461 U.S.A.

17. *The Spiritual Science of Kriya Yoga* by Goswami Kriyananda. The Temple of Kriya Yoga, 2414 North Kedzie, Chicago, Illinois 60647 U.S.A.

18. *Raja Yoga* by Swami Vivekananda. Ramakrisna Vivekananda Center of New York, 17 East Street, New York, N.Y. 10028 U.S.A.

19. *Zen Mind, Beginner's Mind* by Shunryu Suzuki. John Weather Bill, Inc., of New York and Tokyo.

20. *Teachings of Tibetan Yoga.* Translated and annotated by Garma C. Chang. Citadel Press, 120 Enterprises Avenue, Secaucus Avenue, N.J. 07094 U.S.A.

21. *A Practical Guide to Qabbalistic Symbolism* by Gareth Knight. Samuel Weiser, Inc., P.O. Box 612, York Beach Maine 03910 U.S.A.

22. Theosophical Books by Madame Blavatsky, C.W. Leadbeater or by Annie Besant. The Theosophical Publishing House. Adyar, Madras, India.

23. Esoteric Books by Edwin Dingle. Institute of Mental Physics, Yucca Valley, California, U.S.A.

24. Esoteric Books by Robert and Earlyn Chaney. Astara, 800 W. Arrow Hwy., P.O. Box 5003, Upland, California 91785 U.S.A.

25. Esoteric Books by Rudolf Steiner. Harper & Row Publishers, San Francisco, U.S.A.

26. Esoteric Books on Agni Yoga. 319 West 107th Street, New York, N.Y. 10025 U.S.A.

RECOMMENDED READINGS 387

27. Esoteric Books by Alice Bailey. Lucis Publishing Company, 113 University Place, 11th Floor, New York, N.Y. 10003 US.A.

INDEX

A

abrasion, 315-316
acupressure, 6, 233
acupuncture, 6, 41, 42, 44, 126, 319
acute appendicitis, 125, 303
acute glaucoma, 162, 163
adrenal glands, 19, 21, 26
aging, reducing the rate of, 201
air prana. *see* prana.
ajna. *see* chakra, major.
alcohol, 38, 74, 152, 228
allergic reactions, 44, 315
allergy, 44
    nasal, 323
    skin, 119
angels, healing, 242, 247-248
anger, 30, 31, 65, 201, 208, 236, 260, 351
antakharana, 327
appendicitis, 12, 23, 125, 178, 303
appendix, 23, 27, 303
arthritic pain, 297, 313
arthritis, 115, 186-187, 190-191, 200-203, 208, 290, 300-301, 313
asthma, 26, 27, 28, 173
aura,
    health, 13-15, 34, 40, 60-61, 68, 132, 140
    inner, 12-13, 15-16, 19, 36, 54, 56, 60-65, 80, 89, 95, 121, 132, 139, 140, 173, 209, 212, 340-341
    outer, 14-15, 35, 60-61, 68, 91, 132, 164, 203, 206, 222, 340
ayurveda, 319

B

back pain, 295
basic chakra. *see* chakra, major.
bedwetting, 180
bioplasmic body, 2, 3, 5, 39, 41, 42, 128, 241. *see also* energy body.
bioplasmic channels, 6, 12, 39, 42. *see also* meridians.
biosynthetic ki, 23, 155, 223
birth, difficulty in giving, 23, 26
bladder incontinence, 263
bladder infection, 181, 277
bleeding, intradural, 282
blessing the earth, 328, 333, 337, 339
blindness, 162, 273, 286
blood, 5-6, 16, 21, 24-26, 27, 47, 104, 154, 167-169, 174, 175, 181-182, 190, 192-193, 195, 202, 220, 259-260, 272, 282, 285, 288, 290, 306, 308, 313
boils, 120
bone cancer, 21. *see also* cancer.
bones, 21, 26, 46, 101, 103, 154, 174-176, 222, 264-265, 268
bones, broken, 21
brain tumor, 298

INDEX

breast cancer, 296
breathing, chakral, 219-220
breathing, difficulty in, 25, 30, 104, 306, 319
burns, 125, 144, 267

C

cancer, 21, 70, 124, 200-201, 204, 220, 226, 228, 231, 296
carpal tunnel syndrome, 270
cataract, 281
cervical spondylitis, 284
chakra, major,
    ajna, 21, 28, 29, 88, 93-100, 104, 111, 121-122, 160-161, 162, 164, 166-171, 174-175, 184, 194, 198, 199, 202-203, 226, 244, 315, 329
    basic, 19, 21, 103, 106, 108-109, 112, 114-116, 118-122, 155-156, 166-169, 172, 174-176, 180-182, 184, 187, 189, 192-201, 203, 220, 329
    crown, 29, 168-169, 183, 226, 243-244, 326, 328-329, 334-335, 339, 345, 349
    forehead, 28-29
    heart, 25, 28, 91, 100-101, 104, 163-165, 167, 174-175, 202-203, 244, 330
    meng mein, 23, 88, 112, 167-169, 181-182, 190, 195, 202, 204, 207, 221
    navel, 23-25, 103-109, 115, 155, 159, 177-179, 187, 220, 223, 225
    sex, 21, 23, 28, 115, 180-182, 185-186, 194, 198-199, 215, 226, 329
    solar plexus, 16, 24, 25, 27-30, 32, 33, 63, 87, 91, 93-94, 96-97, 99-105, 110, 115, 120, 122-123, 154-155, 159, 161-163, 165-167, 170-171, 174-177, 181-182, 184, 187, 190, 192-195, 202-203, 207, 225, 228-229, 329-330
    spleen, 24, 27, 88, 96, 104, 142, 155, 176, 192-193, 202, 204, 220
    throat, 21, 28, 111, 152, 157-158, 166, 170-171, 195, 198-199, 329
chakra, minor,
    armpit, 113, 185, 186, 188, 191
    back head, 88, 94-95, 161-162, 193, 202
    elbow, 189
    finger, 53, 59, 80, 139
    hand, 19, 103, 154, 176, 189
    hip, 185-186, 188
    jaw, 99, 157-158, 166-167
    knee, 188-189
    secondary navel, 220, 223
    secondary throat, 173, 175

sole, 103, 172, 174-175, 189, 191
character-building, 330, 351
chi, 7, 149, 167, 209, 224, 341. see also life energy.
chi kung, 149, 167, 341
chicken pox, 155
cholesterol level, high, 166
Christ, 236, 358
cleansing, 16, 24, 25, 34, 49, 50, 51, 52, 53, 66, 67, 68, 71, 73, 83, 89, 90, 91, 95, 102, 104, 114, 122, 146, 149, 150, 152, 156, 165, 172, 178, 185, 186, 188, 189, 200, 201, 208, 214, 220, 222, 227, 253, 254, 267. see also sweeping.
cleansing and energizing, 16, 34, 49-51, 91, 114, 122, 150, 152, 185-186, 188, 214, 220, 222, 267
clockwise motion, 57, 148-149
cold, 15, 91, 178, 213, 319
color prana. see prana.
concussion, 125
connecting the tongue to the palate, 54
constipation, 23, 108-109, 282, 319
contusion, 117
correspondence, law of, 15
cough, 7, 15, 16, 104
counterclockwise motion, 57, 147-149
cramps, 275, 285, 321
cross-eyes, 161
crown chakra. see chakra, major.

cuts, 125, 144, 315-316
cysts, ovarian, 277

D

defense system, strengthening the body's, 159
diabetes, 25, 27-28
diarrhea, 285
directability, principle of, 250
diseased energy, 13, 34, 49-51, 53, 64-67, 69, 71, 73-74, 86, 142, 146, 148-149, 151-152, 164-165, 178, 200, 206, 208, 216-219, 222, 224, 226, 229-232, 241, 250, 253-254
disposal unit, 66, 69, 146, 151-152, 206, 208, 214, 216, 222, 253-254
distant healing, pranic, 37, 214, 216, 221, 250, 253, 262
distant scanning, 250, 252, 254
distributive sweeping, 80, 90, 145, 225. see also sweeping.
diversion, principle of, 230. see releasing.
divine energy, 327
dysmenorrhea, 69, 111

E

eczema, 119
emphysema, 172, 302
empty retention, 134
endocrine glands, 19, 23, 27, 28-29, 34. see glands.

energizing, 16, 24-25, 28-30, 34, 49-52, 53-55, 67-68, 74-75, 79-81, 83, 85-97, 99-106, 108-109, 111-123, 136, 138, 142-155, 157-159, 160-174, 176-185, 187-190, 192-199, 202-205, 207-209, 214-216, 220-222, 242-243, 253, 267, 300
   non-parallel double, 145
   parallel double, 143, 145
   with pranic breathing, 142, 146
energy body, 2, 5-6, 12, 15-18, 30-31, 33-34, 36, 41, 49-51, 53, 56, 65, 67, 75, 92, 126, 142, 146-147, 204, 206, 210-212, 224, 226-229, 232, 242, 251, 331, 339-341
energy centers, 3, 18-19, 34, 87. see chakras, major.
epilepsy, 29
etheric body, 2, 5, 38-40, 132, 155, 249-250, 332, 334, 337-338
exercises, physical, 209, 224, 230, 320, 332, 338-339
extraction technique, 150-151
eyestrain, 93-95

F

fainting, 159
fever, 8, 86, 101-103, 108, 155, 172, 176, 293, 303, 306
fistula, anal, 291
forehead chakra. see chakra, major.

forgiveness, law of, 238-239
fracture, 45-46, 292
frozen shoulder, 113

G

Gaikin, Mikhail Kuzmich, 42
gall bladder, 31
gas pain, 8, 86
general cleansing, 24, 220, 222. see general sweeping.
general sweeping, 24, 67, 88-89, 91, 93, 95, 99-105, 107, 114, 118, 122-123, 141, 146, 154-155, 157-158, 162, 164, 168-171, 173, 180-182, 187, 188-189, 192-199, 202-203, 216, 253, 290
generosity, 352
german measles, 155
ginseng, 231
glands, 19, 21, 23, 26-29, 34, 158, 195, 290
glaucoma, 33, 162-163, 330
goiter, 27-28
golden rule, 236-237
gout, 186, 189
ground prana. see prana.

H

hand chakra. see chakra, minor.
hand chakras technique, 55, 84, 134, 243
headache, 8, 69, 93, 152, 159, 181-182, 190, 215, 229, 269, 298

health rays, 13, 15, 34-35, 50-51, 61, 67-68, 72, 141, 164, 203, 208, 217, 222
hearing loss, 285-286
heart, 9, 12, 16, 25, 27, 28-29, 31, 33, 45, 64-65, 88, 91, 100-101, 104, 115, 125, 163-171, 174-175, 202-204, 207, 211, 220, 244, 259, 290, 326, 328-331, 333-336, 339, 346, 349, 352, 356, 358
heart ailments, 25, 27, 91, 163
heart chakra, 25, 28, 91, 100-101, 104, 163-165, 167, 170-171, 174-175, 202-203, 220, 244, 326, 328-331, 333, 335, 339
hemiplegia, 282
hemorrhoid, 270-271
hepatitis, 15-16, 25, 27, 176
herpes zoster, 272, 289
hiccup, 105
high blood pressure, 26, 202, 220, 290, 306. *see also* hypertension.
hoarseness, 318
honesty, 353
hypertension, 24, 45, 88, 96, 104, 115, 155, 167, 176, 192-193, 195, 330-331

I

illumination technique, 326. *see also* Meditation on Twin Hearts.
immune system, 44

impetigo, 267
impotence, sexual, 183
indigestion, 30
industriousness, 354
infection, 7, 14-15, 24, 31-32, 40, 68, 75, 91-102, 104, 125, 144, 154-155, 176, 180-182, 220
infertility, 277
inflammation, 32, 268, 272, 284-285, 312
insomnia, 45, 122, 319, 331
interconnectedness, principle of, 250
internal organs, 19, 22, 26-27, 44, 154, 218
intestine, 23, 104, 178, 285
invocative healing, pranic, 241, 243, 245

J

jaundice, 15-16
jaw, 99, 104, 114, 121, 157-158, 166-167, 268, 312
jaw inflammation, 312
jaw minor chakras. *see* chakra, minor.

K

kaballah, 327
karma, 233-238, 245
ki, 1-2, 5-6, 23, 33, 39, 52-53, 80, 141, 155, 217, 223, 231, 240, 327. *see also* life energy.

ki, heaven, 327
kidney infection, 181
kidney stones, 279, 308-309
kirlian photography, 5
Kirlian, Semyon Davidovich, 41
kundalini, 331, 341

L

lacerations, 264
lag time, principle of 204
large intestine, 23, 26, 104, 178, 285
laryngitis, 99
leather, 93, 146
leukemia, 21, 26, 204, 220, 226, 259
Levo-Dopa, 319
life energy, 1-2, 5-8, 18, 23, 31, 33, 43, 47, 49, 75, 79, 103, 128-129, 143, 154-155, 158-159, 241, 249. see also prana.
life energy, law of, 7
liposuction, 289
liver, 9, 15-16, 25, 27, 32, 44, 64, 115, 119, 120, 154-155, 165-167, 174-176, 187, 192-193, 202, 228-229, 290
liver inflammation, 32
localized sweeping, 67, 69, 70-71, 85, 87, 89, 91, 93-109, 111-124, 141-142, 145-146, 149, 154-204, 208, 215-216, 225-226, 253, 290, 315, 334
loose bowel movement, 8, 30, 50-51, 69, 86, 108, 215

loss of consciousness, 159
loving-kindness, 210, 326, 328-329, 333-335, 337, 339, 349, 351-352
low back pain, 45, 278
low vitality, 21, 23, 26
lump, 294
lungs, 3, 16, 28, 62-63, 100-101, 104, 170-172, 174-175, 211
lymphatic system, 27-28

M

macrobiotic diet, 319
major chakra, 19, 23-24, 28, 30, 34, 63, 89, 121, 140-142, 148, 170-171, 178, 201, 204, 222, 251, 290, 326, 330, 339-340. see also chakra, major.
malnutrition, 32
master chakra, 28
medical qigong, 2, 43
meditation, 31, 167, 221-224, 229, 312, 319-320, 328-329, 331, 334, 336-346, 348-350
Meditation on Twin Hearts, 246, 319, 326, 330-332, 338-339, 341-342, 344, 346, 348-349
Meditation on the White Light, 222, 224
meng mein chakra. see chakra, major.
menstruation, 110
    absence of, 111
    irregular, 111

mercy, law of, 238-239
meridians, 6, 81, 142, 223
migraine, 45, 301, 322
minor chakra, 53, 88, 95, 99, 103, 113, 135-136, 141, 154, 157-158, 160-161, 166-167, 172-177, 184-186, 188-189, 191. *see also* chakra, minor.
minor surgery, 198-199
miscarriage, 197-198, 280
moderation, 354
multiple sclerosis, 278
mumps, 157
muscle pain, 8, 86
muscular system, 187, 189

N

nadis, 6, 39, 41, 142, 211
navel, 21, 23-26, 29, 103-109, 114-116, 119, 121, 123, 155, 159, 161, 165, 172, 176-180, 184, 187, 189, 190, 192-195, 198-199, 202, 220, 223, 225, 273
navel chakra. *see* chakra, major.
negative emotions, 32, 163, 167, 192-193, 201, 208, 228, 232
neuralgia, post herpetic, 289
neuritis, 290
neurologic disorder, 275
night blindness, 286
non-excessiveness, 354
non-injury, 351-353
non-laziness, 354
non-lying, 353
non-stealing, 352-353
nose, 28, 100, 104, 170-171, 315
nose bleeds, 315
numbness, 138, 278, 282

O

om, 329, 336-337
osteoarthritis, 188
ovaries, 184, 277

P

pancreas, 27-28, 195, 290
paralysis, 29, 226, 282, 330
parasitic worms, 109
parathyroid glands, 27-28
parkinson's disease, 319
pillar of light, 327
pimples, 120
pineal gland, 29, 290
pituitary gland, 28
pneumonia, 172, 295, 299
prana, 2-8, 12, 15-16, 19, 23-25, 28-31, 33-36, 38-40, 49-53, 55, 63-64, 67-68, 74-75, 77-88, 90, 92-93, 101, 103, 125-126, 129, 131, 134-138, 141, 143, 145-147, 149-155, 158, 205-207, 209-210, 217-219, 222-224, 228, 231, 233, 240-241, 255, 289, 291, 315, 332, 338
  air, 2-3, 5, 23-24, 75, 138, 147

color, 36, 315
ground, 2, 4, 23, 93, 103, 135-136, 141, 146-147, 228
law of, 7
redistribution of, 150
solar, 2
white, 141, 315
pranic breathing, 131-133, 134-136, 138-139, 141-142, 144, 147, 152-153, 214-222, 224-227, 231, 244, 252-253, 320
pranic congestion, 12, 15, 24-25, 28, 33-34, 50-51, 64-65, 80, 88-90, 93, 125, 144, 159-160, 165, 177, 201, 207, 219-221, 223, 332, 334, 338, 341
pranic depletion, 12, 15, 30, 32, 34, 63-65, 89-90, 93, 98, 140, 145, 163, 165, 206, 208
Prayer, The Lord's, 238
pregnancy, 277, 280
pregnant women, 195
projecting hand, 78, 79
prostate gland, enlarged, 180
psoriasis, 272
pyorrhea, 158

Q

qigong, medical, 2

R

receiving hand, 79, 81
receptivity, 55, 75, 89, 205, 247
recharging, physical and mental, 225
reflexology, 6
reiki, 319
releasing, 230, 246, 319, 334, 337
renal failure, 293
respiratory ailments, 170-172
rheumatism, 187, 202, 213
rheumatoid arthritis, 27, 191, 228. see also arthritis.
root chakra, 21
royal jelly, 200, 228

S

scanning, 12, 16, 43, 54, 59-60, 63, 80, 91, 139-141, 207, 213-214, 216, 250, 252, 254, 315, 340
scoliosis, 192-193, 265
self-distant healing, 218, 220
self-healing affirmation, 246
self-healing, pranic, 213-214, 216, 230, 232, 319-320
self-recovery, law of, 7
self-scanning, 214
sensitizing, 19, 54, 57, 59, 86, 139
sensitizing the fingers, 139
sensitizing the hands, 19, 59, 139
shaman, 66, 147

shingles, 272, 273. see herpes zoster.
sinusitis, 169, 324
skeletal system, 19, 114-115
skin rash, 317
slipped disk, 276
small intestine, 23, 27, 104
smoking, 211, 318, 331
solar plexus chakra. see chakra, major.
solar prana. see prana.
sore eyes, 95
sore throat, 15, 27-28
spine, 19, 21, 57, 63, 88-89, 111-112, 141-142, 168-169, 187, 189, 191, 194, 201, 222, 251, 265, 276, 278, 290
spleen, 24, 27, 29, 44, 88, 96, 104, 142, 155, 176, 192, 193, 202, 204, 220
spleen chakra. see chakra, major.
sprain, 15, 111
sterility, 28
stiff neck, 115
St. Francis of Assisi, prayer of, 238, 333
stomach, 27, 44, 69, 104
stomach pain, 69
stress, 25, 33, 45, 122, 163, 167, 297, 299
stroke, 259, 293, 313
stuffy nose, 100, 104
sunburn, 118
sweeping, 24, 50-51, 54, 66-71, 73-74, 80, 83, 85-91, 93-109, 111-124, 141-142, 145-146, 149, 151, 154-200, 202-206, 208, 215-216, 225-226, 243, 253, 290, 315, 334
swimming, 201

T

tai chi, 209, 224
taoist six healing sounds, 214
tension, 25, 33, 203, 275, 299
testes, 184
throat, 15-16, 21, 27-29, 63, 99-100, 104, 111, 114, 121-122, 152, 155, 157-158, 164, 166-167, 170-171, 173-175, 184, 195, 198-199, 202-203, 275, 282, 318, 329
throat chakra. see chakra, major.
throat pain, 318
thrombocytosis, 259
thymus gland, 25, 27
thyroid glands, 28, 195
tiredness, 124
tonsillitis, 15
toothache, 8, 98, 310
tuberculosis, 172
tumor, brain, 298

U

ulcer, 25, 27, 31
ulcerative colitis, 285
upward sweeping, 71, 73, 122, 141. see also sweeping.
urethral infection, 277
urinary tract infection, 269
urination, frequent, 179-180

INDEX

V

venereal diseases, 204, 226, 228
visualization, 36, 81, 92, 142, 231, 252, 328, 333
vitality, low, 21, 23, 26
vitamins, 200, 228
vomiting, 50, 51, 269, 287, 293

W

walleyes, 161
water and salt, basin of. *see* disposal unit.
water and salt bath, 201
weakness, general, 27, 86, 90, 124, 331
white prana. *see* prana.
wounds, 21, 118, 304-305, 351

Y

yoga, 6, 224, 328, 329, 341, 348
    arhatic, 341
    hatha, 224, 328
    taoist, 224, 327